Critical Observations in Radiology
for Medical Students

Critical Observations in Radiology for Medical Students

Katherine R. Birchard, MD

Assistant Professor of Radiology, Cardiothoracic Imaging
Department of Radiology
University of North Carolina
Chapel Hill
USA

Kiran Reddy Busireddy, MD

Department of Radiology
University of North Carolina
Chapel Hill
USA

Richard C. Semelka, MD

Professor of Radiology, Director of Magnetic Resonance Imaging, Vice Chair of Quality and Safety
Department of Radiology
University of North Carolina
Chapel Hill
USA

WILEY Blackwell

This edition first published 2015 © 2015 by John Wiley & Sons, Ltd

Registered Office
John Wiley & Sons, Ltd, The Atrium, Southern Gate, Chichester, West Sussex, PO19 8SQ, UK

Editorial Offices
9600 Garsington Road, Oxford, OX4 2DQ, UK
The Atrium, Southern Gate, Chichester, West Sussex, PO19 8SQ, UK
350 Main Street, Malden, MA 02148-5020, USA

For details of our global editorial offices, for customer services and for information about how to apply for permission to reuse the copyright material in this book please see our website at www.wiley.com/wiley-blackwell

Library of Congress Cataloging-in-Publication Data

Critical observations in radiology for medical students / [edited by] Katherine R. Birchard, Kiran Reddy Busireddy, Richard C. Semelka.
    p. ; cm.
  Includes bibliographical references and index.
  ISBN 978-1-118-90471-8 (pbk.)
  I. Birchard, Katherine R., 1973– , editor. II. Busireddy, Kiran Reddy, 1983– , editor. III. Semelka, Richard C., editor.
  [DNLM: 1. Radiography. 2. Diagnostic Imaging. WN 200]
  RC78.4
  616.07′572–dc23

                        2014047515

A catalogue record for this book is available from the British Library.

Wiley also publishes its books in a variety of electronic formats. Some content that appears in print may not be available in electronic books.

Cover images: Axial CT image showing acute right temporal subdural hematoma; coronal contrast enhanced image of the abdomen and pelvis demonstrating long-segment small bowel dilatation; coronal T1 image showing left acute invasive sinusitis; PA radiograph image of both hands showing rheumatoid arthritis; coronal CT image in lung window setting showing left pneumothorax. Images by Katharine R. Birchard, Kiran Reddy Busireddy and Richard C. Semelka.

Set in 9/11pt Minion by SPi Publisher Services, Pondicherry, India
Printed and bound in Singapore by Markono Print Media Pte Ltd

1 2015

Contents

Contributors

Mamdoh AlObaidy, MD
Department of Radiology
University of North Carolina
Chapel Hill
USA

Katherine R. Birchard, MD
Assistant Professor of Radiology
Cardiothoracic Imaging
Department of Radiology
University of North Carolina
Chapel Hill
USA

Lauren M.B. Burke, MD
Assistant Professor of Radiology
Division of Abdominal Imaging
Department of Radiology
University of North Carolina
Chapel Hill
USA

Kiran Reddy Busireddy, MD
Department of Radiology
University of North Carolina
Chapel Hill
USA

J.T. Cardella, MD
University of North Carolina
Chapel Hill
USA

Mauricio Castillo, MD, FACR
Professor and Chief of Neuroradiology
Department of Radiology
University of North Carolina
Chapel Hill
USA

Matthew S. Chin, MD
Department of Radiology
University of North Carolina
Chapel Hill
USA

Susan Ormsbee Holley, MD, PhD
Assistant Professor of Radiology
Breast Imaging Section, Mallinckrodt Institute of
Radiology
Washington University School of Medicine
St. Louis, MO
USA

Benjamin Huang
Assistant Professor of Radiology, Neuroradiology
Department of Radiology
University of North Carolina
Chapel Hill
USA

Ari J. Isaacson, MD
Assistant Professor of Radiology
University of North Carolina
Chapel Hill
USA

J. Larry Klein, MD
Clinical Professor of Medicine and Radiology
University of North Carolina
Chapel Hill
USA

Daniel B. Nissman,
MD, MPH, MSEE
Assistant Professor of Radiology
Musculoskeletal Imaging, Department of Radiology
University of North Carolina
Chapel Hill
USA

Joana N. Ramalho, MD
Department of Neuroradiology
Centro Hospitalar de Lisboa Central
Lisboa
Portugal
Department of Radiology
University of North Carolina
Chapel Hill
USA

Miguel Ramalho, MD
Research Instructor
Department of Radiology
University of North Carolina
Chapel Hill
USA

Pinakpani Roy, MD
Radiology Resident
Department of Radiology
University of North Carolina
Chapel Hill
USA

Cassandra M. Sams, MD
Department of Radiology
University of North Carolina
Chapel Hill
USA

Saowanee Srirattanapong, MD
Instructor
Department of Diagnostic and Therapeutic Radiology
Faculty of Medicine Ramathibodi Hospital
Mahidol University
Bangkok, Thailand

Richard C. Semelka, MD
Professor of Radiology; Director of Magnetic
Resonance Imaging; Vice Chair of Quality and Safety
Department of Radiology
University of North Carolina
Chapel Hill
USA

Frank W. Shields IV, MD
Clinical Fellow
Department of Radiology
University of North Carolina
Chapel Hill
USA

Sarah Thomas
Clinical Fellow
University of North Carolina
Chapel Hill
USA

Nicole T. Tran, MD
Assistant Professor of Medicine
Department of Cardiology
University of Oklahoma
Norman, USA

Preface

The intention of this textbook is to provide medical students with a concise description of what is essential to know in the vast field of modern Radiology, hence the expression 'critical observations'. More and more in the modern age of health care, imaging studies occupy a central role in the management, and progressively also the treatment, of patients. It is important that our future doctors have a good, broad understanding of modern Radiology practice, which this book provides. Rather than rehashing old information from old text-books, which typically happens with texts designed for students, we have taken a fresh look at imaging providing state-of-the-art descriptions, discussions and images.

Katherine R. Birchard
Kiran Reddy Busireddy
Richard C. Semelka

About the companion website

Don't forget to visit the companion website for this book:

www.wiley.com/go/birchard

There you will find valuable material designed to enhance your learning, including:

- Interactive multiple choice questions
- Downloadable images and algorithms from the book

Scan this QR code to visit the companion website:

CHAPTER 1

Basic principles of radiologic modalities

Mamdoh AlObaidy, Kiran Reddy Busireddy, and Richard C. Semelka
Department of Radiology, University of North Carolina, Chapel Hill, USA

Introduction

In this chapter, we will describe the features and basic imaging principles of the various modalities employed in radiology. Since many specialties perform these types of studies, "radiology" is often also referred to generically as "imaging." A basic feature of all imaging is that pictures are generated, and the quality of the pictures oftentimes depends on how pathologies stand out compared to normal tissues.

Each of the different modalities uses their own terms to describe pathology, which relate back to how the images themselves are created. In this chapter, brief technical descriptions of each modality will be discussed with special emphasis on image production, image description, factors that influence image quality, and associated imaging artifacts with each modality.

X-ray-based imaging modalities

Plain radiography, mammography, fluoroscopy, and computed tomography (CT) all use X-rays as the source of generating images. All these modalities employ an X-ray tube to generate the images. The controllable factors are tube voltage, measured in kVp; tube current, measured in mA; and total exposure time, measured in seconds.

The X-ray tubes produce X-rays by accelerating electrons to high energies from a filament (cathode) to a tungsten target (anode) by heating the filaments to a very high temperature, which then emits electrons. The flow of electrons from the filament to the target constitutes the tube current (mA). X-rays are produced when energetic electrons strike the target material; electron kinetic energy is transformed into heat and X-rays, which are then filtrated at the X-ray tube window to achieve higher beam quality. The term mAs refers to the product of tube current and time duration.

These X-rays are then directed to the imaged subject (the patient). The number of X-rays produced by the X-ray beam is related to the X-ray beam intensity, measured in terms of air kerma (mGy). X-ray beam intensity (mA) is proportional to the X-ray tube current. X-ray beam intensity is also proportional to the exposure time, which is the total time during which a beam current flows across the X-ray tube. Doubling the tube current, the number of X-rays or the exposure time will double the X-ray beam intensity, but will not affect the average energy of the beam. KVp affects the penetrating power of X-rays and hence tissue contrast.

Image production can be achieved using analog or digital systems. Analog radiography uses films to capture, display, and store radiographic images. Digital systems can be classified as cassette and noncassette systems.

Plain radiography (X-rays)

Image production

X-ray tube voltage varies according to imaged body part. Exposure times range between tens and hundreds of milliseconds.

The typical settings to obtain an erect posteroanterior chest radiograph are a kVp of 100 and mAs of 4. The typical settings to obtain an erect anteroposterior abdominal radiograph are a kVp of 80 and mAs of 40. The typical kVp and mAs settings for imaging the appendicular skeleton are 52–60 and 2.5–8, respectively. Note that there are slight variations between the kVp and mAs for these different regions. This reflects that more current is needed to penetrate regions with more tissue (abdomen compared to chest), and optimal contrast is different to study the disease processes of these different regions as well (abdomen compared to skeleton).

Image descriptors

The most common projections in plain radiography are frontal (anteroposterior or posteroanterior), lateral, oblique, or cross-table, based on the direction of X-ray beam in relation to the patient. Special positions and projections are used in musculoskeletal (MSK) imaging.

Frontal projection images are interpreted as if the patient is sitting in front of the reader; where the left side of the image corresponds to the right side of the patient.

Critical Observations in Radiology for Medical Students, First Edition. Katherine R. Birchard, Kiran Reddy Busireddy, and Richard C. Semelka.
© 2015 John Wiley & Sons, Ltd. Published 2015 by John Wiley & Sons, Ltd.
Companion website: www.wiley.com/go/birchard

The brightness of a structure on plain radiography is related to its atomic number; structures containing material with higher atomic number absorb more photons before they reach the detector or film. In plain radiography, bright areas are described as radiopaque or radiopacity, and dark areas are described as radiolucent. Metals, bones, some stones, contrast materials, and various pathologies appear as radiopaque. Air/gas appears as radiolucent.

Image performance

X-ray-based imaging modalities including plain radiography, mammography, fluoroscopy, and CT share the same parameters that can influence image quality. Combinations of tube voltage, tube current, and exposure time, and focal spot size govern the final image quality.

Optimization of these parameters to achieve a diagnostic quality image with minimum radiation is the principal goal. Plain radiographic studies generally offer the highest spatial resolution, with the subcategory of mammography having the very highest, followed by CT, magnetic resonance imaging (MRI), and then nuclear medicine.

Mammography

Mammography is an X-ray-based imaging modality that uses low-energy X-rays to image the breasts as a diagnostic and screening tool.

Image production

X-ray tubes in mammography units used molybdenum as a target and a much smaller focal spots. The tube voltage in mammography ranges from 25 to 34 kV. The heel effect, described as higher X-ray intensity on the cathode side, is utilized in mammography to increase the intensity, that is, penetration, of radiation near the chest wall where tissue thickness is relatively greater.

Compression is used in mammography to reduce the breast parenchymal thickness, which achieves immobilization and reduction in radiation dose, thereby decreasing blurring and increasing sharpness.

Digital tomosynthesis mammography is a newer form of mammography that offers high resolution and is performed using limited-angle tomography (multiple projections at different angles) at mammographic dose levels. The acquired data set is reconstructed using iterative algorithms.

Stereotaxic localization is achieved by acquiring two images, each 15° from the normal projection. This technique provides good localization of masses and is used to perform core needle biopsies.

Image descriptors

The two routinely used mammography views are craniocaudal (CC) and mediolateral oblique (MLO). Other additional views include true lateral, exaggerated, axillary, and cleavage views. Compression views can also be acquired in cases of where the presence of a tumor is uncertain and to resolve any possible parenchymal overlap.

Images are usually reviewed in pairs to help assess for any asymmetry. Mammographic findings are usually described using the terminology of Breast Imaging Reporting and Data System (BI-RADS) lexicon, which includes the description of breast parenchyma, masses, calcifications, and distortion, followed by the assignment of a BI-RADS score, which is used for patient management and to determine follow-up intervals.

Fluoroscopy

Fluoroscopy is an X-ray-based imaging technique commonly used to obtain real-time images of the internal structures of a patient through the use of a fluoroscope.

Image production

Fluoroscopy units are composed of X-ray generator, X-ray tube, collimator, filters, patient table, grid, image intensifier, optical coupling, television system, and image recording. Fluoroscopy units operate using low tube currents (1–6 mA) and tube voltages (70–125 kV). When the X-ray beam is switched off, last image hold (LIH) software permits the visualization of the last image. Newer fluoroscopy systems use pulsed fluoroscopy to reduce dose by acquiring frames that are less than real time (quarter to half the number of frames per second).

Fluoroscopy systems use a television camera to view the image output of the image intensifiers by converting light images into electric (video) signals that can be recorded or viewed on a monitor. Fluoroscopy allows real-time observation and imaging of dynamic activities. It has many applications in radiology, including gastrointestinal (GI), genitourinary, cardiovascular, neuromuscular, and MSK procedures. It can be used for diagnostic and interventional procedures, whether in the fluoroscopy, cardiology, endoscopy, and interventional suites as well as in the operating room.

Cineradiography refers to real-time visualization of motion with fluoroscopy, and frame rate varies from very fast (30 frames/s) in vascular studies during injection of contrast injection to slower to observe motility of the GI tract.

Digital subtraction angiography (DSA) is a fluoroscopic technique used for imaging the vascular system following intravascular contrast injection. In this technique, subtracting the acquired non-contrast mask image, from subsequent frames following contrast administration, allows the removal of static nonenhancing vascular structures that augments visualization of even the smallest contrast differences. This permits using a much lower intravenous (IV) contrast dose. The mean rate of flow of iodine contrast through a vessel can be determined; the extent of vessel stenosis and the pressure gradients may also be estimated.

Road mapping permits an image to be captured and displayed on a monitor while a second monitor shows live images, which is primarily utilized in vascular applications.

Image descriptors

Fluoroscopy uses the same projections and image descriptions used in plain radiography. Oblique views are extensively used in real time fluoroscopy to detect structures or abnormalities, and the position is described in relation of the beam to the patient and patient orientation to the imaging table. Examples of these views include right anterior oblique, left anterior oblique, and right posterior oblique.

CT

CT is a modality that uses computer-processed X-rays to produce axial, cross-sectional "tomographic" images, allowing for excellent imaging with great anatomical details.

Image production

A CT X-ray tube produces a fan-shaped X-ray beam, which passes through the patient, and is measured by the array of detectors on the opposite side of the patient, the sum of which is referred to as a projection. A number of projections are used for each tube rotation.

The sum of projections is plotted as a sinogram, which is then converted to CT images by a mathematical analysis process using filtered back-projection image reconstruction algorithms and applying different types of filters depending on the clinical indication and structure of interest. The factors adjusted by the CT scan operators are the X-ray tube voltage, current, field of view, collimation, slice thickness, and pitch.

CT scanners have gone through revolutionary changes in the last four decades. The generation of systems that is the most common in current use is the third-generation CT machines. These utilize a wide fan beam and a large array of detectors, which rotate around the patient.

Most modern CT scanners also have multiple rows of detectors, typically between 4 and 64, with the more current systems having a greater number of rows. These multidetector CT (MDCT) systems permit larger anatomical coverage in a shorter time frame.

In helical acquisition mode (also known as spiral CT), the table continuously moves while the X-ray tube rotates around the patient until the desired anatomic area is scanned. This is the most common form of CT acquisition in CT studies.

CT fluoroscopy utilizes continuous X-ray tube rotation with very low tube currents (15–60 mA) to obtain a near-real-time image reconstruction. This technique is primarily used to aid interventional procedures, like fine needle aspiration, biopsies, or drainage procedures.

Dual-energy CT (DECT) employs utilization of two different energies (80 and 140 kVp). This optimizes the detection of substances that have greatly different X-ray absorptions (densities). This technique offers various advantages including improved temporal resolution (as short as 83 ms), improved tissue characterization, ability to generate virtual nonenhanced data sets, improved subtraction of bones, pulmonary ventilation and perfusion imaging, and improved detection of iodine-containing substances on low-energy images.

Image descriptors

All CT examinations begin with acquisition of two projection radiograph (frontal and lateral), referred to as topographic or scout images.

Newer MDCT scanners use volumetric data acquisition in the axial plane with slice thickness of 0.625 mm, which can then be reconstructed into slice thickness of 3–5 mm, which are then submitted to PACS or printed on films (hard copies).

The original data set can be reformatted into coronal or sagittal reformats. They can also be postprocessed on dedicated workstation for multiplanar reformation (MPR), maximal intensity projection (MIP) imaging, minimal intensity projection (MinIP) imaging, and volume rendering (VR) imaging.

CT images are composed of maps of the relative attenuation values of the imaged tissues (4096 gray levels), expressed as CT numbers or Hounsfield units (HU). HU value of zero is by default assigned to water. These values are approximate values that can be used to characterize tissues.

CT images are viewed as if the patient is being looked at from below, where the left side of the image corresponds to the right side of the patient and vice versa. The terms "density" and "attenuation" are used to semiquantify tissues where bright structures are described as hyperdense or high attenuating and darker structures are described as hypodense or low attenuating.

Artifacts

Artifacts in CT imaging can be related to mechanical malfunction or related to patients. The most common artifact is motion artifact that is generally secondary to bulk patient motion or organ motion (e.g., heartbeat, breathing). Motion artifact is becoming less of a problem with the advent of newer MDCT machines that acquire images with faster acquisition.

One of the most important artifacts is streak artifact, which is encountered when imaging high-density structures, such as metallic implants, dental fillings, surgical clips, or dense contrasts within the GI tract. This creates a starburst effect of radiating bright lines, which can lead to significant image degradation.

Another common artifact is volume averaging, which arises when structures that are adjacent to each other along the long axis of the patient appear as if they are of the same entity or that they arise from the same entity. This occurs as a function of slice thickness; the thicker the slices, the more likely this effect will be observed.

Ultrasound

Ultrasound (US) is a nonionizing imaging modality that utilizes US waves to provide imaging of anatomical structures with excellent spatial resolution and to study vascular flow dynamics.

Image production

US is a widely available, compact, portable, and relatively inexpensive modality capable of providing real-time imaging. It does not use any ionizing radiation and has no known long-term side effects. Additionally, US Doppler/duplex allows for quantitative measurement of absolute blood velocity. US can be used for diagnostic and interventional procedures.

US probes contain a specific type of crystals, made from specialized materials, which convert voltage oscillations to US waves by changing shape and pressure (piezoelectric effect). Gel is always applied between the transducer and skin to displace air, permitting better transducer–skin contact to minimize interference with US transmission into the patient. After the US beam interacts with soft tissue, the reflected beam is received by the probe crystals, and the crystals record the change in pressure of the reflected beam. This is then converted back to electrical current, which is then processed by the computer board to produce an image.

There are different types of transducers, including linear, curved, and sector transducers, which also have variable frequencies. US transducers are commonly used on the skin surface for scanning. However, endoluminal techniques obviate many of the problems of surface scanning and include endovaginal, endorectal, endointestinal, and endovascular.

US images can be displayed by a variety of methods. The most commonly used mode is the brightness (B) mode, which can be seen as shades of gray, which offers real-time imaging with a high frame rate.

Color Doppler is used to display moving red blood cells (RBCs) according to their direction of flow in reference to the US probe. Power Doppler is a variation of this method, which has better sensitivity for detecting moving objects, but without the ability to assess the direction of flow.

Duplex scanning combines real-time B mode imaging with Doppler imaging. Spectral analysis displays frequency shift as a function of time that can provide information regarding blood flow pulsatility, direction, and absolute flow velocity (quantitative evaluation).

US can also be used intraoperatively by applying a transducer with a sterile probe cover or sheath in direct contact with the organ being examined. It can also be used to guide interventional procedures, such as biopsy, drainages, or tube placement.

High-intensity focused ultrasound (HIFU) is used as a hyperthermia therapy, a class of clinical therapies that use temperature to treat diseases. Clinical HIFU procedures are typically performed in conjunction with an imaging study, an example of which is HIFU treatment of uterine fibroids localized with MRI.

Image descriptors

The interpretation of US images relies on recognizing anatomical relationships and level of pixel brightness, the latter referred to as echogenicity.

Structures are described according to their echogenicity compared to adjacent structures as hypoechoic (low), hyperechoic (high), isoechoic (similar), or anechoic (almost no reflection).

The direction of flow is described according to the direction of the flow as toward (red) or away (blue) from the US probe on color Doppler and as toward (above) or away (below) from the baseline on spectral Doppler images. Images are described based on the orientation of the probe in relation to the human body as longitudinal, when the axis of the probe is parallel to the body, or axial, when the axis of the probe is perpendicular to the body.

Image performance

The quality of the US image is based on resolution, which can be divided into axial, lateral, and elevational resolution. Axial resolution is the ability to separate two objects lying along the axis of the beam and is determined by the US probe frequency. Lateral resolution is approximately four times worse than axial resolution, and it decreases at a longer distance from the probe. Elevational resolution is equivalent to slice thickness and is proportional to US probe width.

Artifacts

Artifacts in US imaging are very common and should be recognized to avoid diagnostic errors. Some artifacts can be utilized to enhance diagnostic performance such as acoustic shadowing, acoustic enhancement, aliasing, twinkle, and ring-down artifacts. Some artifacts however negatively impact diagnostic performance such as mirror image and side-lobe artifact.

MRI

MRI is a nonionizing imaging modality that uses the body's natural magnetic properties (imaging of protons) to produce detailed images with excellent anatomical details and exquisite, unmatched soft tissue contrast images from any part of the body.

Image production

Hydrogen nuclei have the largest nuclear magnetization, and these occur abundantly in humans in the form of water, which contains two hydrogen molecules (protons), and fat, which contains multiple protons. In the absence of an applied magnetic field, these hydrogen protons are randomly aligned with no net magnetization.

MRI machines are based on powerful magnets, which can generate a strong and stable magnetic field. The magnetic field strength is measured in tesla (T). The magnets used may be resistive, permanent, or superconducting. The vast majority of current magnetic resonance (MR) scanners use superconducting magnets, which contain a wire-wrapped cylinder and a constantly circulating electric current of hundreds of amps to generate the uniform magnetic field. The encircling wire that forms the magnetic core is composed of specialized material that must be kept very cold (using liquid helium as a refrigerant), in order that the electrons flowing in the wire experience extremely low friction or impedance. This permits creation of a very powerful current that generates a strong magnetic field strength, a process termed superconduction.

Unlike most other imaging modalities (such as CT and US) that are only "on" when the patient is being imaged, the MR system magnet is always "on." This explains why with MRI health-care professionals have to be very careful not to bring ferromagnetic (iron-containing) objects into the MR room that can be drawn into the magnet at high velocity giving a missile effect, which can lead to injury of the patients and personnel, as well as cause unnecessary downtime of the MR system.

Other essential components of an MRI system are three gradient coils, which are used to code the spatial location of the MR signal by superimposing a linear gradient on the main magnetic field (this causes protons at different locations to have different precession frequencies), and the radiofrequency (RF) coils, which consist of various configurations of radio wave antenna and are used to transmit and receive electromagnetic radio waves. There are different coils including volume coils, specialized coils, and surface coils. Phased array coils are a combination of many surface coils (elements) and are required for parallel imaging, which is most commonly employed for imaging most regions on modern MR systems.

When a person is placed inside the powerful magnetic field of the scanner, the magnetized protons (spins) align with the external magnetic field either along (spin up) or opposite (spin down) the direction of the magnetic field, a phenomenon referred to as the Zeeman effect. The spin-down position has higher energy than the spin-up. The principle of MRI depends on this small difference between the spins, which is influenced by the main magnetic field strength and estimated to be around 3 spins/million protons at 1 T.

When applying a 90° RF pulse, the net magnetization vector will produce longitudinal and transverse components. The time it takes the longitudinal magnetization to go exponentially from 0% to 63% of full magnetization (equilibrium value) is referred to as T1 relaxation time or spin–lattice relaxation. When the RF pulse is switched off, the longitudinal magnetization will return exponentially to zero in a time equal to T1. Different tissues have different T1 relaxation times (long for fluids, with the result that they appear dark on T1-weighted images, and short for fat, with the result that they appear bright on these images). Gadolinium-based contrast agents (GBCAs) cause T1 shortening, which renders tissues brighter.

When the RF pulse is switched off, the transverse magnetization will exponentially decay; when it reaches 37% of its original value, the time duration is referred to as T2 relaxation time or spin–spin relaxation. Different tissues have different T2 relaxation times (long for fluids, bright on T2-weighted images, and short for solid tissues, darker on T2-weighted images). Tissue T2 values, unlike T1 values, are not affected significantly by magnetic field strength.

The acquisition of the image requires the execution of a preselected predefined set of RF and gradient pulses at certain time intervals, known as pulse sequences, to generate an MR image of certain characteristics. These pulse sequences are computer commands that control all hardware aspects of the MRI measurement process.

The time required between each pulse is termed the time to repeat (TR). The time between the start of a pulse sequence and maximum signal is termed the echo time (TE). The time between a 180° inversion pulse and 90° excitation pulse in inversion recovery pulse sequences is termed inversion time (TI). TR and TE are always employed in MR sequences (and TI, if utilized), are used to describe basic MR pulse sequences, and are all measured in milliseconds.

A combination of TR and TE is used to generate different image weighting. Short TR and TE provide T1 weighting, long TR and TE provide T2 weighting, and long TR and short TE provide proton density (PD) weighting.

The basic pulse sequences include conventional spin echo, fast spin echo, gradient-recalled echo, and inversion recovery sequences. More advanced MRI sequences include MRA sequences, echo-planar imaging/diffusion-weighted imaging sequences, magnetization transfer sequences, MR spectroscopy, and functional imaging.

Fat suppression applied to some acquisitions is an integral part of nearly all routine MR examinations, and this function is employed for tissue characterization and for emphasizing contrast agent enhancement. There are many fat-suppression techniques used in routine MRI, each with its own advantages and disadvantages. These include Dixon techniques, spectral fat saturation, water excitation, and fast suppression with inversion recovery (SPAIR and STIR).

The principle of parallel imaging is that different coils detect the signal from the same body part with different signal strengths due to their locations in space by applying the sensitivity maps of individual elements. Acceleration factor is a term used to denote the speed improvement achieved by combining the signal reception from imaging coils, where an acceleration factor of 2 represents a decrease in time of study of approximately 50%. Parallel imaging leads to significant reduction of scan time at acceleration factors of 2–3 while still achieving acceptable image quality with good signal-to-noise ratio (SNR) and minimal artifacts.

Image descriptors

MR images can be acquired in different planes: axial, coronal, and sagittal. Additionally, obliques planes can be planned based on these basic planes including long-axis and short-axis images. Similar to CT, three-dimensional (3D) MR data sets can be postprocessed on dedicated workstation to reformat the images in different planes termed MPR, MIP, and VR images.

Axial MR images are also interpreted as if the patient is being viewed from below, and coronal images are interpreted as if standing in front of the patient, where the left side of the image corresponds to the right side of the patient, and vice versa.

The appearance of structures on MR is described based on their intensities: hypo-, iso-, or hyperintense on T1- or T2-weighted images and hypo-, iso-, or hyperenhancing on postcontrast images, based on their level of enhancement compared to the background tissues/organs.

T1-weighted images can be recognized by the signal of different normal body tissues. Fluids show low T1 signal and high T2 signal intensities. Fat shows high T1 and intermediately high T2 signal intensities and suppresses on fat-suppression sequences, but not on opposed-phase T1-weighted images. Opposed-phase T1-weighted images can be used to detect intracellular, microscopic, intravoxel fat. Other common substances that can give high T1 signal (T1 relaxation time shortening) include gadolinium, protein, and methemoglobin.

Gray matter demonstrates lower T1 and higher T2 signal intensities compared to white matter. CSF demonstrates low signal on T1- and FLAIR-weighted images and high signal on T2-weighted images. T2 gradient-weighted images are very sensitive to susceptibility and are used to detect subtle blood degradation products and superparamagnetic substances, that is, iron.

Image performance
Contrast resolution

Contrast resolution depends on variations between the different tissues and is dependent on T1 and T2 times of these tissues. Flow also affects image contrast, and this property can be utilized in noncontrast-enhanced MR angiography. Gadolinium can also alter tissue contrast through T1 time shortening. PD imaging shows little intrinsic contrast because of the small variations in PD for most tissues.

Spatial resolution

Spatial resolution describes how sharp the image looks and is a product of pixel size. Pixel size equals the field of view divided by the data acquisition matrix size. In routine imaging, the spatial resolution is half that of CT. Higher-resolution imaging can be achieved in MRI, but at the expense of SNR.

SNR

SNR is the critical determinant for MR image quality. General factors like higher magnetic field and use of small-diameter surface coils (which are often aligned into a matrix of multiple coils, termed phased array) increase the SNR. SNR is also increased by increasing the slice thickness and/or decreasing the matrix size. Increasing the number of excitations, signal averages, or acquisitions increases the SNR but at the expense of increased scanning time.

Artifacts

Imaging artifacts in MRI can be divided into equipment-related or patient-related artifacts. One of the most important artifacts in MRI is motion related.

Motion appears as ghosting and blurring of the image along the phase-encoding direction, which is one of the directions of data acquisition in the XY plane (the other is frequency encoding). Motion artifacts can be the result of gross patient movement (nonperiodic) or secondary to respiratory or cardiac motion (periodic) motion. Nonperiodic movement is the most problematic, and it causes smearing across the image, and these types of artifacts may render studies uninterpretable. Periodic movement causes coherent ghosting, which are generally not so challenging.

Other artifacts include zipper, susceptibility, chemical shift, aliasing (wraparound), standing-wave, magic angel, cross-talk, and truncation artifacts.

Nuclear medicine

Nuclear medicine is a medical specialty that involves the application of radioactive material to either diagnose or treat diseases. Nuclear medicine primarily reflects physiological information, which on occasion can precede anatomical changes that are seen by other modalities.

Image production

Very heavy nuclei tend to be unstable. Unstable nuclides are called radionuclides. The transformation of a parent unstable nuclide into daughter nuclides is called radioactive decay. During that transformation, the mass number, electric charge, and total energy are unchanged.

Gamma rays (photons) are form of high-energy electromagnetic radiation that is emitted during radioactive decay and occasionally accompany the emission of alpha or beta particles. They have no mass or charge and interact less intensively with matter compared to ionizing particles. Gamma rays are comparable to X-rays both in their imaging capabilities, and also in their potential to cause biologic radiation damage.

Image acquisition usually takes several minutes for full acquisition. Images can be viewed in real time on a display monitor during the acquisition, to monitor for gross motion, in addition to viewing the static images after the completion of a study data acquisition. Analog-to-digital converters (ADCs) are used to generate the digital information.

Nuclear medicine can be used for diagnostic (gamma rays) and interventional (beta particles) applications. Beta particles have higher energy but shorter traveling distances compared to gamma rays.

Most noncardiac applications in nuclear medicine utilize planar imaging. The exception is single-photon emission computed tomography (SPECT) imaging that provides computed tomographic views of the 3D distribution of radioisotopes in the body. SPECT imaging can be combined with CT (SPECT/CT). Low-dose CT scans are used for coregistration and attenuation correction only. Higher-dose CT scans can be acquired for diagnostic imaging.

In PET imaging, a ring of detectors (scintillators) surrounding the patient is used coupled with photomultiplier tubes to detect light produced in each detector. The detectors are thicker to allow the registration of incidence gamma photons. The positron travels for a distance of 0.4 mm and then collides with an adjacent electron, resulting in annihilation and emission of two 511 keV gamma ray photons at nearly opposite directions (coinciding photons). The simultaneous detection of coinciding photons allows for the identification of line of response and creation of a sinogram, which may be reconstructed using iterative reconstruction algorithms. The most commonly used agent in PET imaging is fluorine-18 fluorodeoxyglucose (18F-FDG), which has a half-life of 110 min. 18F undergoes beta minus decay with the emission of a positron.

PET/CT uses a hybrid of PET and CT imaging. The principle is similar to SPECT/CT. Most recently, systems have been developed in which PET can be simultaneously acquired in combination with MRI (MR/PET).

Image descriptors

Nuclear medicine images are divided into planar, SPECT, or PET images. Most applications require the acquisition of whole-body images from two cameras while the patient is lying supine on the imaging table, which results in two images (anterior and posterior projections).

Planar images are usually displayed in pairs with two different windows and sent to PACS or printed on films. Additionally, spot images can be acquired as part of routine imaging or as a problem-solving addition. Spot images can have different projections. On the anterior projection images, the left side of the image corresponds anatomically to the right side of the patient. On the posterior projection images, the left side of the image corresponds anatomically to the left side of the patient.

SPECT and PET images are obtained in axial plane and can be reconstructed into coronal and sagittal plane images. SPECT and PET images are displayed in the same fashion as CT and MRI where the left side of the image corresponds to the right side of the patient.

Terms used to describe imaging findings in nuclear medicine are different from those used to describe other radiologic studies. Areas of increased activity are described as areas of increased uptake. Areas with decreased activity are referred to as areas of decreased uptake. Areas with no activity are often referred to as photopenic areas.

Image performance

Spatial resolution in nuclear medicine is the ability to distinguish two adjacent radioactive sources. The most common method to measure resolution is to measure the full width half maximum of the imaged line source of activity. It depends on the width of the camera and the collimators. SPECT has the lowest spatial resolution.

Image contrast is the difference in intensity (counts) between a specific tissue or organ and background and depends on the concentration of the radiopharmaceutical in the targeted tissue (target-to-background ratio). The background count is proportional to collimator septal penetration and scatter.

Noise, also called quantum mottle, is much higher in nuclear medicine compared to X-ray imaging because the number of photons used to generate an image is low. SPECT imaging has the highest noise due to the low number of photons used to reconstruct each voxel.

Artifacts

Motion artifact, as in all radiological modalities, is the most common artifact in nuclear medicine. The most problematic, as with other modalities, is gross patient motion.

Image defects can be of different appearances. The appearance of the defect can be characteristic for malfunction of a specific component within the imaging system. Common defects related to external effects include metallic implants or dense contrast material (e.g., barium).

Contrast agents

A radiological contrast agent (or contrast media) is a substance used to emphasize the appearance of structures within the body and is commonly used to enhance the visibility of blood vessels, GI tract, or disease process.

Radiographic contrast agents

Radiographic contrast agents may be used with all imaging techniques to enhance the differences between body tissues. Ideally, contrast agents should achieve a high concentration in the body without producing any adverse effects. Unfortunately, this target has not yet been achieved, and all contrast agents have potential adverse effects.

They are classified into positive and negative agents. Positive contrast agents can be divided into water and nonwater soluble. Air is often referred to as a negative contrast agent, which can be used alone or in addition to other positive contrasts to achieve a double contrast effect.

Non water-soluble agents consist of a suspension of insoluble barium. These agents are only used for GI tract imaging and are not absorbed.

Iodine-based contrast agents are water soluble and are based on a molecular structure of three-iodine atom attached to a benzene ring (tri-iodinated benzene ring). Based on the number of tri-iodinated benzene rings, these agents are classified into monomers and dimers.

Iodine-based contrast agents can be classified into ionic and nonionic based on their electrical structure. They can be further classified based on their osmolality into hypo-, iso-, and hyperosmolar agents. They can be given intravenously or orally or injected into different abdominopelvic cavities.

Iodine-based contrast agents have different viscosities, which is a function of solution concentration, molecular structure, and interactions with water molecules.

Iodine-based contrast agents are distributed throughout the extracellular space when administered intravenously. They enhance the diagnostic performance of CT and conventional diagnostic angiographic procedures. They can also be administered directly into the body cavities, for example, the GI tract and the urinary tract.

Ultrasonographic contrast agents

Contrast agent can also be used to enhance the diagnostic value of US. These agents are composed of microbubbles that persist in the bloodstream for several minutes, which in combination with specialized US techniques (harmonics) allow a definite improvement in the contrast resolution and suppression of signal from stationary tissues.

These agents are commonly used to enhance the conspicuity of solid organ lesions, either for diagnostic or interventional purposes, and to offer enhancement characterization of these lesions. They can also be used to augment the diagnostic value of Doppler US to assess solid organ perfusion, especially following transplantation.

MR contrast agents

Contrast agents in MRI are divided into positive (paramagnetic) and negative (superparamagnetic) contrasts.

Negative agents are iron based and cause significant T2/T2* shortening; these agents can cause significant T1 shortening during their vascular phase, but once internalized within the reticuloendothelial system, they have negligible effect on T1 relaxation time. Currently, none of these agents are commercially available, apart from an oral preparation.

Positive agents are gadolinium based (the great majority), and they cause T1 and T2 shortening, with the most prominent effect, which is employed in most clinical applications, being the T1-shortening effect. T1 enhancement is best shown on T1-weighted images, with the appearance of tissue brightening. Gadolinium is a heavy metal and is very toxic in its free form. In Gadolinium-based contrast agents (GBCAs), the gadolinium ion is bound to ligand forming a chelate to minimize toxicity.

There are a variety of ways to classify GBCAs based on various properties that they possess. One common classification is based on the molecular structure of the agent, where more stable (hence often "safer") structures are macrocyclic and less stable structures are linear and as an independent property ionic (more stable) and nonionic (less stable). GBCAs can also be classified into extracellular agents or mixed extracellular/organ-specific (hepatocyte) agents.

Extracellular GBCAs do not show appreciable binding to protein and are solely excreted by the kidneys, while agents with protein-binding property are excreted to a varying extent through the bile as well as the kidneys.

The following GBCAs in clinical usage are described with their structure: gadoterate meglumine (Dotarem) is an ionic macrocyclic agent, gadoteridol (ProHance) and gadobutrol (Gadavist) are non-ionic macrocyclic agents, and gadopentetate dimeglumine (Magnevist) and gadobenate dimeglumine (MultiHance) are ionic linear agents.

Ionic linear GBCAs with dual elimination are gadobenate dimeglumine (MultiHance) and gadoxetate disodium (Eovist/Primovist), which also exhibit high relaxivity (greater tissue brightening).

Different GBCAs have different r1 and r2 relaxivities, also termed T1 and T2 relaxivity. Protein binding often results in heightened relaxivity, with the net effect that enhancement is more intense on T1-weighted images.

Immediately after IV injection, extracellular and protein-bound agents behave the same and exhibit the same extracellular distribution and excretion as iodine-based agents. However, protein-binding agents are taken up by hepatocytes and excreted into the bile in addition to their renal excretion. Protein binding also allows for longer intravascular dwell time in some of these agents.

Nuclear medicine radiopharmaceuticals

Radionuclides are combined with existing pharmaceutical compounds to form radiopharmaceuticals. They are designed to mimic a natural physiologic process and localize in the organ or tissue of interest by different mechanisms including compartmentalization, active transport, simple exchange, phagocytosis, or capillary blockage.

Technetium (^{99m}Tc) is a radiotracer used in approximately 80% of all nuclear medicine examinations. It is considered an ideal radiotracer because it has gamma ray energy of 140 keV and a convenient t half-life of 6 h. Pertechnetate (^{99m}TcO$_4$) is produced directly from a shielded generator containing ^{99}Mo using a saline eluant. A ^{99m}Tc generator is normally eluted daily over the course of a week and then replaced.

There are many radiopharmaceuticals used for different clinical applications with different chemical properties.

Biological effects

Ionizing radiation modalities

Ionizing radiation results in ejection of an electron from a neutral atom, which becomes positively charged. X-rays, gamma rays, and ultraviolet radiation are all considered ionizing radiations. Table 1.1 demonstrates the effective dose of common radiological examinations.

X-ray-based modalities

Although large doses of ionizing radiation are known to cause cancer, there has been controversy whether lower doses, in the range observed with CT scans (5–50 mSv), pose a risk.

Sponsored by several federal agencies, the seventh Biological Effects of Ionizing Radiation (BEIR) report [1] updated the health risks from low linear energy transfer radiation (≤100 mSv), which deposits little energy in a cell and thus tends to cause little damage. It was stated that there is no threshold below which there is no risk, and that as exposure increases, so does the health risk (linear-no-threshold model).

Table 1.1 Radiation dose estimates for common radiological techniques in mSv.

Diagnostic examination	Effective dose (mSv)[†,‡]
Chest X-ray (PA film)	0.02
Lumbar spine X-ray	1.8
Extremity X-ray	0.001
Mammogram (two views)	0.36
CT head	2
CT coronary angiography	5–32
Cardiac CT for calcium scoring	3
CT chest	10
CT abdomen	10
18F-FDG PET/CT	25
Cardiac 201Tl chloride	41
Coronary angiography (therapeutic)	15
Transjugular intrahepatic portosystemic shunt (TIPS) placement	70

[†]The effective doses are typical values for an average-sized adult. The actual dose can vary substantially, depending on a person's size as well as on differences in imaging practices.
[‡]The use of effective dose for assessing the exposure of patients has severe limitations that must be considered when quantifying medical exposure.

The linear-no-threshold model predicts that any dose, no matter how small, may produce health effects based on the hypothesis that a single ionizing event can result in DNA damage. From a practical standpoint, low-dose procedures such as chest X-rays (0.10 mSv) are treated differently from high-dose procedures such as CT (2–20 mSv), as risk related to individual low-dose procedures is likely largely nonexistent.

Much of the data for radiation risk has been derived from atomic bomb survivors from Japan, and until relatively recently, reliable data on the risks related to CT imaging have been lacking.

In 2012, two important studies were published describing more direct evidence of risk of malignancy development. Pearce et al. [2] reported a study on pediatric patients who underwent CT examination in Great Britain. They showed that the use of CT scans in children that delivered cumulative doses in the range of 50 mGy might almost triple the risk of leukemia and doses of about 60 mGy might triple the risk of brain cancer. Mathews et al. [3] reported on 680,000 Australians who underwent a CT scan when aged 0–19 years and showed that malignancy incidence was increased by 24% (95% CI: 0.20–0.29) compared with the incidence in over 10 million unexposed people. Their study also showed that the proportional increase in risk was evident at short intervals after exposure and was greater for persons exposed at younger ages. They reported that absolute excess cancer incidence rate was 9.38 per 100,000 person-years at risk and that the incidence rates were increased for most individual types of solid cancer and for leukemias, myelodysplasias, and some other lymphoid tumors.

A third large-scale study, reported by Eisenberg et al. [4] involving 82,861 patients who had an acute myocardial infarction and no history of cancer, described 64,000 patients who underwent at least one cardiac imaging or therapeutic procedure in the first year after acute myocardial infarction. They reported that for every 10 mSv of low-dose ionizing radiation, there was a 3% increase in the risk of age- and sex-adjusted cancer over a mean follow-up period of 5 years.

Nuclear medicine

Radiation exposure is extremely high with a number of nuclear medicine studies, notably thallium studies and CT/PET. CT/PET is reported to have an exposure of 25 mSv, but much of that radiation is attributable to the CT part of the study, and approximately 5 mSv from PET.

Nonionizing radiation modalities
US and MRI

Present data have not conclusively documented any deleterious effects of cancer induction or fetal defects secondary to either US or MRI.

Contrast-related adverse events

Contrast reactions are classified into acute, subacute, and chronic reactions based on the interval between contrast administration and development of side effects.

Acute adverse reactions are defined as reactions occurring within an hour up to 48 h following contrast medium injection. There is increased risk for developing acute adverse events in patients with history of asthma or history of allergy to other contrast agents.

Allergic acute reactions have been classified as mild, moderate, or severe. Mild reactions usually do not need treatment and include nausea, vomiting, urticaria, and itching. Moderate reactions include severe vomiting, marked urticaria, bronchospasm, facial or laryngeal edema, and vasovagal reactions. Severe reactions include hypotensive shock, pulmonary edema, cardiopulmonary arrest, and convulsion.

The management of acute adverse reactions is identical whether they are caused by iodine- or gadolinium-based agents or by US agents. Nausea, vomiting, hives, and pruritus are usually self-limited. However, patients should be observed closely for systemic symptoms while IV access is maintained. If the urticaria is extensive or bothersome to the patient, antihistamines, such as Benadryl, may be given.

Bronchospasm without coexisting cardiovascular problems should be treated with high rate oxygen (6–10 L/min) and inhaled beta-2 agonist bronchodilators (two to three deep inhalations).

Isolated hypotension is best managed initially by rapid IV fluid replacement rather than vasopressor drugs. Large volumes may be required to reverse the hypotension. Vagal reactions are characterized by the combination of prominent sinus bradycardia and hypotension. Treatment includes patient leg elevation and rapid infusion of IV fluids. The bradycardia is treated by IV administration of atropine to block vagal stimulation of the cardiac conduction system.

Anaphylactoid reactions are acute, rapidly progressing, systemic reactions characterized by multisystem involvement. Initial treatment includes maintenance of the airway, administration of oxygen, rapid infusion of IV fluids, intramuscular adrenaline (0.3–0.5 mL of 1:1000), electrocardiogram (ECG) monitoring, and slow administration of adrenaline.

Iodine-based contrast agents
Acute adverse events

Acute adverse reactions (as described in the section "Contrast-related adverse events") to iodine-based contrast media are almost always associated with intravascular administration. Prompt recognition and treatment are essential.

Contrast medium-induced nephropathy

Contrast medium-induced nephropathy (CIN) is defined as an onset of diminished renal function that occurs shortly after contrast agent administration without other predisposing causes. Current practice for preventing CIN still relies on identifying patients at increased risk.

Preexisting renal impairment, defined as an effective glomerular filtration rate (eGFR) of less than 60, is the most important risk factor for CIN. CIN has been seen with all stages of chronic renal disease, but most often with stages 3–5. CIN has been reported in patients with normal renal function in 0.6–2.3%, but this is most often a transient effect on renal function.

The risk of developing CIN in patients with renal impairment is about 3–21% when contrast is administered intravenously and 3–50% when given intra-arterially. The risk of CIN is greater if renal impairment is associated with diabetes mellitus, hypertension, and concurrent use of metformin or nephrotoxic medications. The risk of requiring dialysis in patients developing CIN is 3%, with a 1-year mortality rate of 45% for these patients.

A number of measures have been proposed to reduce the incidence of CIN, but the most important, and consistently observed as beneficial, patient preparation is to ensure good hydration, which may require IV administration of fluid.

Dialysis is effective for eliminating iodine-based contrast media.

Contrast extravasation

Extravasation of contrast medium during injection is a common problem. The mechanism of injury is related to chemical and tissue compression effects. The clinical picture varies from trivial pain and redness at the site of injection to (rarely) skin ulceration and compartment syndrome.

When extravasation is identified, the injection should be immediately terminated. The injection site should be carefully inspected. The patient should be advised to elevate the involved limb. Alternating hot (to induce vasodilatation and promote absorption of the extravasated material) and cold (to induce vasoconstriction and limit inflammation) compresses, performed a few times per day for the first few days, is recommended.

Gadolinium-based contrast agents (GBCAs)
Acute adverse events
Acute adverse reactions may occur after administration of GBCAs; however, their rate is much lower compared to iodine-based agents. There may be no difference in the rate of acute adverse events between the different GBCAs. Acute adverse event and their medical management are similar to those of iodine-based contrast agents.

Nephrogenic systemic fibrosis
Nephrogenic systemic fibrosis (NSF) is an important subacute adverse reaction to nonchelated gadolinium, with onset typically occurring between 2 months and 2 years after GBCA administration.

Patients who are at high risk to develop NSF are those with stage 4–5 chronic kidney disease (CKD), in particular stage 5, and those with severe acute renal failure. The type of GBCA used also plays an extremely important role in NSF, with linear nonionic agents having the highest causal association.

Agents with low risk include MultiHance, Eovist/Primovist, and Ablavar/Vasovist (which are ionic linear agents that possess additional hepatobiliary elimination), and ProHance, Dotarem, and Gadavist (which are macrocyclic agents).

In efforts to avoid causing NSF, guidelines for the utilization of GBCAs have been developed and generally employed at all institutions. The bases of these guidelines include avoiding the use of nonionic linear agents in patients with renal impairment and avoiding repeated doses of GBCAs in patients with poor renal function. Routine determination of eGFR is generally advised in patients at risk of having poor renal function.

Summary
Remarkable advances in radiology have been achieved in the last three decades. In addition to the strengths, it is imperative to understand associated risks and biological effects. It is the responsibility of the radiologist and requesting physician to consider the risk and benefit of each radiological investigation and to choose the appropriate, yet sufficiently safe, technique based on the available data of probabilistic risk assessments (Table 1.2).

Table 1.2 Probabilistic risk estimates of contrast agents' adverse effects.

Event	Incidence
CIN in patients with renal impairment	1 in 5
NSF from Omniscan in patients with renal impairment	1 in 25
CIN in patients with normal renal function	1 in 50
Cancer from 10 mSv of radiation (1 body CT)	1 in 1,000
NSF from Omniscan	1 in 2,500
NSF from Magnevist	1 in 40,000
Death from anaphylactoid reaction to nonionic iodine-based contrast	1 in 130,000
Death from anaphylactoid reaction to gadolinium-based agents	1 in 280,000
NSF from MultiHance, ProHance, Gadavist, and Dotarem	<1 in 10,000,000 for each

The use of nonionizing radiation modalities should always be considered, especially in more radiosensitive populations. Physicians should also avoid requesting redundant examinations and unnecessary short-term follow-ups. Specific considerations have been provided in this chapter that allow the understanding of basic imaging principles and safety practices.

Reference
1 National Research Council (US) Committee on the Biological Effects of Ionizing Radiation (BEIR V). *Health Effects of Exposure to Low Levels of Ionizing Radiation: BEIR V*. Washington, DC: National Academies Press (US), 1990. Available at http://www.ncbi.nlm.nih.gov/pubmed/25032334. Accessed October 31, 2014.

2 Pearce, M. S., Salotti, J. A., Little, M. P., McHugh, K., Lee, C., Kim, K. P., et al. (2012) Radiation exposure from CT scans in childhood and subsequent risk of leukaemia and brain tumours: a retrospective cohort study. *Lancet, 380*(9840), 499–505. doi:10.1016/S0140-6736(12)60815-0

3 Mathews, J. D., Forsythe, A. V., Brady, Z., Butler, M. W., Goergen, S. K., Byrnes, G. B., et al. (2013) Cancer risk in 680,000 people exposed to computed tomography scans in childhood or adolescence: data linkage study of 11 million Australians. *BMJ (Clinical Research Ed.), 346*, f2360.

4 Eisenberg, M. J., Afilalo, J., Lawler, P. R., Abrahamowicz, M., Richard, H., & Pilote, L. (2011) Cancer risk related to low-dose ionizing radiation from cardiac imaging in patients after acute myocardial infarction. *CMAJ : Canadian Medical Association Journal = Journal De l'Association Medicale Canadienne, 183*(4), 430–436. doi:10.1503/cmaj.100463

Suggested reading
ACR Committee on Drugs and Contrast Media ACR Manual on Contrast Media (V9). ACR Manual on Contrast Media (9 ed.), 2013. Retrieved from http://www.acr.org/quality-safety/resources/contrast-manual. Accessed October 31, 2014.

Amis, E.S., Jr & Butler, P.F. (2010) ACR white paper on radiation dose in medicine: three years later. *Journal of the American College of Radiology, 7* (11), 865–70.

Allisy-Roberts, P.J. & Williams, J. (2008) *Farr's Physics for Medical Imaging*. Saunders, Edinburgh, New York.

Huda, W. (2010) *Review of Radiologic Physics*. Lippincott Williams & Wilkins, Baltimore, MD.

Westbrook, C., Kaut Roth, C. & Talbot, J. (1998) *MRI in Practice*. Blackwell Science, Malden, MA.

CHAPTER 2

Imaging studies: What study and when to order?

Kiran Reddy Busireddy, Miguel Ramalho, and Mamdoh AlObaidy

Department of Radiology, University of North Carolina, Chapel Hill, USA

Radiology at present is the key diagnostic tool for numerous disease processes and has also an important role in monitoring treatment and predicting outcome. It is well recognized that imaging achieves a great proportion of diagnosis in daily clinical practice and changed the way how medicine is performed. The improved image resolution and tissue differentiation in a number of conditions dramatically augment the range of diagnostic information and in many cases the demonstration of pathology without the requirement of invasive tissue sampling. New knowledge in imaging is being developed at an increasingly rapid rate, and the field of radiology has expanded dramatically.

There are a number of imaging modalities with differing physical principles of varying complexity. Despite the recent technological advances, different imaging investigations have strengths and weaknesses, and development of appropriate integrated imaging algorithms to maximize clinical effectiveness is recommended. The referring physicians need a clinical interface with the imaging specialist, ensuring the best use of assets and health-care resources.

The imaging tests that the health-care team recommends depend on a number of factors, such as what type and where the pathology is, as some imaging studies work better for certain organs or tissues; whether or not a biopsy (tissue sample) is needed; the balance between any risks or side effects and the expected benefits; and overall cost.

In this chapter, we describe the role of specific imaging methods for different organ systems and recommend the modalities for common disease processes, maximizing the use of resources. Also, we have included imaging workup algorithms for the few most commonly found clinical scenarios. These are very similar to the American College of Radiology (ACR) appropriateness criteria, which is recognized as the best compendium of recommendations of imaging exams and can be found at http://www.acr.org/quality-safety/appropriateness-criteria. Overall, the recommendations listed here provide additional weighting to magnetic resonance imaging (MRI) for many indications, reflecting heightened MR image quality of new MR systems and the intrinsic safety of MRI.

Respiratory system

Plain radiography (PXR) and computed tomography (CT) are the predominant imaging modalities used to evaluate the respiratory system.

Plain radiography is often used as a first imaging modality to evaluate signs and symptoms related to the respiratory, cardiac, and bony structures of the thorax.

CT is used for further evaluation when PXR is normal or equivocal and when there is a high suspicion of a clinically significant disease. Other indications of PXR are preoperative evaluation and follow-up of known thoracic disease processes to assess for improvement, progression, or resolution.

High-resolution computed tomography (HRCT) is the examination of choice to evaluate suspected small and large airway diseases, to demonstrate and differentiate the diffuse pulmonary diseases (especially interstitial lung disease), to assess the extent of diffuse disease pathology, and to determine the best site for biopsy.

MRI has a limited role in evaluating respiratory diseases because of the low proton density of normal lung, the decrease of signal by susceptibility artifacts induced by the air–soft tissue interfaces within the lung, and the consequences of cardiac and respiratory movement. One possible indication of chest MRI is suspicion of pulmonary embolism (PE) if radiation and intravenous (IV) iodinated contrast medium need to be avoided.

Ventilation/perfusion (V/Q) scintigraphy is a noninvasive technique for assessing the probability of acute or chronic pulmonary thromboembolic disease. Pulmonary scintigraphy is also indicted for evaluating the effect of congenital heart diseases or pulmonary arterial pathologies on pulmonary perfusion and regional lung function pre- and postoperatively, including post-lung transplant patients. Ionizing radiation is delivered with this modality in the form of gamma rays.

Critical Observations in Radiology for Medical Students, First Edition. Katherine R. Birchard, Kiran Reddy Busireddy, and Richard C. Semelka.
© 2015 John Wiley & Sons, Ltd. Published 2015 by John Wiley & Sons, Ltd.
Companion website: www.wiley.com/go/birchard

Imaging role and workup algorithms for selected clinical scenarios

Chest trauma

- PXR remains the initial diagnostic modality for all chest trauma patients.
- CT possesses high sensitivity and specificity and is often helpful in rapid assessment of emergency patients presenting with chest trauma.

Hemoptysis

Chronic bronchitis, pneumonia, bronchiectasis, malignancy, fungal infections, and tuberculosis are the most common causes of hemoptysis. Refer to the imaging workup algorithm for hemoptysis:

- CT imaging should be considered for further evaluation in patients who are active or ex-smokers with a chest radiograph showing no abnormalities.
- Patients with greater than 40 years of age or greater than 40 pack-year smoking history with a negative PXR, CT scan, and bronchoscopy should be followed with PXR or CT imaging for the next continuous 3 years as they are considered to be at high risk for lung cancer.

Acute respiratory illness

The presence of one or more of the following symptoms such as cough, sputum production, chest pain, or dyspnea with or without associated fever is known as acute respiratory illness (ARI). The choice of imaging study also depends on many factors, such as patient's age, clinical history, physical examination, the presence of other risk factors, severity of illness, and the presence of fever or increased white blood cell count or hypoxemia. Refer to the ARI imaging workup algorithm:

- In patients presenting with ARI, the workup usually involves PXR and CT.
- In patients presenting with chronic obstructive pulmonary disease (COPD) and asthma exacerbations, PXR is not indicated unless there is a suspected complication such as pneumonia or pneumothorax or in the presence of one or more of the following:

chest pain, leukocytosis, history of coronary artery disease, or congestive heart failure.

- PXR is also considered in adult patients with a clinical suspicion of pneumonia, although some clinicians may not choose to request any imaging if clinical suspicion of respiratory infection is sufficiently high to initiate treatment.
- PXR is indicated early in the evaluation of immunocompromised patients presenting with ARI, and further CT imaging is not warranted if a plain radiograph shows a single, focal airspace abnormality in a patient with acute bacterial pneumonia symptoms.
- CT without contrast is indicated in patients with nonresolving pneumonia or severe pneumonia with multilobar involvement or if any intervention is contemplated. Further imaging with CT may not be needed.

Dyspnea

Asthma, emphysema, PE, pneumothorax, upper airway obstruction, and interstitial lung disease are the most common causes of dyspnea. Dyspnea is classified into acute, lasting a few minutes to a few hours, or chronic, lasting greater than a month:

- In the setting of chronic dyspnea, a negative chest PXR does not rule out diffuse pulmonary disease and should be followed with HRCT imaging.
- HRCT is also indicated in a situation where PXR reveals an abnormality, but no definitive diagnosis can be made.
- Transesophageal echocardiography (TEE) and transthoracic echocardiography (TTE) are widely performed procedures that play a significant role in evaluating patients with dyspnea suspected from cardiac diseases.

Solitary pulmonary nodule

Solitary pulmonary nodule is defined as a rounded opacity less than or equal to 3 cm in diameter, surrounded by a normal lung parenchyma with no associated abnormalities such as atelectasis or hilar lymphadenopathy. These nodules are usually followed by CT. Refer to the solitary pulmonary nodule imaging workup algorithm.

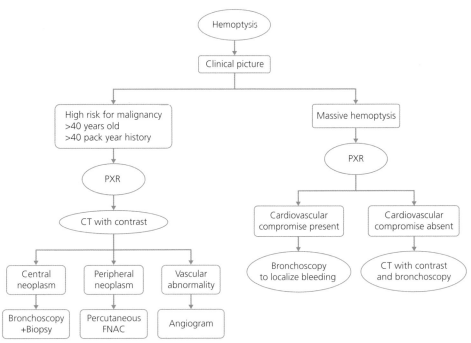

PXR, plain X-ray; CT, computed tomography; FNAC, fine needle aspiration cytology.

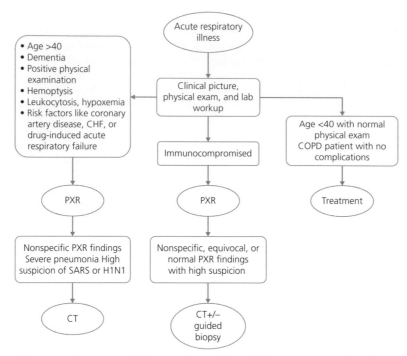

PXR, pain X-ray; CT, computed tomography; CHF, congestive heart failure; COPD, chronic obstructive pulmonary disease; SARS, severe acute respiratory syndrome; +/– with or without.

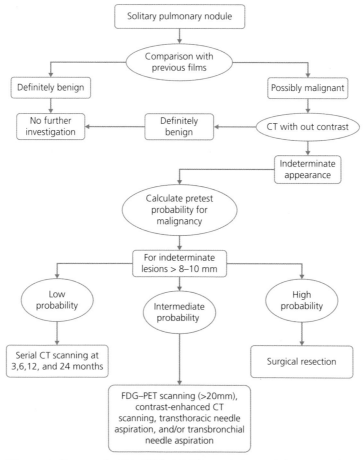

CT, computed tomography; FDG–PET-fludeoxyglucose–positron emission tomography

Lung cancer

Histologic confirmation of the lung cancer is mandatory in all patients, unless there is a clear-cut evidence of multiple sites of metastatic disease:

- Lung cancer staging employs a number of imaging modalities such as PXR, CT, MRI, and fluoro-2-deoxy-D-glucose positron emission tomography (FDG PET). Small cell lung cancer staging involves imaging of CT chest and abdomen, FDG PET, and imaging of the central nervous system (CNS), preferably with MRI.
- Non-small cell lung cancer staging consists of chest CT and FDG PET, whereas CNS imaging with MRI is considered only in symptomatic and high-risk cases.

Cardiovascular system

PXR is indicated for evaluating signs and symptoms potentially related to the heart and is considered the initial modality for clinically suspected conditions such as heart enlargement, heart failure, and pulmonary edema and for monitoring treatment for these conditions.

Cardiac CT in addition to evaluating the anatomy and pathology can also assess the central great vessels and cardiac valves including the cardiac function.

ECG-gated unenhanced cardiac CT may be indicated for detecting and quantifying coronary artery calcium, that is, calcium score, and for localizing myocardial, pericardial, valvular, and aortic calcium. Pericardial effusion, masses, the position of the implants, and postoperative complications such as focal fluid collections can be readily seen on an unenhanced cardiac CT. The use of IV contrast medium allows better evaluation of the cardiac chambers and adjacent vascular anatomy.

CT is used to screen for, diagnose, or characterize the great vessel pathology (atherosclerosis, arterial dissection, intramural hematoma, aneurysms, and vascular infection, vasculitis, and collagen vascular diseases), cardiac abnormalities, ventricular function, myocardial viability, myocardial perfusion, and coronary artery anatomy including narrowing and stenosis.

Cardiac magnetic resonance (C-MR) imaging is well known for its increasing value in the initial assessment and monitoring of a wide range of cardiac diseases, including cardiomyopathy, congenital heart disease, congestive heart failure, valvular heart disease, and cardiac tumors as well as the evaluation of the surrounding anatomy. However, in some patients with implantable devices, CT imaging is indicated as artifacts due to metal are less of a problem in CT compared with C-MR.

Contrast-enhanced magnetic resonance angiography (CE-MRA) is comparable to conventional angiography in the assessment of the

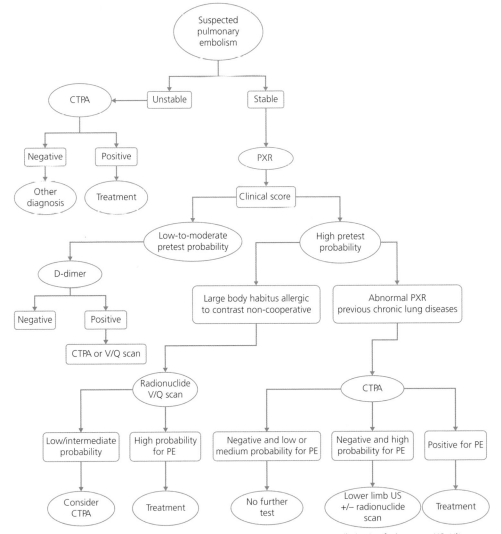

PXR, plain X-ray; CTPA, computed tomography pulmonary angiogram; V/Q scan, ventilation/perfusion scan; US, Ultrasonography.

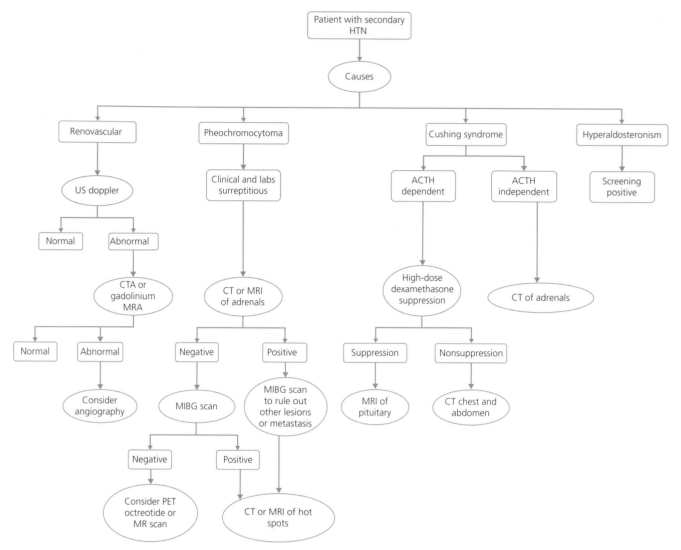

US, Ultrasonography; CTA, computed tomography angiography; MRA, magnetic resonance angiography; CT, computed tomography; MRI, magnetic resonance imaging; ACTH, adrenocorticotropic hormone; MIBG, metaiodobenzylguanidine scan.

vascular system and the associated diseases and thus helpful for pretreatment planning. CE-MRA is increasingly used to evaluate myocardial perfusion and evaluation of infarcts.

The main goal of cardiac scintigraphy is to assess myocardial perfusion and/or function, to detect physiologic and anatomic abnormalities of the heart, and to determine the prognosis.

Imaging role and workup algorithms for selected clinical scenarios
PE

- CT angiography (CTA) of the chest is now the first-line approach in the assessment of suspected PE.
- V/Q scanning is indicated only if contrast-enhanced CT is contraindicated in the evaluation of suspected PE.
- MRA is an alternative method, which has an additional advantage of nonionizing radiation side effects.
- Patients evaluated for PE in the emergency department are frequently young and often present with other disease processes that may mimic symptoms of PE. There is an incidence of about 5% of PE in young patients. If available, MRA should be regarded as a first choice for the evaluation of young patients.

Refer to the imaging workup algorithm for pulmonary embolism.

Secondary hypertension
Hypertension with an underlying, potentially correctable or reversible cause is termed as secondary hypertension. A secondary etiology can be suggested by findings such as flushing and sweating suggestive of pheochromocytoma, a renal bruit suggestive of renal artery stenosis, or hypokalemia suggestive of aldosteronism. Secondary hypertension should also be considered in patients with hypertension resistant or refractory to treatment, in young patients, and in patients with a history of renal disease. Refer to the imaging workup algorithm for secondary hypertension.

Deep venous thrombosis
The initial screening workup for a suspected deep venous thrombosis (DVT) includes clinical risk score (i.e., Wells criteria) along with plasma D-dimer assessment. Both Wells scoring and D-dimer assessment, however, have limitations, and imaging is ultimately required for the confirmation of DVT and to plan for a proper treatment:

- Ultrasonography (US) is the most cost-effective imaging performed to diagnose DVT.
- In the setting of pelvic and thigh DVT, MRI and CT are the choice of imaging to evaluate pelvic and thigh DVT if US is nondiagnostic.

Gastrointestinal system

Plain abdominal radiographs are still commonly performed for the initial assessment of the clinically acute abdomen, which include evaluation for suspected bowel perforation in unstable patients, bony fractures in blunt trauma, pneumoperitoneum, possible toxic megacolon, and follow-up of bowel obstruction, nonobstructive ileus, and abdominal distension.

Modified barium swallow is a procedure performed for evaluation of the oral and pharyngeal phases of swallowing and is used mainly for evaluation of oropharyngeal dysphagia and disorders affecting swallowing (e.g., neurological, myopathy conditions, masses) and for oral feeding assessment in stroke, trauma, and ventilator-dependent patients.

Single-contrast and double-contrast upper gastrointestinal (GI) series are procedures performed for evaluating signs and symptoms of the esophagus and the upper GI tract, such as dysphagia, odynophagia, suspected gastroesophageal reflux, epigastric distress or discomfort, dyspepsia, and upper GI bleeding.

Small bowel follow-through and enteroclysis. The small bowel follow-through is a fluoroscopic procedure performed to evaluate the small bowel that requires the patient to drink a substantial volume (typically >1 l) of water-soluble contrast. Examination for the clinical suspicion of Crohn's disease is still one of the most common indications.

Enteroclysis is a radiologic examination of the small intestine in which barium is infused through a transnasally placed enteric catheter with the tip positioned distal to the ligament of Treitz. Its main advantage is optimal distention of the small bowel lumen that facilitates fine delineation of mucosal detail and permits the evaluation of ulceration, small polypoid filling defects, constricting lesions, and adhesive bands. The patient discomfort, technical difficulty of placing the nasoenteric tube, and evaluation limited to only lumen are some of its shortcomings. Furthermore, small bowel follow-through and enteroclysis have been replaced to a larger extent by CT and MRI enterography, as these latter techniques evaluate not only the lumen but also the bowel wall and extraintestinal findings.

Lower GI series is a radiographic examination of the colon using single-contrast or double-contrast technique, known to have a role in the detection and evaluation of diverticular disease and inflammatory bowel disease, colon cancer screening, and evaluation of surgical anastomosis sites for stenosis and/or any leakage. Lower GI series has been replaced by colonoscopy for detecting intraluminal masses, and CT and MRI, because of their ability to detect mural and extraintestinal findings in addition to the luminal-based lesions.

US is indicated for patients presenting with signs or symptoms that may be referred from the abdomen and pelvis, especially gallbladder or female pelvis, palpable abnormalities such as abdominal masses or organomegaly, and abnormal laboratory values. US plays a major role in detecting free or loculated peritoneal and/or retroperitoneal fluid and/or blood in the emergency setting, including aortic rupture and unstable abdominal trauma. To plan for and guide an invasive procedure and follow-up of known or suspected abnormalities are other indications.

CT remains the first-line imaging modality for evaluating stable patients with abdominal trauma, detecting solid organ injury, and evaluating patients presenting with acute abdominal pain including evaluation of suspected pancreatitis, appendicitis, and diverticulitis. Bowel obstruction and abdominal aortic aneurysms are conditions that are readily assessed and diagnosed with CT. CT is also helpful in evaluating primary or metastatic malignancies, including lesion characterization, and assessing for tumor recurrence following surgical resection. CT has a role in evaluating abdominal inflammatory processes, like inflammatory bowel disease, infectious disease, and their complications such as abscess. CT enterography has a role in visualizing small bowel mucosa and has become the first-line examination in the diagnosis of Crohn's disease.

Computed tomographic colonography, also termed as virtual colonoscopy, may be used as a primary imaging modality for evaluation of colon polyps or in circumstances where colonoscopy is contraindicated.

MRI is the primary imaging modality used for the evaluation of a wide range of liver disorders. Most pancreatic diseases, especially tumors, are also well studied with MRI. In addition, this modality is also able to evaluate the full range of abdominal diseases. In general, the advantages of MRI over CT include higher soft tissue contrast resolution and safety, as it does not require ionizing radiation, thus making it most preferred examination in the evaluation of young adults and children.

Scintigraphy involves the administration of a radionuclide that transits or localizes in the salivary glands, GI tract, peritoneal cavity, or vascular system followed by gamma camera imaging. The GI scintigraphy is also often performed to assess the salivary gland function and tumors, presence and site of acute GI bleeding, and quantification of the rate of emptying from the stomach and transit through the small and large intestine.

Hepatobiliary scintigraphy has a role in the diagnosis of acute cholecystitis, evaluation of common bile duct (CBD) obstruction, and demonstration of biliary leaks.

Imaging role and workup algorithms for selected clinical scenarios
Blunt abdominal trauma
- The initial workup for hemodynamically unstable patients following blunt abdominal trauma includes chest radiographs, focused assessment with sonography for trauma (FAST) scans, and kidney–ureter–bladder abdominal radiography (KUB). Hemodynamically stable patients presenting with blunt abdominal trauma are best evaluated using MDCT with IV contrast.
- Bladder perforation or urethral injury should be ruled out in hemodynamically stable patients presenting with pelvic fracture and/or gross hematuria following a blunt or penetrating trauma to the abdomen or pelvis. This is readily performed with CT cystography after the initial assessment of the abdomen and pelvis using contrast-enhanced MDCT.

Acute GI bleeding
Upper GI bleeding from lower GI bleeding can be distinguished to a certain extent on the basis of history and nasogastric tube lavage if necessary. Refer to the imaging workup algorithm for acute GI bleeding:
- In a patient with continued GI bleeding with no identified cause on colonoscopy and endoscopy, MDCT enterography is the best imaging method to detect small obscure GI bleeding.
- Nuclear imaging and angiography are the other options considered to determine the cause of bleeding. Radionuclide scans with

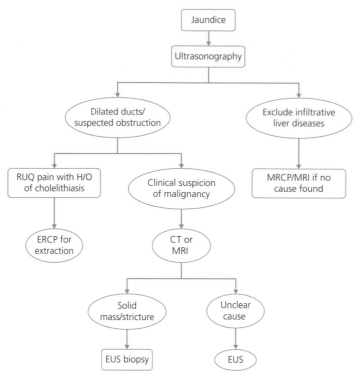

CT, computed tomography; MRI, magnetic resonance imaging; RUQ, right upper quadrant pain; MRCP, magnetic resonance cholangiopancreatography; EUS, endoscopic Ultrasonography.

technetium-99m-labeled red cells are a sensitive, noninvasive technique for detecting both arterial and venous GI bleeding. However, in patients with obscure GI bleeding, it detects only if bleeding is at a rate of greater than 0.1 ml/min.

- Angiography identifies lesions with bleeding at a rate of greater than 0.5 ml/min and is superior in localizing the source of bleeding than nuclear scans, in addition to the main advantage of embolization during the time of the procedure.

Right upper quadrant pain

In the acute setting, imaging should be performed only if clinically indicated:

- CT with IV contrast provides a comprehensive assessment of the pancreas and complications related to the pancreatitis. In acutely ill patients, CT is often preferred because of its more prompt and motion-resistant data acquisition. Centers with specialized motion-resistant strategies for MRI are able to study acutely ill patients as well.
- Contrast-enhanced MRI with magnetic resonance cholangiopancreatography (MRCP) possesses higher sensitivity for detecting subtle edema or fibrotic chronic pancreatitis changes over CT.
- US is currently considered the preferred initial imaging technique for patients who are clinically suspected of having acute calculous cholecystitis. The diagnosis of acute cholecystitis is usually confirmed or excluded with ultrasonography.
- CT has higher sensitivity and specificity for the diagnosis of acute calculous cystitis but is usually reserved for doubtful cases. One limitation of CT is the consistent demonstration of CBD stones.
- MRI is overall the best imaging modality to evaluate cholecystitis because of its unmatched ability to show acute calculous and acalculous cholecystitis and importantly because of the outstanding evaluation of the CBD and intrahepatic biliary tree; however, the lack of widespread availability of MRI and the

relatively high cost prohibit its primary use in patients with acute calculous cholecystitis.

- Scintigraphy has a high sensitivity and specificity in patients who are suspected of having acute cholecystitis and is occasionally used. Due to a combination of reasons, including drawbacks, broad imaging capability, and clinician referral pattern, its use is limited in clinical practice.

Right lower quadrant pain

Appendicitis can be clinically diagnosed; however, sensitivity and specificity for diagnosis are substantially increased by imaging, reducing the number of white appendectomies. Refer to the imaging workup algorithm for right lower quadrant pain:

- CT is the most accurate imaging modality for evaluating suspected appendicitis and alternative etiologies of right lower quadrant abdominal pain.
- In children and thin adults, US is the preferred initial examination, as it is nearly as accurate as CT for diagnosis of appendicitis while avoiding the exposure to ionizing radiation. In pregnant women, MR is the examination of choice. At experienced centers, MRI is an excellent test to study appendicitis in all subjects.

Left lower quadrant pain

- Female patients of reproductive age group are evaluated with transabdominal pelvic US with or without transvaginal US.
- CT is most commonly used for evaluating suspected acute diverticulitis for its high sensitivity and specificity, its ability to define the presence and extent of disease that might need a percutaneous catheter drainage or surgery, and its ability to show any associated extracolonic diseases.
- MRI has similar features to CT and shows inflammation with similar sensitivity.

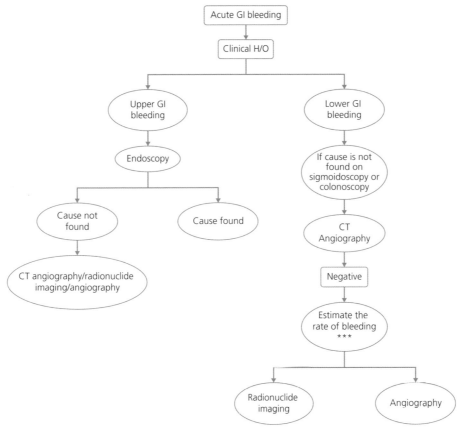

CT, computed tomography.

Jaundice

The primary aim of imaging in jaundice is to detect whether there is a mechanical obstruction of the bile ducts. Refer to the imaging workup algorithm for jaundice:

- US is usually the first-line modality that helps to determine bile duct dilatation and to confirm or exclude the presence of stones.
- If there is ductal dilatation with a high suspicion for stone disease associated with right upper quadrant pain, MRI and MRCP may be performed as the second modality.
- If there is ductal dilatation with a high suspicion of malignancy, then MRI with MRCP or CT with thin reconstructions is helpful in defining the point of obstruction, assessing for resectability, and staging a metastatic disease.
- If no mechanical cause for jaundice is identified by the first-line modality of US with no dilatation of the ducts, it is important to exclude infiltrative hepatocellular disease before performing invasive testing such as liver biopsy. The superior tissue characterization offered by MRI in this situation may help further the diagnosis and help direct biopsy.

Pancreatic cancer

The selection of appropriate candidates for potentially curative surgical resection is the major role of imaging in the patients newly diagnosed with pancreatic cancer:

- Overall, the imaging technique that is best able to detect and stage pancreatic cancers, especially the most important ones, small potentially surgically curable, is high-quality MRI on state-of-the-art MR equipment.
- CT is a method that is most often used in the setting of pancreatic cancer but may miss small potentially curable cancers.

- Endoscopic US (EUS) is an excellent method to confirm a mass lesion, best suited for evaluation of the head of the pancreas, but also dependent on local resources and expertise.

Colorectal cancer

Staging processes for colon cancer and rectal cancer are different. In colon cancer, regional staging is indicated only when advanced disease is suspected:

- In colon cancer, CT/US/MR of the abdomen and chest XR/chest CT may be performed if surgical or management decisions are likely to change.
- In rectal cancer, accurate preoperative staging is indicated, as chemoradiotherapy has been proved to be effective in certain groups of the population.
- MRI and endorectal US are the preferred methods to evaluate the rectal wall and invasion of the mesorectal fascial envelope; however, MRI has the advantage to better define the presence of perirectal and iliac lymph nodes.

Genitourinary system

X-ray kidneys, ureters, and bladder (KUB). X-ray kidneys, ureters, and bladder also known as X-ray KUB is rarely used nowadays to evaluate for presence of stones, as noncontrast CT is overwhelmingly superior in detecting stones. The KUB may be used as a follow-up to evaluate the changes in stones that have been localized on CT. KUB may be used to determine the positioning of indwelling devices such as ureteral stents, central lines, and catheters.

Intravenous urogram (IVU). An IVU is a radiographic study that allows to study both anatomic and functional information of

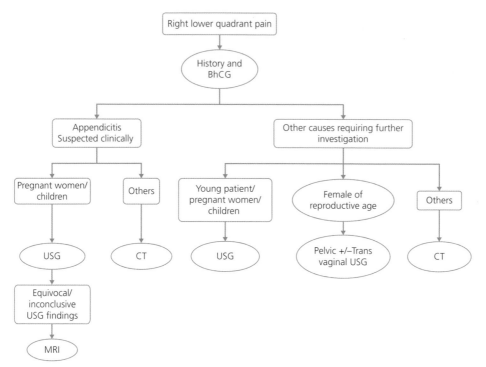

BhCG, beta-human chorionic gonadotropin; CT, computed tomography; MRI, magnetic resonance imaging; USG, ultrasonography.

the urinary tract by using IV contrast. To determine the integrity of urinary tract following trauma or therapeutic interventions, to assess the urinary tract for any lesions in the setting of hematuria, and to evaluate for suspected ureteral obstruction or congenital anomaly are some of the major indications to perform an IVU. Contrast-enhanced CT urography (CTU) has largely replaced IVU because of its greater ability to localize stones and to identify other urinary tract processes, such as urothelial cancer, and its ability to directly visualize the adjacent tissue around the collecting system.

Cystography and urethrography. Cystography and urethrography are plain radiographs of the bladder and urethra, respectively, obtained by fluoroscopy, following retrograde contrast media administration into the distal urethra using Foley catheter. Bladder and urethra imaging may involve various procedures by either combining the aforementioned studies or performing individually, such as cystography, cystourethrography, voiding cystourethrography, and urethrography (antegrade and retrograde). The most common indication is suspicion of urethral trauma suggested by one or more of the following: abdominal pain, inability to void urine, the presence of blood at the urethral meatus, scrotal hematoma, or free-floating prostate on rectal examination. Congenital urethral abnormality is the next most common indication.

In voiding cystography, fluoroscopy is performed at rest and/ or during voiding following contrast. It plays a significant role in detecting abnormalities of the bladder or urethra, in documenting the presence of vesicoureteral reflux, and in demonstrating extravasation of contrast from the bladder or urethra as well as mass effects on them by adjacent abnormalities.

CT cystogram is an imaging technique for trauma evaluation, in which contrast media is instilled into the urinary bladder prior to CT of the pelvis and a CT cystogram is obtained at the same time as the pelvis is examined. CT cystogram also helps to determine the presence of any bladder and urethral abnormalities, including vesicoureteral reflux.

Ultrasonography KUB. US is an optimal imaging in patients with unexplained increased creatinine level or recent onset of renal dysfunction in the evaluation of an abdominal or flank bruit, in the detection and evaluation of nephrocalcinosis, and in the diagnosis, evaluation, and follow-up of cyst and in patients with suspected masses within the renal collecting system. Renal artery color Doppler is primarily indicated in the evaluation of patients with suspected renovascular hypertension and for follow-up of patients with known renovascular disease who have undergone renal artery stent placement.

Prostate ultrasonography. US examination of the prostate and surrounding structures is performed in the diagnosis of prostate cancer, benign prostatic enlargement, prostatitis, prostatic abscess, congenital anomalies, and male infertility. For prostate cancer screening, a combination of digital rectal examination and a test for serum prostate-specific antigen (PSA) level usually serves as the initial screening procedure. Ultrasound-guided biopsy of the prostate is best reserved for evaluating those patients who have abnormal digital rectal examinations or an abnormal serum PSA level.

Pelvic ultrasonography. US is the initial modality in the evaluation of pelvic masses, pelvic pain, and abnormal bleeding. A pelvic US can also be performed to evaluate for uterine anomalies or to monitor for the development of ovarian follicles in infertility patients. The typical scanning techniques are transabdominal or endovaginal. It is the primary imaging modality in assessing the normal growth of the fetus and evaluating congenital abnormalities and abnormal bleeding during pregnancy. Sonohysterography involves cervical fluid injection by transcervical route followed by US examination of the endometrial cavity. The main goal of sonohysterography is to depict the endometrial cavity in a greater detail, to access the tubal patency, and to delineate endometrial masses, beyond the routine transvaginal US.

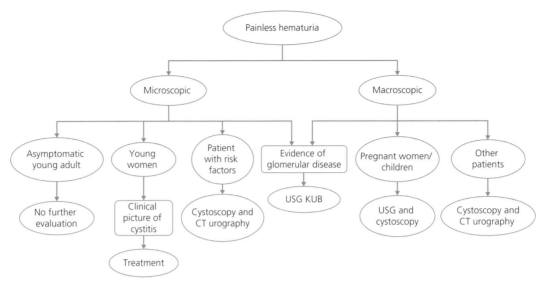

CT, computed tomography; MRI, magnetic resonance imaging; USG, ultrasonography; KUB, kidney ureter bladder.

CTU. CTU has become the modality of choice in imaging the urinary tract. CTU is a comprehensive examination whereby the kidneys and upper collecting system, ureters, and urinary bladder can be evaluated in one setting for evaluating urological symptoms and conditions. This study is often performed as a noncontrast study followed by taking arterial and later phase images.

MRI. MRI application in urology includes evaluation of adrenal, renal, and urinary pathology such as adrenal hyperplasia and adrenal tumors, diagnosis and staging of renal cell carcinoma, renal vascular assessment, evaluation of ureteral abnormalities, retroperitoneal lymphadenopathy, and retroperitoneal fibrosis. In the pelvis, MRI performs well at diagnosis and staging of malignancy in the urinary bladder and prostate gland and produces superior staging information for seminal vesicle involvement compared to all other imaging techniques. MRI is the best overall imaging modality to evaluate female pelvic pathology, including detection and local staging of gynecological malignancies; evaluation of pelvic pain; detection and characterization of the masses such as adenomyosis, endometriosis, and fibroids; characterization of adnexal cystic lesions and other ovarian and tubal diseases; and evaluation of Müllerian anomaly.

Imaging role and workup algorithms for selected clinical scenarios

Lower urinary tract trauma

CT abdomen and pelvis with bladder contrast (CT cystography) are the preferred imaging study for suspected lower urinary tract injury due to trauma to lower abdomen and/or pelvis. Retrograde urethrography should be considered when pelvic fracture is present and also in the setting of gross hematuria to exclude a urethral injury before bladder catheterization.

Urinary tract symptoms: Refer to the imaging workup algorithm for common urinary tract symptoms.

Hematuria

In patients with hematuria that is determined to be due to glomerular disease, there is no defined role for imaging except for US KUB. Refer to the imaging workup algorithm for hematuria:

- Complete radiologic workup of microscopic hematuria is unnecessary in younger women with a clinical picture of simple cystitis and whose hematuria resolves after successful therapy.

- Most adults with micro- or macrohematuria require urinary tract imaging, with CTU being considered the preferred method.
- MRI is an excellent technique to evaluate the renal parenchyma for masses and other abnormalities and good for evaluating the urothelium and detecting early subtle urinary masses.

Acute flank pain

Non-contrast-enhanced CT is the quickest and most accurate technique for evaluating flank pain suspected for urinary stones. Otherwise, healthy patients with suspected uncomplicated pyelonephritis will typically need no radiologic workup if they respond to antibiotic therapy within 72 h:

- If there is no response to therapy in suspected acute pyelonephritis, CT abdomen and pelvis are the imaging study of choice.
- Diabetics or other immunocompromised patients who have not responded promptly to antibiotic treatment should be evaluated with precontrast and postcontrast CT within 24 h of diagnosis.
- MRI would perform equally well because of its high sensitivity to fluid (T2-weighted images) and adequate appreciation of inflammatory enhancement of postcontrast images.
- If there is uncertainty about whether a calcific density represents a ureteral calculus or a phlebolith, which rarely happens when interpreted by an experienced radiologist, IV contrast material can be administered and excretory-phase images obtained for definitive diagnosis.
- In pregnant patients with flank pain, US is preferred. This is also a good indication for MRI, which provides more comprehensive information.

Abnormal vaginal bleeding

Imaging procedures cannot replace definitive histologic diagnosis, and tissue sampling may be the most appropriate initial step in evaluating a woman with abnormal vaginal bleeding, depending on the clinical situation. Imaging can play an important role in assessing endometrial thickness, staging, and following up after treatment or intervention. Refer to the imaging workup algorithm for abnormal vaginal bleeding:

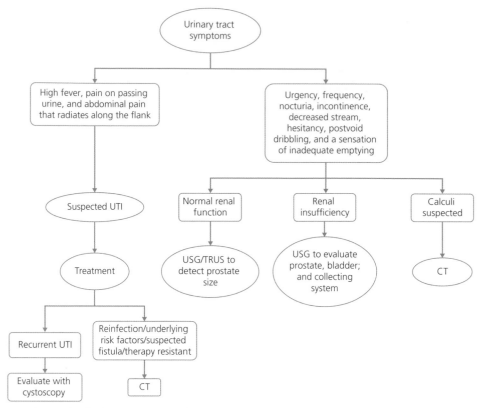

UTI, urinary track infection; TRUS, trans rectal Ultrasonography; CT, computed tomography.

- US or MRI is preferred for screening, characterizing structural abnormalities, and directing appropriate patient care, often preventing inappropriate diagnostic procedures.
- Endovaginal US is the initial imaging procedure for evaluating abnormal vaginal bleeding, and endometrial thickness is a well-established predictor of endometrial disease in postmenopausal women.
- Transabdominal US is generally an adjunct to endovaginal US and is most helpful when endovaginal US cannot be performed or limited due to poor visualization due to uterine position or poor penetration due to uterine pathology such as fibroids or adenomyosis. Overall, MRI might be the most accurate method to evaluate all forms of abnormal vaginal bleeding.
- Occasionally, hysterosonography is used to identify focal abnormalities within the endometrial cavity, which may then lead to hysteroscopically guided biopsy or resection.

Clinically suspected adnexal lesions

US has been often the initial study for evaluating a woman with a clinically suspected adnexal mass. Refer to the imaging workup algorithm for adnexal lesions:

- Most adnexal masses can be characterized using US with or without color Doppler examination. Both MRI and CT are useful for further evaluation. Patients may often be directly sent for surgical evaluation.
- Overall, MRI provides the most comprehensive information for the evaluation of adnexal and surrounding structures due to its unmatched soft tissue contrast resolution.

Renal mass

- CT is the modality most commonly used for evaluating indeterminate renal lesions that are suspicious for malignancy.

- MRI with gadolinium contrast performs equally well and may be a better choice in individuals under 40 years of age because of radiation concerns.

CNS

Plain radiography is seldom used nowadays and has been replaced by axial imaging methods such as CT and MRI but may still be used on occasions.

CT is often used as a baseline imaging in neuroradiology especially in the setting of head trauma, headache, and suspected stroke to rule out hemorrhage or a tumor and to rule out brain metastasis in a patient with known malignancy.

Brain *MRI* is a well-established and the most accurate imaging modality due to its high sensitivity in detecting characteristic contrast differences of tissues, providing a wide range of utility in the evaluation of the CNS disease process.

Vascular imaging such as *CTA*, *MRA* and *angiography* is often used to depict vascular injuries in the setting of penetrating or blunt head and neck injury and skull base or cervical spine fracture. A wide spectrum of vascular diseases of the cervicocerebral system are best evaluated using MRA.

Single-photon emission computed tomography (SPECT) imaging uses a lipophilic radioisotope that crosses the blood–brain barrier and localizes in normal brain tissue, which is of value to define the regional distribution of brain perfusion, evaluate a variety of brain abnormalities, and corroborate the clinical impression of brain death in appropriate situations.

Few major indications include monitoring and assessing vascular spasm following subarachnoid hemorrhage, evaluating patients with suspected dementia and transient ischemic attacks (TIA), differentiating lacunar from nonlacunar infarctions, localizing

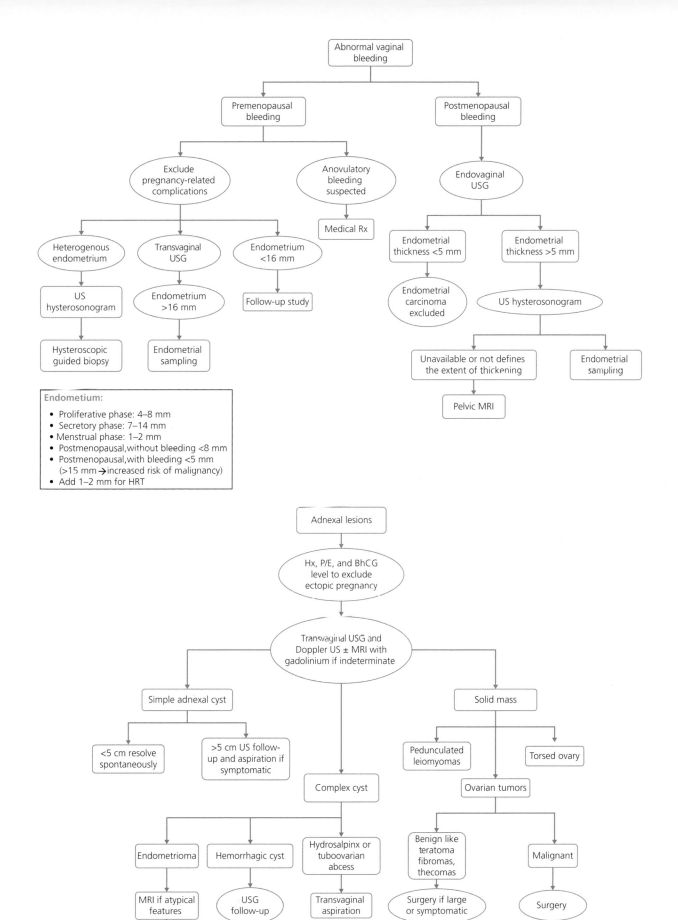

BhCG, beta-human chorionic gonadotropin; MRI, magnetic resonance imaging; USG, ultrasonography.

epileptic foci preoperatively, and predicting the prognosis of patients with cerebrovascular accidents.

Imaging role and workup algorithms for selected clinical scenarios
Suspected head trauma

- CT is the most appropriate initial study for emergent evaluation of the head-injured patient, who may have lesion(s) that requires immediate neurosurgical intervention. Certain clinical findings like focal neurological deficit, patients on anticoagulation or suffering with a bleeding diathesis, penetrating skull injury, depressed skull fracture, Glasgow Coma Scale (GCS) less than 13 at any time since injury, posttraumatic seizure, and unstable vital signs with major trauma require an immediate CT.
- Further risk evaluation based on clinical findings should be done for patients with a history of loss of consciousness (LOC), amnesia/disorientation, and a GCS greater than 13 and is usually followed by observation or CT head may be indicated. Cervical spine imaging is indicated and appropriate in head-injured patients.
- MR has a role in subacute or chronic brain injury for its sensitivity in detecting and characterizing nonneurosurgical lesions such as hypoxic ischemic encephalopathy (HIE) and diffuse axonal injury (DAI) and may also help in determining the prognosis.

Headache

Screening of patients presenting with an isolated, nontraumatic headache by use of CT or MRI is usually not warranted, but in some settings, imaging may be required depending on the clinical circumstances. Thunderclap headaches, headaches radiating to the neck, and temporal headaches in an older individual are examples of headaches for which imaging procedures may be helpful.

Patients with suspected meningitis and those presenting with headaches in pregnancy also often pose important diagnostic challenges. HIV-positive individuals, cancer patients, or other populations at high risk of intracranial disease also should be screened when presenting with new-onset headaches. Refer to the imaging workup algorithm for headache:

- CT is often the initial imaging modality of choice. Further imaging with MRI with or without MRA or magnetic resonance venography (MRV) is done based on the clinical settings.

Suspected stroke

Imaging in the setting of suspected stroke serves a number of purposes: (i) to determine if the patient has had a stroke, (ii) to determine the vascular territory of the stroke, and (iii) to determine the etiology of the stroke:

- Noncontrast CT is the initial imaging modality of choice in suspected stroke. The main value of CT in the acute setting is to exclude hemorrhage or tumor.
- Further imaging is dictated by the clinical situation and includes MRI with Diffusion-Weighted Index (DW-I) with or without MRA or CTA.

TIA

- Noncontrast CT is the initial imaging modality of choice in suspected TIA.
- Carotid Doppler US should be performed to assess for extracranial arterial stenosis or plaque. If the carotid arteries are normal on US, alternative sources of cerebral emboli should be considered (echocardiogram/Holter).

- If there is uncertainty regarding the degree of carotid stenosis, further noninvasive imaging with CTA or MRA should be done. Refer to algorithm on TIA.

Musculoskeletal system

The initial modality indicated for the evaluation of signs and symptoms potentially related to the musculoskeletal (MSK) system is *plain radiography*. Radiography plays a major role in evaluating trauma, pain, instability, impingement, neurologic symptoms, infection, degenerative disorders, osteoporosis, and neoplastic (benign and malignant) lesions.

Fluoroscopy. Fluoroscopy is a portable form of X-ray specially used to perform studies that visualize the ongoing movement. This can be used to assess joint motion. Fluoroscopy is commonly used to monitor the placement of hardware during orthopedic surgeries. It may also be of assistance in positioning patients for unusual conventional radiographic views.

Ultrasonography. US is increasingly used more frequently for the detection of soft tissue injuries involving tendons, ligaments, nerves, and muscles. US can also be used in the assessment of soft tissue masses because of its ability to distinguish solid from cystic and guide injections into the joints, soft tissue biopsies, and aspirations.

CT. In patients following a major trauma, a rapid evaluation of bony anatomy is performed using PXR and CT to confirm or exclude a diagnosis of fracture. CT is routinely used to evaluate for spine stability in the trauma patient. Additionally, CT allows imaging of coexistent visceral injury, hemorrhage, and full depiction of fractures involving complex bony anatomy such as the face, spine, and pelvis in settings where plain radiographs are not able to clearly define the fractures. CT is also considered to be superior in detecting cortical fractures. Reconstructed CT images in the coronal and sagittal planes are critical to evaluate a fracture in planes of section that cannot be achieved in the primary view, which helps the orthopedic surgeon to plan an operative intervention.

The other major use of CT is an evaluation of bone tumors or tumorlike diseases and evaluation of congenital or developmental spine abnormalities, such as scoliosis or spondylolysis with or without spondylolisthesis.

MRI. MRI procedure uses a variety of pulse sequences for the diagnosis of musculoskeletal trauma. Soft tissue injuries are best studied with MRI technique for its unique ability to visualize the ligaments, cartilages, tendons, and muscles. Compared to other imaging modalities, MRI is the only one that facilitates evaluation of soft tissue and bone injury concurrently and thus helpful in identifying stress fractures and coexistent tendinous and ligamentous injuries. Due to its superior contrast resolution, MRI offers the best delineation of anatomy to determine the tumor extent within bone marrow or muscle or other soft tissues.

MRI of the spine is a powerful tool that allows direct visualization of the spinal cord, nerve roots, and discs and has a prominent role in detecting anatomic abnormalities of the spine and adjacent structures, especially spinal cord disease such as multiple sclerosis or tumors.

MRI is the cornerstone for local staging and assessing the operability of primary bone tumors and also planning routes of biopsy that will allow diagnosis and treatment plans for patients with primary bone, secondary bone, and soft tissue tumors. MRI is also

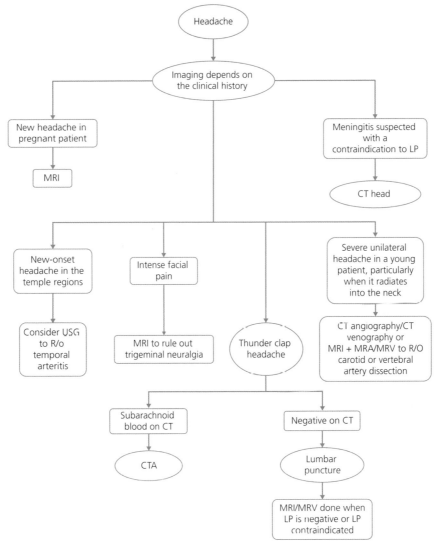

CT, computed tomography; CTA, computed tomography angiography; MRI, magnetic resonance imaging; MRA, magnetic resonance angiography; MRV, magnetic resonance venography.

outstanding at detecting bone metastases as well as multiple myeloma.

Radionuclide imaging. Skeletal scintigraphy has shown to be a sensitive method for detection of a variety of anatomic and physiologic abnormalities of the MSK system such as primary and metastatic bone tumors; stress/occult fractures involving the wrist, scaphoid, femoral neck, and ankle; infection; and inflammation.

The two most common nuclear studies are the technetium bone scan and technetium- or indium-labeled white blood cell scan. Activity on the bone scan is based on the detection of osteoblastic activity, but diseases that do not generate substantial osteoblastic activity may not be visible. Bone scans are commonly used for screening bone metastases in patients with a known malignancy. PET/CT, a combination of FDG PET with CT, has currently shown to be an excellent tool in detection of skeletal metastases by identifying increased glucose metabolism of metastases in the bone marrow that also simultaneously permits to correlate with CT findings.

Imaging role and workup algorithms for selected clinical scenarios
Shoulder problems

In the setting of shoulder trauma, plain radiography is the initial imaging of choice as it provides a quick, inexpensive evaluation of any fracture and/or dislocation present:

- US with good expertise is an excellent tool in the depiction of rotator cuff and biceps long head pathology in the evaluation preoperative and postoperative shoulder.
- Occult fractures and the shoulder soft tissues such as tendons, ligaments, muscles, and labrocapsular structures are best studied with MRI.
- Fluoroscopic arthrography is indicated only in patients with suspected rotator cuff disease who have a contraindication to MRI and when shoulder US is normal.
- CT with the use of reconstruction is especially helpful to demonstrate the complexity of the fracture, displacement, and angulation, thus illustrating fractures and providing more information preoperatively.

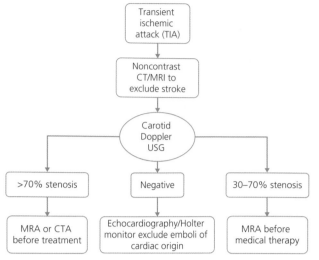

USG, ultrasonography; CT, computed tomography; CTA, computed tomography angiography; MRI, magnetic resonance imaging; MRA, magnetic resonance angiography; MRV, magnetic resonance venography.

Hip pain

In the setting of hip and knee pain, triage of patients to the most appropriate imaging is based on the initial clinical assessment:

- For nontraumatic hip pain, radiographs are obtained as the first imaging study, and most often MRI is indicated as the next imaging study, except in cases of suspected osteoid osteoma or labral tear. Osteoid osteoma is best diagnosed with CT.
- Direct MR arthrography is performed in suspected cases of acetabular labral tear and in patients with clinical evidence of femoroacetabular impingement.
- A bone scan is helpful in identifying widespread bone metastases and is also useful in the evaluation of suspected infected hip prostheses.
- US is useful in diagnosing bursitis and tendinopathy, but the user dependence and the insufficiency for imaging articular or osseous structures are its main limitations.
- MRI is the imaging modality of choice if suspicion of occult hip fracture continues.

Knee pain

Most individuals who present with acute knee injuries have soft tissue rather than osseous injuries, and where fracture is present, it is often accompanied with soft tissue injury. Refer to the imaging workup algorithm for hip or knee pain:

- Because of the soft tissue components of injury, MRI is of paramount importance. MRI is also useful for the detection of ongoing knee instability following trauma to the knee, as it is able to accurately delineate the soft tissues of the joint.
- CT has a lesser role in the assessment of posttraumatic knee pain, though it is useful in demonstrating subtle bony injury and loose bodies within the knee joint and for preoperative planning.
- MRI is preferred in most cases of nontraumatic knee pain to evaluate for suspected osteomyelitis, avascular necrosis, osseous or soft tissue mass, chondral lesions, and ligamental or meniscal derangements.

Low-back pain

Low-back pain (LBP) in patients presenting with an acute uncomplicated LBP without any "red flags" is considered to be a benign, self-limited condition in which imaging evaluation is not recommended.

Imaging is prompted in patients presenting with LBP associated with "red flags" such as recent significant trauma; unexplained weight loss; fever; history of malignancy or immune compromise; age less than 22 or greater than 55 years; IV drug use; suspicion of ankylosing spondylitis, osteoporosis, or glucocorticoid use; and compensation or work injury issues. In the absence of "red flags," imaging is only indicated after a period of conservative therapy:

- CT is indicated in the setting of major trauma, as the spine and surrounding tissues of the chest, abdomen, and pelvis can all be simultaneously assessed. CT is advantageous in patients with surgical fusion/instrumentation or with bony structural abnormalities and in whom MRI is contraindicated.
- MRI is superior to CT and myelography and is the initial imaging modality of choice in complicated LBP; the use of IV contrast is helpful in the diagnosis of malignant tumors and infection and postoperative evaluation.
- MRI is indicated for patients with neurologic deficits as when clinical suspicion is high despite a normal plain film and/or normal CT scan.

Suspected acute osteomyelitis

PXR is the initial imaging modality of choice, but it may demonstrate normal findings in the early stages of disease. "Normal" PXR does not exclude osteomyelitis:

- MRI is considered the next best imaging modality in the evaluation of suspected osteomyelitis and associated soft tissue abnormalities.
- Nuclear medicine studies are indicated, when there are no localizing signs or symptoms in suspected osteomyelitis, when MRI is contraindicated or unavailable, or in suspected periprosthetic infection patients. They can also be obtained to monitor response to treatment.

Breast imaging

Mammography is an examination employed for both screening and diagnostic purposes.

Annual screening mammography is recommended starting at:

1. Age 40 for general population
2. Ages 25–30 for BReast CAncer 1 (BRCA1) carriers and untested relatives of BRCA carriers
3. Ages 25–30 or 10 years earlier than the age of the affected relative at diagnosis (whichever is later) for women with a first-degree relative with premenopausal breast cancer or for women with a lifetime risk of breast cancer greater than or equal to 20% on the basis of family history
4. 8 years after radiation therapy but not before the age 25 for women who received mantle radiation between the ages of 10 and 30
5. Any age for women with biopsy-proven lobular neoplasia, atypical ductal hyperplasia (ADH), ductal carcinoma *in situ* (DCIS), or invasive breast cancer

Diagnostic mammography is indicated as the initial examination in the evaluation of a palpable breast finding for women aged 40 and older. Because of the theoretical increased radiation risk of mammography and the low incidence of breast cancer (<1%) in younger women, their imaging evaluation differs from that performed for older patients, according to most investigators. As with all age-related guidelines, pertinent clinical factors such as family history should be used to determine appropriate patient care.

Breast *Ultrasonography* is commonly used to further evaluate a palpable abnormality and to characterize a mammographic finding or an abnormality. It is preferably used in women less than 30 years

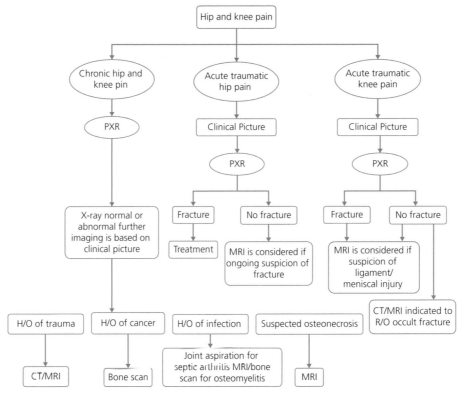

CT, computed tomography; MRI, magnetic resonance imaging.

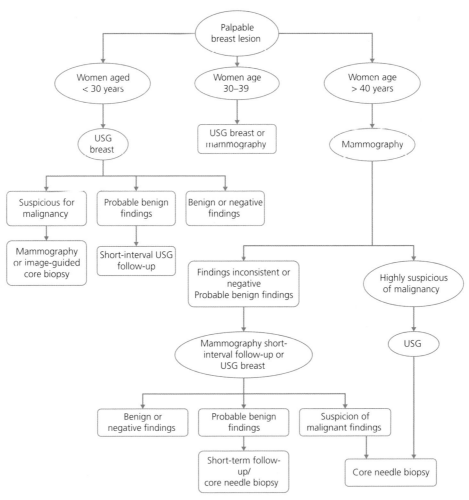

USG, ultrasonography.

of age who are at low risk of developing breast cancer and in pregnant and lactating women. It is also helpful to guide breast biopsy and other therapeutic interventional procedures, for the evaluation of complications associated with breast implants, and in treatment planning for radiation therapy.

Most benign lesions in young women are not visualized on mammography, and US is therefore used as the initial imaging modality in younger women. The criteria for "young" have historically been considered as younger than age 30. However, the risk of breast cancer remains relatively low for women in their fourth decade. The sensitivity of US may be higher than mammography for women younger than age 40. It is therefore reasonable to use US as the initial imaging modality for women younger than age 40, with a low threshold for using mammography if the clinical examination or other risk factors are concerning.

If US demonstrates a suspicious finding in a younger woman, bilateral mammography is recommended to evaluate for additional ipsilateral and contralateral lesions.

Breast *MRI* is performed either for evaluation of the integrity of breast prostheses (implants) or for evaluation of breast cancer. Breast cancer evaluation can further be subdivided into screening of high-risk patients, diagnosis, staging, and posttherapy monitoring. Often, a patient may undergo breast MRI for a combination of reasons, such as staging the local extent of known cancer in one breast while also simultaneously screening for an occult cancer in the other breast.

Imaging role and workup algorithms for selected clinical scenarios
Palpable breast lesion

Due to the fact of inconsistencies in clinical examination, a thorough imaging workup of a palpable breast mass is essential prior to biopsy. Refer to the imaging workup algorithm for palpable breast lesion:

- US is the preferred initial examination of choice in women less than 30 years old, while diagnostic mammography is the initial imaging modality of choice in women aged 40 or older for evaluating a clinically palpable breast mass.
- Either US breast or mammography may be used as an initial examination in women aged from 30 to 39 years. Any highly suspicious breast mass either found clinically or detected by imaging should be biopsied even if the findings essentially do not correlate with the imaging and clinical examination, respectively.

Suggested reading

ACR Appropriateness Criteria, 2014. http://www.acr.org/Quality-Safety/Appropriateness-Criteria

ACR Radiology Safety, 2014. http://www.acr.org/Quality-Safety/Radiology-Safety

American Society of radiology (ACR) Practice Guidelines by Organ or Body System, 2013. http://www.acr.org/Quality-Safety/Standards-Guidelines

Canadian Association of Radiologists (CAR) Practice Guidelines (by Organ System), 2012. http://www.car.ca/en/standards-guidelines/standards.aspx#2

CAR CAR Diagnostic Imaging Referral Guidelines, 2012. http://www.car.ca/en/standards-guidelines/guidelines.aspx

CHAPTER 3

Chest imaging

Saowanee Srirattanapong[1] and Katherine R. Birchard[2]

[1]Department of Diagnostic and Therapeutic Radiology, Faculty of Medicine Ramathibodi Hospital, Mahidol University, Bangkok, Thailand
[2]Department of Radiology, University of North Carolina, Chapel Hill, USA

Imaging of diseases of the chest forms a central component of radiologic practice, with chest imaging being one of the most common radiologic procedures performed. There are a number of differing types of imaging modalities used to evaluate chest disease. Each modality has different strengths, limitations, indications, and contraindications for each clinical circumstance. The purpose of this chapter is to provide an overview of imaging common chest diseases.

Normal anatomy

The lung is made up of numerous anatomical units smaller than a lobe or segment. The pulmonary acinus is the smallest functioning unit, is defined as the portion of the lung distal to a terminal bronchiole, and is supplied by a first-order respiratory bronchiole or bronchiole. Since respiratory bronchioles are the largest airways that have alveoli in their walls, an acinus is the largest lung unit in which its airway participates in gas exchange. Acini usually range from 6 to 10 mm in diameter. The secondary pulmonary lobule, as defined by Miller, is the smallest unit of lung structure marginated by connective tissue septa that contains pulmonary vein and lymphatics (interlobular septa). The secondary pulmonary lobules are irregularly polyhedral in shape and vary in size, measuring from 1 to 2.5 mm in diameter in most location. Each secondary lobule is supplied by a small bronchiole and pulmonary artery branch. Secondary pulmonary lobules are usually made up of a dozen or fewer acini.

Normal peripheral airways are not visualized on chest radiographs because the mural tissue is thin and they are surrounded by air in the alveolar sacs. Filling of alveolar spaces with material such as fluid, pus, inflammatory cells, protein, or hemorrhage creates opacity in the alveolar spaces, and air in the bronchi can be visible on chest radiograph (air bronchogram).

The lung interstitium is a network of connective tissue that supports the lungs and is formed of three components: peribronchovascular interstitium (tissue along the bronchi and pulmonary arteries), subpleural interstitium (tissue immediately beneath the visceral pleura and that penetrates into the lung, which is refers to

interlobular septa), and intralobular interstitium (tissue network within the secondary pulmonary lobule).

Normal interstitial tissue has too thin structure to be visible on plain radiographs or computed tomography (CT), so when interstitial markings become apparent, it reflects the presence of disease involving the interstitium. These patterns are more clearly defined on CT.

Imaging modalities

Plain radiography

The primary tool used for imaging chest disease is the plain chest X-ray. Chest radiography is a diagnostic tool that is widely available, noninvasive, inexpensive, and often sufficiently diagnostic and is therefore usually the initial examination in individuals suspected of having chest disease of any cause. To obtain optimized detection and localization of disease on chest radiography, two orthogonal upright views of the chest, frontal posteroanterior and lateral views, are needed. On the normal study, various structures are demarcated when they have different densities from adjacent structures: some of which are dramatic, such as air–soft tissue interface (e.g., left ventricle and adjacent left lower lobe); others are of moderate distinction, such as fat and nonfat soft tissues (e.g., mediastinal fat and superior vena cava); and others still are more subtle, such as different nonfat soft tissue structures (e.g., paratracheal lymph nodes and superior vena cava). The outline of the mediastinum should be well demarcated because there are substantial differences of densities between mediastinal soft tissues (which are denser and termed more radiopaque) and air-containing lungs (which are much less dense and termed radiolucent). If a disease process in the lungs results in increased opacity and it is situated such that it abuts any part of the mediastinum, the demarcation or border of the affected mediastinum will be lost, which is termed the silhouette sign. This permits localization of the process because of its approximation to a certain mediastinal structure, which has a known location.

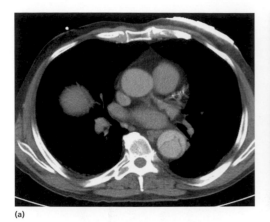
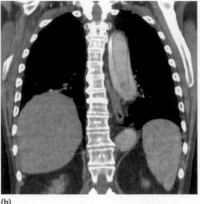
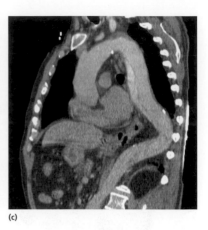

(a) (b) (c)

Figure 3.1 *Aortic dissection:* axial (a) and coronal CT images (b) and oblique sagittal (c) contrast-enhanced CT of the chest show aortic dissection, its origin slightly distal to the left subclavian artery and extending inferiorly. The origin of the false lumen, from a rent in the descending aorta intima, is noted at the level of the left atrium.

CT

A variety of modifications of CT are performed to image different types of chest disease: plain CT with or without intravenous contrast, CT pulmonary or aortic angiography, and high-resolution CT (HRCT). The goal of HRCT is to enhance spatial resolution to detect small and subtle abnormalities. The thinnest possible slice thickness (usually 1–1.5 mm) should be used to optimize spatial resolution. Standard HRCT is a sampling technique, and interspacing between each section is usually 10 mm. A window level of −500 to −800 Hounsfield units (HU) and a width of between 1100 and 2000 HU are generally satisfactory for lung window setting. Most HRCT scans are obtained with the patient in the supine position and at full inspiration. Prone scans are required when there is dependent opacity, to differentiate dependent atelectasis from other abnormality, which will be persistent in prone position.

The introduction of MDCT scanners has revolutionized HRCT technique. MDCT scanners are capable of rapid, contiguous, or even overlapping high-resolution 1 mm images throughout the chest in a single breath hold by using volumetric imaging technique and allowing retrospective reconstruction of thin sections from data used for routine thick-slice imaging and reconstructed images in any desired plane.

Nuclear medicine

The most commonly employed nuclear medicine study for diseases in the chest is the ventilation/perfusion (V/Q) scan. This technique is employed in the setting of suspected pulmonary embolism (PE).

Critical observations

In this subsection, we highlight with illustrative examples findings in chest disease that are critical to observe, either because of the seriousness of the conditions or because of their common occurrence. Greater details about these entities are described in the following text of the chapter:

1 *Traumatic aortic injury/aortic dissection* (Figure 3.1)
  ◦ Widening of the mediastinum due to mediastinal hematoma and loss of aortic outline on plain radiograph raise the suspicious of this entity.
  ◦ The CT findings of aortic injury include intimal flap, pseudoaneurysm (change of aortic caliber), contour irregularity, lumen abnormality (resulting from intraluminal thrombus), and extravasation of contrast material.

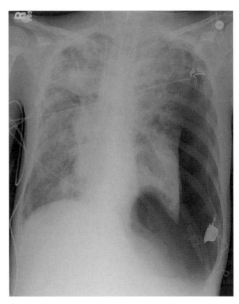

Figure 3.2 *Tension pneumothorax:* semiupright portable chest radiograph shows large left pneumothorax with mediastinal shift to the right. Note the collapsed left lung, the depression of ipsilateral hemidiaphragm, and the hyperlucent left hemithorax.

2 *Tension pneumothorax* (Figure 3.2)
  ◦ Radiographic findings of tension pneumothorax include evidence of pneumothorax on the chest radiograph (white pleural line) with mediastinal shift to the opposite site.
3 *PE* (Figure 3.3)
  ◦ Most radiographic findings are nonspecific for diagnosis or exclusion of this entity. The main purpose of a chest radiograph, in patients suspected of PE, is to exclude diagnoses that clinically mimic PE.
  ◦ Multidetector CT pulmonary angiography has a very high sensitivity and specificity to detect PE. Direct CT findings are occlusion or filling defect of pulmonary arteries or their branches.
4 *Pneumonia*
  ◦ Pneumonia is an infection of the lung caused by an infective organism, bacterial, viral, or fungal. Radiographic patterns of abnormal pulmonary opacities are basically categorized into

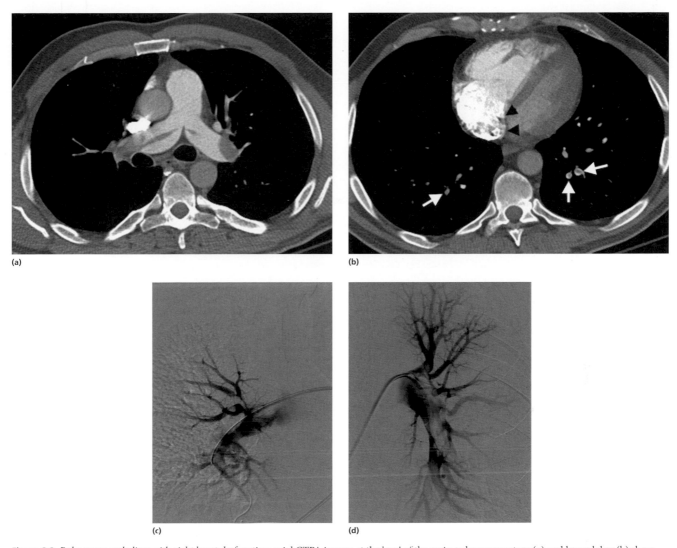

Figure 3.3 *Pulmonary embolism with right heart dysfunction:* axial CTPA images at the level of the main pulmonary artery (a) and lower lobes (b) show bilateral pulmonary emboli in the distal main pulmonary arteries and a small saddle embolus. The emboli extend into segmental and subsegmental branches of the lower lobes (arrows). There is flattening of the interventricular septum, leftward bowing of the interatrial septum (arrow heads), and enlargement of the right atrium and right ventricle, indicative of right heart dysfunction. Right and left pulmonary angiography (c and d) during thrombectomy shows filling defect of bilateral pulmonary arteries and their branches.

airspace disease or interstitial disease based on the radiographic appearances and localization in the lungs.

5 *Lung cancer*
  ○ There are two major radiographic presentations of lung cancer: peripheral lung cancers, which usually present as a solitary pulmonary nodule or mass, and central lung cancers, which may present with hilar enlargement and consolidation or collapse of peripheral lung due to tumor bronchial obstruction or invasion.
  ○ Plain radiographs have limited ability to detect early-stage cancer. CT plays an important role to evaluate and stage lung cancer.

Congenital disease

Cystic fibrosis

Cystic fibrosis (CF) is an autosomal recessive genetic disorder of the secretory glands and is most common in the Caucasian population. Patients with CF have a thick and sticky mucus instead of the normal watery and slippery mucus. The sticky mucus causes blockage of small airways and tubes and ducts of other affected organs, leading to repeated infections and subsequent organ damage. The common affected organs are the lungs, pancreas, liver, bowel, and sex organs. The common clinical presentations include repeated pulmonary infection, pancreatic insufficiency, sinusitis, malnutrition, and male infertility. The most common infective organisms in the lungs are staphylococcus and pseudomonas species:

• The radiographic abnormalities may not be apparent for months or years after birth. The early radiographic findings are nonspecific, including diffuse bronchial wall thickening, recurrent pneumonia, or atelectasis. The parenchymal changes generally progress over time.
• The chest radiographic findings are bronchial thickening and bronchiectasis, atelectasis and focal consolidation, hilar lymphadenopathy, enlarged pulmonary arteries, and hyperinflation due to chronic airway obstruction (Figure 3.4).
• Severe disease can lead to mucus plugging, pneumothorax, pneumomediastinum, hemoptysis, and pulmonary hypertension (PH). Air–fluid levels in cystic bronchiectasis may be seen in

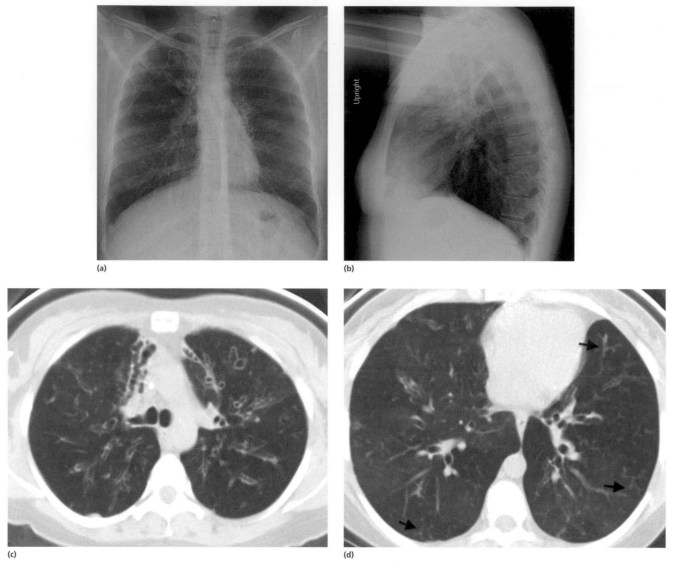

Figure 3.4 *Cystic fibrosis*: PA upright (a) and lateral (b) chest radiographs show hyperinflation of both lungs with evidence of bronchial wall thickening and bronchiectasis, prominent in the upper lobes. Axial CT images at the level of carina (c) and lower lung fields (d) show bronchiectasis, bronchial wall thickening, tree-in-bud appearance (arrows), and mosaic attenuation, suggestive of air trapping due to mucous plugging in small airway.

acute exacerbation. In advanced cases, bronchiectasis tends to be more severe in the upper lungs.

- CT provides more accurate parenchymal lung change than chest radiography because of its overall topographic display. CT findings include cylindrical or cystic bronchiectasis, predominantly in the upper lobes; diffuse bronchial wall thickening; mucus plugging (tree-in-bud pattern, bronchocele); mosaic attenuation; consolidation or atelectasis; bullae; and pleural thickening.
- In patients with advanced disease, HRCT may be useful to evaluate specific lung changes, when more aggressive treatment such as surgical intervention is indicated.

Bronchial atresia

Bronchial atresia is a congenital anomaly representing focal obliteration of a proximal segmental or subsegmental bronchus, with the normal development of distal structures. The atretic distal segment leads to accumulation of mucus within the distal bronchi or

bronchocele. The majority of patients are asymptomatic. Symptomatic patients may present with recurrent chest infection or chronic cough:

- The radiologic findings are central branching opacity (bronchocele) surrounded by an area of hyperlucency (due to collateral air drift).
- CT can clearly demonstrate central bronchocele and hyperlucency of the affected segment. The left upper lobe (LUL) is the most commonly affected. CT is also useful for demonstrating absence of the bronchus of the affected segment.

Trauma/emergency

Aortic and great vessel injury

Traumatic aortic injuries are a major cause of morbidity and mortality in the setting of motor vehicle accidents (MVAs). Death is immediate in 80–90% of individuals who experience this injury, and in the remaining 10–20% of individuals, the mortality rate is

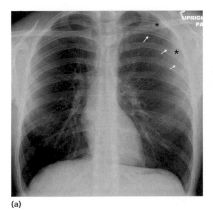 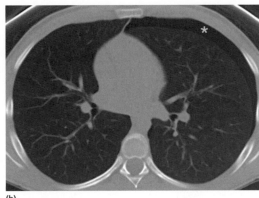 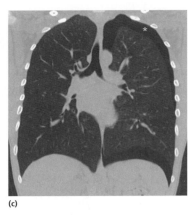

(a)   (b)   (c)

Figure 3.5 *Pneumothorax:* (a) PA upright chest radiograph shows a thin white pleural line (arrows) parallel to the chest wall of left hemithorax. Note absent of lung markings beyond the white pleural line (*). (b and c) Axial and coronal CT images in lung window setting shows clearly evidence of air in left pleural space (*). Note pneumothorax in the anterior part of hemithorax on CT image, which is the highest part in supine position.

high. The most common location of aortic injury is the aortic isthmus, within 2 cm of the origin of the left subclavian artery.

Clinical sign and symptoms of aortic injury are often nonspecific and related to distension or stretching of mediastinal tissue from the ensuing mediastinal hematoma. Patients may present with chest pain and dyspnea:

- A plain chest radiograph is usually the first imaging study performed on patients with blunt trauma. Approximately 93% of these patients have an abnormal mediastinum on initial chest radiographs obtained in the emergency department. The most sensitive radiographic sign is widening of the mediastinum due to mediastinal hematoma and loss of the aortic outline. Other findings on chest radiograph are relatively nonspecific and include pleural effusion/hemothorax, rightward deviation of nasogastric (NG) tube/trachea/endotracheal tube, left apical pleural cap, and first and/or second rib fractures.
- When chest radiograph is indeterminate or suspicious, CT scan with IV contrast is indicated. Contrast-enhanced thin-section CT scan has been adopted over the last decade as the preferred method to evaluate for aortic injury and has largely replaced conventional angiography in this setting. The CT findings of aortic injury include intimal flap, pseudoaneurysm (change of aortic caliber), contour irregularity, lumen abnormality (resulting from intraluminal thrombus), and extravasation of contrast material.
- In addition to diagnosing aortic injury, CT can also evaluate other structures for associated injury, such as lung injury, bone fracture, pneumothorax, and hemothorax.
- Pitfalls of CT include motion artifacts from heartbeat and respiration, prominent ductus arteriosus remnant, and atherosclerosis plaque.
- Conventional aortography is generally reserved for the cases with uncertain CT findings or for therapeutic purposes, such as stent graft placement. Intravascular ultrasound may have a role to confirm or clarify subtle aortic abnormalities.

Pneumothorax

Pneumothorax is defined as air in the pleural space. It may occur spontaneously, after blunt trauma or penetrating trauma of a chest, or secondary to rupture of alveoli (in asthmatic patient). Clinical signs and symptoms of tension pneumothorax are chest pain, tachypnea, dyspnea, hypoxia, and hypotension. Pneumothorax occurs

when there is leakage of air into the pleural space from a lung injury or entry of air into the pleural space from events outside the body:

- Plain chest radiograph is the initial imaging modality to evaluate pneumothorax and ideally should be obtained in an upright position to maximize the detection of pleural air. On an upright film, approximately 100 mL of air in pleural space may be detected and is shown by visualizing a white line of visceral pleura along the lateral and superior aspect of the lung parallel to the curvature of chest wall, with absence of lung markings peripheral to this pleural line (Figure 3.5).
- In contrast, in the supine position, air in the pleural space usually locates in the inferior portion of the hemithorax, which is the most anterior location in supine position (and air rises to the most anterior location). Approximately 500 mL of pleural air must be present in order to definitively diagnose, and air outlines the inferior costophrenic angle, observed as inferior displacement of the lateral costophrenic angle (deep sulcus sign).
- In clinical studies by Beres et al., pneumothorax has been reported to be detected 21% more often on upright radiograph than in lateral decubitus view. These results suggest that when clinically feasible, the expiratory upright chest radiograph is the imaging study of choice for the initial evaluation of small pneumothoraces. The combination of air and fluid in the pleural space is termed as hydropneumothorax, and it appears as an air–fluid level in the pleural space.
- Potential pitfalls in radiographic interpretation include overlying skin folds over the lung field, large bullae, and medial border of scapula mimicking a white pleural line.
- Chest ultrasonography (US) has garnered attention in critical care and emergency medicine during the last few years. Ultrasound can detect pneumothorax by demonstrating the loss of "comet-tail artifact" along the anterior chest wall when the patient is supine. These reverberation artifacts are lost due to air accumulating within the pleural space, and air hinders the propagation of sound waves and eliminates the acoustic impedance gradient necessary to visualize the "comet-tail artifact."
- CT is the gold standard to diagnose pneumothorax and is able to detect even very small volumes of air in the pleural space (5–10 mL) by using a lung window setting. CT is occasionally performed when the diagnosis is uncertain, for example, to distinguish pneumothorax from a large bulla or when the lung field is obscured by subcutaneous emphysema.

Tension pneumothorax

In the circumstance where air continues to enter the pleural space without egress, progressive increased pressure develops in the pleural space that causes pressure effect on the ipsilateral lung. As the process continues, high pressure in the pleural space causes shift of the trachea and the mediastinum to the opposite side. If treatment does not occur, the pressure effect on the heart and IVC leads to decreased systemic venous return, ultimately decreasing cardiac output resulting in cardiovascular collapse:

- On imaging, there is evidence of pneumothorax and shifting of the mediastinum to the opposite site.

Diaphragmatic rupture

Diaphragmatic rupture is usually associated with a motor vehicle collision. Left-sided rupture is the most common, accounting for 65–88%, right-sided rupture occurs in 21–32%, and bilateral rupture occurs in 2–6%. The diagnosis is often delayed because of severe concurrent injury, a lack of specific clinical signs, and simultaneous lung disease that may mask or mimic the diagnosis. Patients may complain of chest pain, abdominal pain, dyspnea, or tachypnea or present with signs of complications from the rupture, such as bowel obstruction:

- Plain chest radiography is commonly the first imaging study obtained to evaluate diaphragmatic rupture, and a high index of suspicion is the key factor in early diagnosis. The radiographic findings include normal appearance of diaphragm, elevation of the hemidiaphragm, obscured or discontinuous diaphragmatic outline, contralateral mediastinal shift, rib fracture, pleural effusion, lung contusion, atelectasis, pneumothorax, abnormal displacement of abdominal viscera, and abnormal course of NG tube (Figure 3.6).
- When the chest radiograph is indeterminate or suspicious, CT is the next imaging modality, and it is advisable to perform CT studies in all patients who have undergone major trauma. Multidetector CT has increased diagnostic accuracy, with a sensitivity of 54–78% and specificity of 86–100%. The direct signs of diaphragmatic rupture on CT include focal diaphragmatic defect and the dangling diaphragm sign, in which the free edge of the torn hemidiaphragm curls inward from its normal course parallel to the body wall.

- The indirect signs related to hernia include herniation of visceral organs into the hemithorax, waist-like constriction of the bowel (collar sign) at the level of the diaphragmatic tear in the setting of bowel herniation, and dependent visceral sign due to direct contact of visceral organs with the posterior chest wall.
- MRI is used only in doubtful cases and in hemodynamically stable patients. The MRI features are identical to those observed with CT.

Vascular

PE

PE is a blockage of pulmonary arteries by blood-borne particulate matter, most commonly blood clot. It is the third most common acute cardiovascular disease, after myocardial infarction and stroke. A venous clot most often originates from legs and migrates centrally to the right heart and pulmonary arteries. Risk factors include, but are not limited to, obesity, chronic obstructive pulmonary disease, anemia, post knee procedure, and history of deep venous thrombosis. The clinical signs and symptoms are nonspecific and variable. Patients may present with sudden shortness of breath, chest pain, cough, hemoptysis, tachypnea, and unexplained hypoxia.

Acute PE

- In imaging modalities used for the diagnosis of PE, the main purpose of a chest radiograph is to exclude diagnoses that clinically mimic PE and to aid in the interpretation of the V/Q scan; however, it does not provide adequate information to accurately establish or exclude the diagnosis. Most common radiographic findings are atelectasis and/or parenchymal areas of increased opacity, other findings include oligemia (the Westermark sign), prominent central pulmonary artery (the Fleischner sign), pleural-based area of increased opacity (the Hampton hump), vascular redistribution, pleural effusion, and elevated diaphragm.
- All patients with signs and symptoms of deep vein thrombosis (DVT) should undergo duplex ultrasound evaluation of the deep venous system of both lower extremities. If DVT is detected in a patient with acute-onset chest symptomatology and a relatively

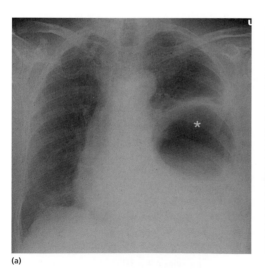
(a)

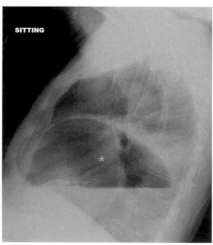
(b)

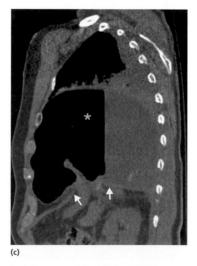
(c)

Figure 3.6 *Traumatic rupture of the diaphragm*: chest radiographs in AP sitting (a) and lateral (b) views show marked elevation of the left hemidiaphragm with mediastinal shift to the right and abnormal location of gas-filled stomach (*). Sagittal reformation of the chest CT (c) shows discontinuity of the left hemidiaphragm (arrows) with intrathoracic herniation of a dilated stomach (*).

unremarkable chest X-ray, the individual is presumed to have PE and usually do not require further investigation. If duplex US is negative and the patients do not have lung disease to explain chest symptoms, the next step should proceed to CTPA.

- Prior to the development of multidetector CTPA, catheter pulmonary angiography was the gold standard to diagnose PE. Patients with a high-quality, negative CTPA do not require further investigation. Because of the high sensitivity and high specificity of CTPA and the invasive nature of pulmonary angiography, pulmonary angiography is now only rarely used, often in patients who have indeterminate CTPA. On imaging, the common findings are:
  1 Filling defect on contrast CTPA and central filling defect with acute angle between embolus and vessel wall
  2 Enlargement of the right descending pulmonary artery/occluded artery
  3 Peripheral wedge-shaped opacity of pulmonary infarction
  4 Sign of right heart dysfunction (right ventricular dilatation, reflux of contrast into hepatic veins, straightening/bowing of ventricular septum toward the left ventricle)
- A fundamental criterion for the diagnosis of acute PE using V/Q scan is a V/Q mismatch in more than one subsegment that conforms to the pulmonary vascular anatomy, with the pattern of preserved ventilation and absent perfusion within the bronchopulmonary segment(s) affected by PE.
- The basic criteria of V/Q for absent PE are normal perfusion pattern, matched V/Q defects, and mismatch that does not have a lobar, segmental, or subsegmental pattern. Patients who have inconclusive or nondiagnostic V/Q scans should undergo further CTPA. Recent studies have shown a superior sensitivity and specificity when using V/Q single-photon emission computed tomography (SPECT) in diagnosing PE.

Chronic PE

The clinical presentation of chronic PE is often insidious, and morbidity and mortality are related to pulmonary arterial hypertension. Diagnostic testing is important to distinguish chronic PE from other causes of PH and to assess the feasibility of pulmonary endarterectomy. V/Q scan plays an important role in patients suspected of having chronic PE. The direct CT findings of chronic PE include:

1 Eccentric filling defect/web or band-like filling defect on CTPA
2 Obtuse angle between embolus and vessel wall
3 Decreased diameter of affected artery
4 Mosaic attenuation
5 Signs of pulmonary arterial hypertension (discussed in the section "Pulmonary Hypertension")
6 Signs of right heart dysfunction

When an embolus blocks the main pulmonary arteries, vascular flow to the affected lung decreases, pulmonary arterial pressure increases, and subsequent pressure overload of the right ventricle occurs resulting in right heart dysfunction. The morphologic abnormalities suggesting right heart dysfunction are right ventricular dilatation with or without reflux of contrast to hepatic veins and straightening or deviation of the interventricular septum toward the left ventricle. The CT findings of heterogeneous lung attenuation (mosaic attenuation due to nonuniform arterial perfusion) and enlargement of the main PA are indirect signs of chronic PE. If no identified cause of PH is observed on CT, V/Q scan is the follow-up imaging technique to rule out chronic PE.

To date, in most centers, MRI has played a limited role in the diagnosis of PE; however, advantages of MRI include absent radiation. Unenhanced MRA technique can be employed to evaluate proximal PE in patients who have contraindication to CT or CT or MR contrast agent; and concurrent MR venography of the lower extremities can be performed in combination with the PE study to evaluate for DVT in the same study.

Recent developments of MRI technique have shown a sensitivity of contrast-enhanced perfusion and MR angiography for detection of PE of 89.7%, and MR may be considered a second-line technique if contraindications to CT are present.

PH

PH has been defined as a resting mean pulmonary arterial pressure (mPAP) greater than 25 mm Hg or mPAP with exercise greater than 30 mm Hg. Causes of PH are categorized as precapillary and postcapillary.

Groupings include:

1 Pulmonary arterial hypertension (PAH) with a family history or patients with idiopathic PAH with germ-line mutation
2 PH secondary to left heart disease
3 PH secondary to lung disease and/or hypoxia
4 Chronic thromboembolic pulmonary hypertension (CTEPH)
5 PH with unclear multifactorial mechanism

The symptoms associated with PH are nonspecific, and diagnosis requires a high index of clinical suspicion. Dyspnea is the most common initial complaint, followed by syncope, near syncope or lightheadedness, fatigue, chest pain, and leg edema. Evaluation of patients with suspected PH requires four stages of diagnostic approach: suspicion, detection, classification, and functional evaluation.

Because treatment for patients with PH depends on the cause, accurate classification is critical. Imaging plays an important role in the diagnostic workup of PH to identify diseases contributing to PH:

- Chest radiographic findings in PAH include right ventricular enlargement and enlargement of the main pulmonary arteries with narrowing or pruning of the peripheral pulmonary arteries, but these findings are usually evident only in the late stage of disease (Figure 3.7).
- CT can provide greater accuracy to measure pulmonary artery diameter. On CT, findings include:
  1 Enlarged main and central pulmonary arteries with narrowing or pruning of peripheral branches
  2 Right ventricular enlargement
  3 Diameter of main PA greater than 29 mm or ratio of main PA diameter/ascending aorta diameter greater than 1
  4 Evidence of PE (filling defect or occlusion of PA)
  5 Enlarged bronchial arteries
  6 Mosaic attenuation
- CT plays an important role in the evaluation of PH. CT can demonstrate many diseases contributing to PH such as PE, diffuse parenchymal lung disease, chronic left to right shunt, and left-sided cardiac disease.
- Cardiac MRI may be used in the functional analysis of the right ventricle and pulmonary circulation at baseline and follow-up.
- The gold standard for the diagnosis of PH is right heart catheterization to measure PAP. However, this is an invasive procedure, involves radiation exposure, and does not provide morphological information.

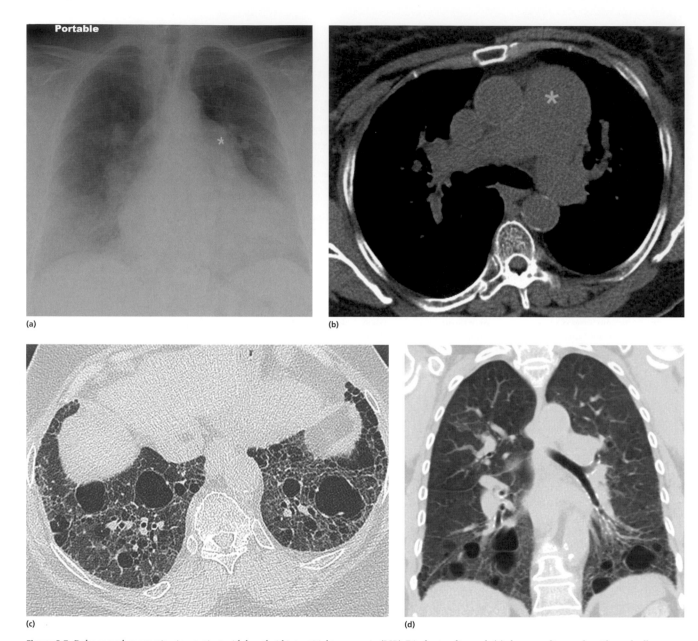

(a)

(b)

(c)

(d)

Figure 3.7 *Pulmonary hypertension in a patient with lymphoid interstitial pneumonia (LIP):* PA chest radiograph (a) shows cardiomegaly with markedly enlarged main pulmonary artery (MPA, *) and bilateral central pulmonary vessels with pruning distally, consistent with pulmonary hypertension. Noncontrast CT at the level of MPA (b) shows markedly enlarged MPA (*). Ratio of MPA diameter/ascending aortic diameter greater than 1 is suggestive of pulmonary hypertension. Axial CT (c) and coronal CT (d) in lung window setting show multiple thin-walled cystic lesions in lung bases, consistent with LIP.

Infection/inflammation

Pneumonia

Pneumonia is a very common disease and one of the most common causes of death worldwide. Causative organisms may be bacterial, viral, or fungal, and the likely organism in a particular individual is strongly influenced by the patient's immune status, underlying diseases, and demographic circumstances. Symptoms of pneumonia are varied from mild to severe, reflecting host factors and type of organism. Common symptoms include fever, chill, cough, and tachypnea. Severe symptoms and complications from pneumonia, such as parapneumonic effusion, empyema, and lung abscess, affect individuals with immature or deficient immunity, including young children, elderly, immuno-compromised hosts, and patients with chronic illness:

- The initial investigation for individuals suspected of having pneumonia should be a plain chest radiograph. The purposes of this study include to detect disease, evaluate the extent, detect potential complications, and follow up after treatment. However, in a number of cases, disease may be subtle and chest radiography may be negative.
- CT has a role in those patients who have high clinical suspicion for pneumonia, but an "unremarkable" chest radiograph, or in patients with clinically severe disease or complicated X-ray study to elucidate the full extent of disease. Airspace opacities of various causes possess ill-defined borders due to the filling of alveolar spaces with material. Multiple airspace opacities may coalesce, and vascular and bronchial margins may be obscured. If the margins of vessels or bronchi are obscured, the term consolidation

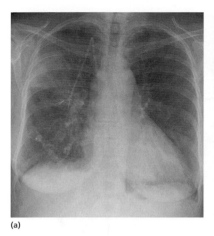
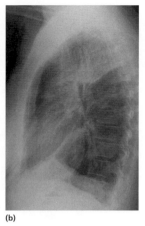
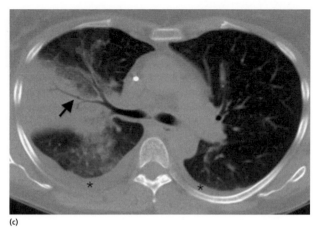

(a)   (b)   (c)

Figure 3.8 *Bacterial pneumonia:* PA upright (a) and lateral (b) chest radiographs show airspace opacity in the posterior segment of the right upper lobe. Axial noncontrast CT with lung window setting (c) shows consolidation of the posterior segment of the right upper lobe with air bronchogram (arrow). Note ground-glass opacity in the anterior segment of the upper lobe and the superior segment of the right lower lobe and small bilateral pleural effusion (*).

is used. Partial filling of alveoli results in ground-glass opacity on chest radiograph and CT, and margins of vessels or bronchi are still preserved.

- Radiographic patterns of abnormal pulmonary opacities are basically categorized to airspace disease and interstitial disease based on the radiographic appearances and localization in the lungs. By categorizing the patterns of opacities, the differential diagnoses are narrowed. However, a mixture of airspace and interstitial opacities is present for a variety of diseases and therefore will have overlapping radiographic manifestations. Clinical history is therefore always critical in evaluating diseases of the lungs.

In pneumonia (particularly bacterial), alveolar spaces are filled with organisms, inflammatory cells, and pus. The distribution may be lobar, focal, or multifocal. Lobar consolidation containing air bronchograms is the classic appearance seen in bacterial pneumonia (Figure 3.8). The filling of alveolar spaces with material may result in a relatively nonspecific pattern so fluid (e.g., pulmonary edema), infection (e.g., bacteria, white cells), tumor (e.g., bronchoalveolar cell carcinoma/adenocarcinoma), hemorrhage (e.g., trauma), or protein (alveolar proteinosis) will appear to have similar opacities. Examples of how clinical information is very important to guide more accurate diagnosis are as follows: differentiation of causes of airspace opacities may be ascertained by the rate of opacity change on serial studies and by the acuity or chronicity of disease process. In pneumonia, if there are no complications, the opacities usually clear within 7–10 day after treatment. In pulmonary edema, the opacities are usually bilateral perihilar in distribution and clear rapidly after treatment within 48 h. If the opacities persist and especially increase over time, especially in the absence of clinical signs such as fever, tumor is suspected.

Opacities representing interstitial disease are seen as reticular (mesh-like or netlike), nodular (small round opacities), or reticulonodular (mixed reticular and nodular pattern). Interstitial patterns of disease involvement in the setting of infectious pneumonia are more unusual than airspace opacities (which are seen with most bacterial pneumonias), and their identification suggests that the infecting organisms may be "atypical," and these patterns may be found in viral, mycoplasma, or fungal pneumonias (Figure 3.9). These organisms may also present with a mixed pattern of interstitial and airspace disease, which often reflects that the disease is more severe.

Pulmonary viral infection

- Radiographic features in pulmonary viral infection are usually nonspecific and overlap with other disease entities, which consist of diffuse or patchy ground-glass opacities with or without consolidation, reticular regions of increased opacity, poorly defined nodules (airspace nodules of 4–10 mm in diameter), and bronchial wall thickening. Lobar consolidation and air bronchograms are uncommon in viral pneumonia.
- CT is currently the imaging modality of choice for evaluating pulmonary viral infection. The CT appearances also vary and include bilateral ground-glass opacities with random distribution, multiple small nodules, tree-in-bud opacities, interlobular septal thickening, and bronchial wall thickening.

Pulmonary tuberculosis

Tuberculosis (TB) is an infectious disease caused by *Mycobacterium tuberculosis*, which typically affects the lungs but can affect other part of body as well. It remains a major global health problem.

Primary TB is increasingly a disease of adults, and the most characteristic feature is lymphadenopathy, which is observed in almost all patients. Lymphadenopathy is generally unilateral with the hilar and paratracheal regions most often affected, and less frequently the subcarinal nodes. Parenchymal consolidation is a common association and is seen in any pulmonary lobe or segment. The lymphadenopathy usually resolves slower than the pulmonary lesions, with no residual features. In one third of cases, the lung infiltrates leave some form of parenchymal residua, such as a nodule (tuberculoma), which can calcify, forming the Ghon focus or an area of fibrosis. The association of a parenchymal calcification with calcified hilar nodes is known as a Ranke complex, a finding highly indicative of prior primary TB.

Postprimary TB or reactivation TB typically manifests as a patchy, poorly defined consolidation in the apical and posterior segments of the upper lobes and the superior segments of the lower lobes, and about 50% of cases have a cavitary lesion, and lymphadenopathy is more uncommon at this stage (Figure 3.10). Cavitation implies a highly contagious disease and is associated with numerous complications including endobronchial spread, tuberculous empyema, hematogenous dissemination, and pulmonary artery pseudoaneurysm. Tuberculous pleurisy is more common in primary than postprimary disease, and effusions are usually unilateral, large,

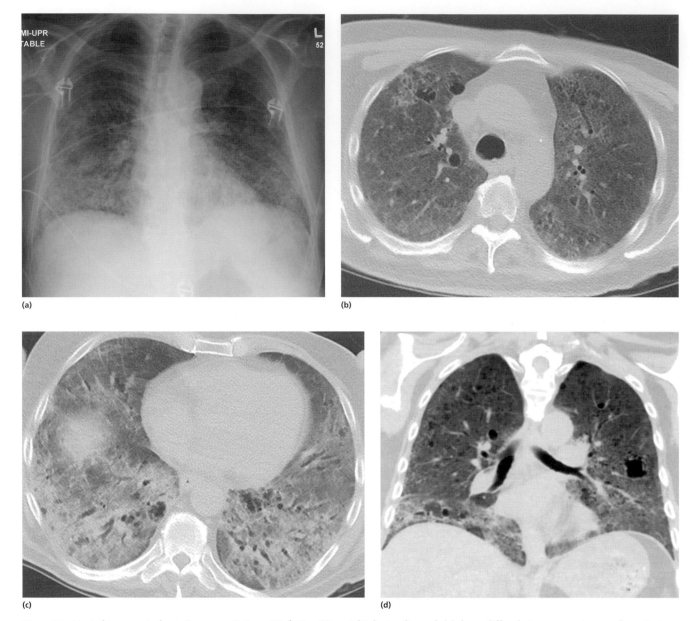

(a)

(b)

(c)

(d)

Figure 3.9 *Atypical pneumonia due to Pneumocystis jirovecii infection:* PA upright chest radiograph (a) shows diffuse heterogeneous increased opacity in both lungs. Axial CT at the upper lung field (b) and lung bases (c) and coronal (d) images in lung window setting show extensive ground-glass opacity in both lungs with component of consolidations in lung bases. Note multiple small thin-walled air cysts scattering in bilateral lung parenchyma.

and self-limited. The pleural fluid is usually a serous exudate with a marked lymphocytosis. Miliary TB is a hematogenous dissemination of infection, also more common in primary than postprimary TB, and is described as innumerable 2–3 mm nodules uniformly involving the lung parenchyma. Chest radiography is the most common study for the assessment of pulmonary TB and is usually sufficient in most cases. CT provides diagnostic findings in cases where the chest radiograph is normal or inconclusive, and to detect complications.

Pulmonary nontuberculous mycobacteria

Nontuberculous mycobacteria (NTM), also known as atypical mycobacteria, represent organisms that are widely distributed in the environment, especially in wet soil. Examples of these groups of species are *Mycobacterium avium complex* (MAC), *Mycobacterium kansasii, and Mycobacterium fortuitum.* Definitive diagnosis of

pulmonary NTM infection is challenging. Because the organisms are often saprophytes, they may colonize airways rather than infect them. Cultures can be falsely positive in patients with chronic lung disease and falsely negative in infected patients without cavities. The clinical and radiologic manifestations of pulmonary NTM infection are protean and include the cavitary ("classic") form, bronchiectasis ("nonclassic") form, infection in immunocompromised patients, nodules or mass-like opacities, infections with deglutition problems, and hypersensitivity pneumonitis. However, these manifestations are not mutually exclusive; several forms can be seen in an individual patient. The cavitary and the bronchiectasis forms are responsible for most NTM infections in the immunocompetent patient.

The clinical and radiologic manifestations of the cavitary (classic) form are quite similar to those of postprimary TB (Figure 3.11). This form of the disease is more prevalent among older white men

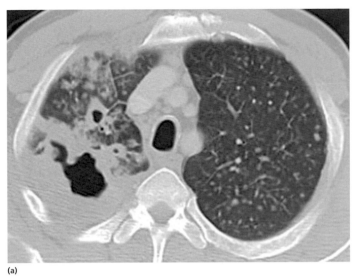

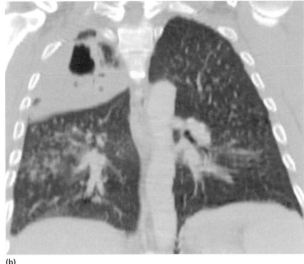

(a)   (b)

Figure 3.10 *Postprimary TB with miliary dissemination:* axial (a) and coronal CT (b) in lung window shows consolidation with cavitary lesion in the right upper and midlobes. Note that there are multiple small nodular opacities scattering in both lungs, indicative of miliary dissemination.

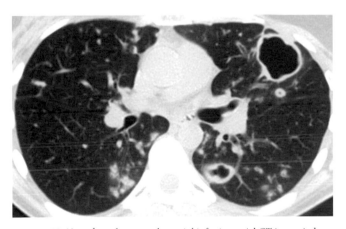

Figure 3.11 *Nontuberculous mycobacterial infection:* axial CT image in lung window setting shows multiple thick-walled cavitary lesions in the left upper lobe. There are multiple small nodular opacities scattering in both lungs, indicative of endobronchial spread of infection. Radiographic findings are indistinguishable from pulmonary TB.

with underlying chronic pulmonary disease (e.g., chronic obstructive pulmonary disease):

- Findings include upper lobe cavitary lesions and endobronchial spread evidenced by nodules adjacent to foci of disease, cicatricial atelectasis, and pleural thickening. In bronchiectasis (nonclassic) form, the infection is more commonly seen among elderly white women with no predisposing factors. Radiographic findings include randomly distributed nodular opacities; cavitation is uncommon.
- CT characteristically shows small centrilobular nodules or tree-in-bud opacities, with cylindric bronchiectasis, usually in the same lobe. Right middle lobe and the lingula are most commonly affected, although any segment can be involved.

Pulmonary fungal infection

Pulmonary fungal infections are less common than bacterial and viral infections. The diseases mainly affect people living in certain endemic areas or present as an opportunistic infection in immunocompromised hosts. The major endemic fungal diseases in North America are histoplasmosis, blastomycosis, and coccidioidomycosis. Their prevalence varies by region. The majority of infected individual have an asymptomatic, self-limiting disease. Clinical pneumonia occurs in those with exposure to a large number of infecting spores. Radiographic findings include solitary or multiple nodular opacities with or without cavity and consolidation, pleural effusion, and lymphadenopathy. Resolution of the pneumonia often leaves calcified pulmonary nodules, calcified mediastinal lymph nodes, or splenic calcifications.

Aspergillosis-related lung disease

Aspergillosis is a mycotic disease caused by *Aspergillus* species. The histologic, clinical, and radiologic manifestations of pulmonary aspergillosis are determined by the number and virulence of the organisms and the patients' immune response. Pulmonary aspergillosis can be subdivided into five categories:

- *Saprophytic aspergillosis* is characterized by *Aspergillus* infection without tissue invasion, such as colonization of preexisting cavity or cystic lesions in the lungs (e.g., cavitary lesions in TB, NTM, sarcoidosis, or bronchiectasis), resulting in fungal ball or aspergilloma.
- Chest radiograph and CT show a moderately thick-walled cavity containing a mobile round or oval soft tissue mass of fungal ball (resulting in the "air crescent" sign) and adjacent pleural thickening (Figure 3.12).
- *Allergic bronchopulmonary aspergillosis (ABPA)* is a form of hypersensitivity reaction to inhaled *Aspergillus* and is seen most commonly in patients with long-standing asthma. This form of aspergillosis is characterized by the presence of mucous plugs containing *Aspergillus* organisms and eosinophils. This results in bronchial dilatation typically involving the segmental and subsegmental bronchi.
- Radiographic and CT findings include tubular, finger-in-glove areas of opacity in a bronchial distribution, usually with predominantly upper lobe distribution (Figure 3.13).
- *Semi-invasive or chronic necrotizing aspergillosis* is characterized by the presence of tissue necrosis and granulomatous infection similar to that seen in reactivation TB. This form usually occurs in patients with mildly impaired immune system such as chronic illness, diabetes mellitus, malnutrition, alcoholism, or chronic steroid usage.

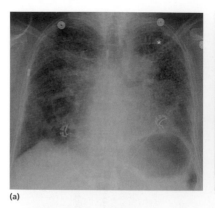
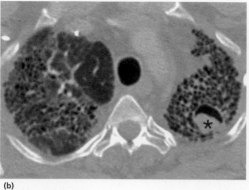
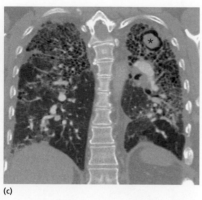

(a)   (b)   (c)

Figure 3.12 *Mycetoma*: PA chest radiograph (a) in sarcoidosis patient shows coarse reticulonodular opacities in both lungs, predominantly in the upper lobes. There is a soft tissue nodule (*) in the LUL outline by crescent of air. Note enlarged central pulmonary arteries suggestive of pulmonary arterial hypertension. Axial CT image (b) and coronal CT image (c) of the chest show a 2.5 cm cavitary lesion in the LUL containing an internal soft tissue mass, consistent with mycetoma (*). Note bilateral diffuse upper lobe cystic changes.

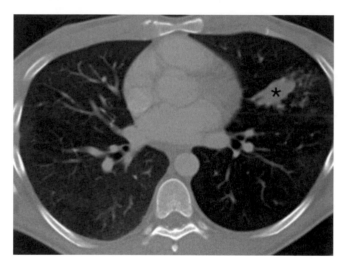

Figure 3.13 *Allergic bronchopulmonary aspergillosis (ABPA):* axial CT image in lung window setting shows a tubular branching opacity (*) in a lingular lobe, consistent with mucous plugging in dilated bronchus. Note mosaic attenuation in both lungs representing air trapping.

- The radiographic findings include indolent mass or focal consolidation and multiple nodular opacities, indistinguishable from TB. It may cavitate and develop a mycetoma. These findings progress slowly over months or years.
- *Airway-invasive aspergillosis* is characterized by the presence of the *Aspergillus* organism deep to the airway basement membrane. It occurs most commonly in immunocompromised neutropenic patients and in patients with AIDS. Clinical manifestations include acute tracheobronchitis, bronchiolitis, and bronchopneumonia.
- The radiographic findings of acute tracheobronchitis are usually normal or occasionally show tracheal or bronchial wall thickening. CT findings include centrilobular nodules and branching linear or a "tree-in-bud" appearance.
- The characteristic CT findings mimic those in ABPA and consist of bilateral bronchial and bronchiolar dilatation, large mucoid impaction (mainly in the lower lobes), and diffuse lower lobe consolidation due to postobstructive atelectasis.
- *Angioinvasive aspergillosis* is the most aggressive form of aspergillosis and occurs in immunocompromised patients with severe neutropenia characterized by the invasion and occlusion of small- to medium-sized pulmonary arteries by fungal hyphae.

- Chest radiographic findings include ill-defined solitary nodule or ill-defined multiple nodular opacities. Characteristic CT findings consist of nodules surrounded by a halo of ground-glass opacity (halo sign) representing hemorrhagic nodule or pleural-based consolidation representing hemorrhagic infarctions (Figure 3.14).

Acute inhalation injury

By virtue of the lung parenchyma experiencing direct contact with the outside environment through respiration, a large and complex category of pulmonary disease reflects inhalational exposure. The most common types are thermal (typically fire-related heat and smoke exposure), chemical, and particulate.

Smoke and fire injury

Smoke inhalation defined as airway or pulmonary injury resulting from the inhalation of toxic combustion products, presents with a wide range of severity in patients with or without skin burn. Extensive and severe cutaneous burn may lead to sepsis, pulmonary edema, or acute respiratory distress syndrome (ARDS).

Radiographic findings may be divided into three phases: acute, subacute, and chronic:

1 The acute phase occurs within 24 h after injury and reflects direct inhalation damage to the lungs and mucosal edema of the upper airways including chemical pulmonary pneumonitis and pulmonary edema. Bronchial wall thickening and subglottic edema are common early findings.
2 In the subacute phase, which occurs between 2 and 5 days after injury, findings include pulmonary edema, atelectasis, pulmonary microembolism, and ARDS.
3 Delayed or chronic complications are seen after the fifth day and include PE, pneumonia, and ARDS.

The correct diagnosis of chest abnormalities in burn victims depends upon correlation of radiologic, clinical, and laboratory findings. In severe disease, pulmonary opacities from various causes may occur in combination. The most common complications are consolidation and ARDS mainly due to inhalation injury and/or following septicemia.

Asthma

Asthma is a common inflammatory airway disease due to abnormal reactivity of the airways to various stimuli, leading to airflow obstruction and mucus hyperproduction. Persistent airway inflammation leads to structural changes known as airway remodeling

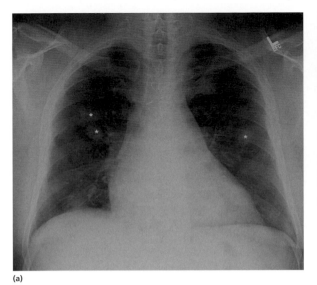
(a)

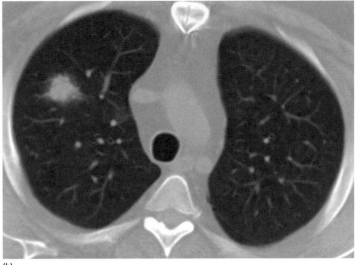
(b)

Figure 3.14 *Angioinvasive aspergillosis*: posteroanterior view of a chest radiograph (a) showed multiple ill-defined nodular opacities (*) in both lungs. Axial CT at the level of the upper lobes (b) in window setting shows a pulmonary nodule in the RUL surrounded by a halo of ground-glass opacity.

and consequently airway obstruction, which is partly reversible. Clinical signs and symptoms of asthma are wheezing, chest tightness, shortness of breath, and coughing:

- Most patients with acute exacerbation usually improve after medical treatment and do not require a chest radiograph. However, in a minority of cases, a chest radiograph is obtained to identify other causes of wheezing or complications, such as pneumothorax, atelectasis, and superimposed pneumonia.
- Hyperinflation of the lungs can be seen in relapse or remission phases. Other findings are bronchial wall thickening, mucoid impaction, focal consolidation (secondary to infection), subsegmental or lobar atelectasis, bronchiectasis, and rarely pneumothorax.
- CT is not routinely used in the management of asthma. However, many studies have documented a number of features that reflect airway remodeling in asthma. Direct findings include direct measurement of airway wall thickness, and evaluating bronchiectasis, using a ratio of bronchial diameter to adjacent pulmonary artery or lack of bronchial tapering. Indirect signs include mosaic attenuation due to air trapping and centrilobular nodules due to mucoid impaction.

Pleural effusion

Parapneumonic effusions are present in about 40–50% of patients with bacterial pneumonia, although only a minority of these will become a complicated parapneumonic effusion or empyema and require intervention.

In the normal situation, the visceral pleura and pleural space are not visible on radiograph or CT and only become visible when there is disease or abnormality:

- An uncomplicated pleural effusion is usually small in volume and flows freely along the dependent portions of the pleural space. In the upright position, approximately 50 mL of pleural fluid may be detected on the lateral radiograph, seen as increased opacity and obliteration of the posterior costophrenic angle, but at least 150 mL must be present to be visualizable on the frontal PA view.
- On the PA view, pleural effusion is evident as an increased density in the dependent portion of the thoracic cavity obscuring the

lateral costophrenic angle creating a concave upper margin (meniscus sign) (Figure 3.15).
- In selected settings, such as tapping a pleural effusion, ultrasound can be a useful procedure, and it is also able to detect a small volume of pleural effusion.

Complicated pleural effusion/empyema

When infection spreads to pleural space, the pleural fluid becomes loculated (i.e., no longer exhibits free flow in the pleural space) due to fibrin formation. The process can progress to frank pus or empyema. The distinction between pleural effusion, loculated pleural fluid, and other pleural abnormalities is often best performed with CT:

- CT findings of empyema are visualization of thickened, separated visceral and parietal pleural surfaces (split pleural sign) and compression of adjacent lung (Figure 3.16).
- CT and ultrasound are also useful modalities to provide guidance to obtain pleural fluid samples for laboratory evaluation, and thoracostomy tube placement, in complicated pleural effusions or empyemas, to avoid potential complications.
- Complicated/loculated pleural fluid may be trapped in dependent and nondependent compartments of the pleural space including interlobar fissures and may be associated with pleural thickening.
- MR features are similar to those described for CT, although the intensity of enhancement of inflamed tissue is greater on MRI.

Lung abscess

Lung abscess is defined as a localized area of necrotic or suppurative tissue due to infection, associated with localized destruction of lung parenchyma. The etiology can arise from primary infection of the lungs, such as necrotizing pneumonia or aspiration, or secondary to other conditions, such as direct extension from adjacent structures, septic emboli, bronchial obstruction, and bronchiectasis.

The clinical presentation is usually indolent, with features that evolve over a period of weeks to months. The common signs and symptoms are fever, productive cough, and weight loss:

- On chest radiographs, a lung abscess is a cavity containing an air–fluid level that tends to be round in morphology on frontal and lateral views, as opposed to empyema, which is usually lenticular in shape (Figure 3.17). These features may overlap on

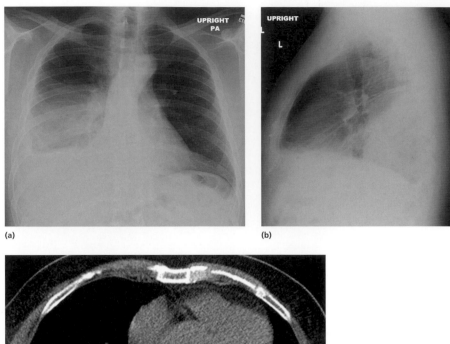

(a)

(b)

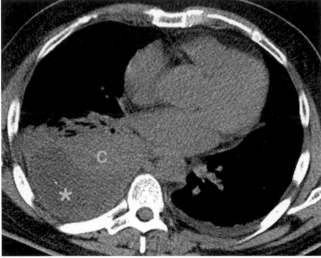

(c)

Figure 3.15 *Pleural effusion*: PA upright (a) and lateral chest (b) radiographs show increased lung density of the right lower lobe obscuring the right hemidiaphragm with blunting of the right costophrenic angle, suggestive of right pleural effusion. Axial noncontrast CT at the level of the lower lungs (c) shows evidence of bilateral pleural effusion (*), right greater than left. Note consolidation (c) of the right lower lobe adjacent to right pleural effusion.

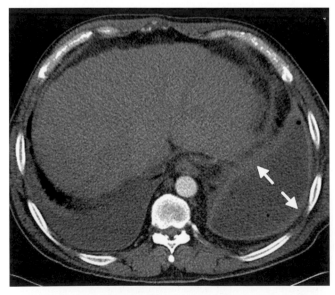

Figure 3.16 *Empyema thoraces*: axial postcontrast CT image shows moderate right pleural fluid collection with thickening of the parietal and visceral pleura (arrows) of the left side (split pleural sign), suggestive of infection/inflammatory process. Small air bubble within the left pleural collection is secondary to postpleural tapping. Note right pleural fluid without pleural thickening.

plain radiographs. It is very important to differentiate lung abscess and empyema, because in general lung abscess does not require intervention, but is managed with antibiotic treatment alone, whereas empyema requires drainage with a chest tube in addition to antibiotic therapy for optimal management.

• CT can accurately diagnose a lung abscess, which shows a thick-walled cavity in area of destroyed lung with irregularity of the luminal margin. Note that clinical features of infection are important since neoplasms may also show central necrosis and cavity formation. Abscess forms an acute angle with the costal or pleural surface, while empyema has an obtuse angle.

Atelectasis

As increased opacity in the lung parenchyma is a nonspecific finding of pneumonia, features that distinguish it from another common lung parenchymal abnormality that is not serious, atelectasis, are especially important:

• Radiographic and CT findings of atelectasis include increased lung opacity with evidence of volume loss and crowding of pulmonary vessels, displacement of interlobar fissure, elevation of the hemidiaphragm of the affected lung, hilar or mediastinal displacement, focal obscuration of the heart or diaphragm border.

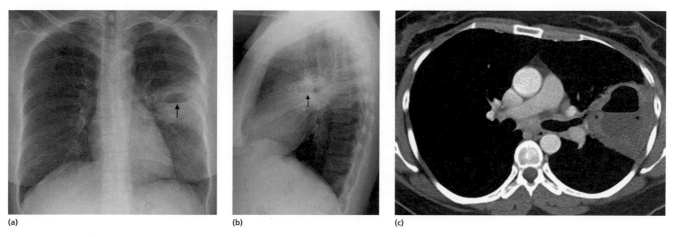

Figure 3.17 *Lung abscess:* PA upright (a) and lateral (b) chest radiographs show a cavitary lesion with internal air–fluid level (arrow), which is round in shape in PA and lateral views. Note consolidation surrounding a cavitary lesion. Axial noncontrast CT image (c) shows a thick-walled cavitary lesion containing air–fluid level, consistent with lung abscess. Note a lesion forms an acute angle with the costal surface.

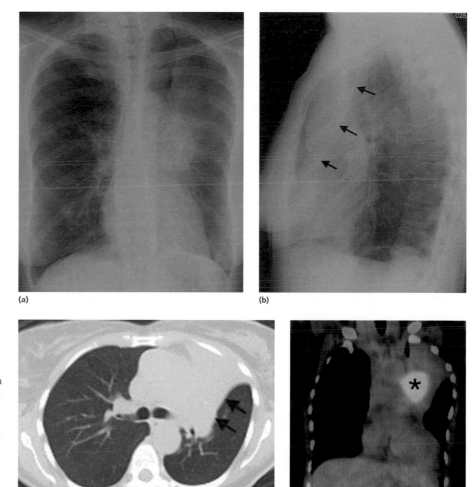

Figure 3.18 *Central mass at the LUL with LUL atelectasis:* PA chest radiograph (a) shows a veiling density of the left hemithorax with volume loss and obliteration of the left upper cardiac outline. Lateral chest radiograph (b) shows increased lung opacity anteriorly due to LUL collapse and anterosuperior displacement of minor fissure (arrows). Axial CT lung window setting (c) shows total collapsed LUL indicated by increased attenuation and anterior displacement of the major fissure (arrows). Coronal PET (d) shows a FDG-avid mass at the LUL (*).

- Air bronchograms, which are classic for pneumonia, may uncommonly also be seen in atelectatic lung and reflect the absence of a central obstructing process. Atelectasis generally shows more prominent volume loss associated with the increased lung opacity and, on arterial phase CT and MR images, more intense enhancement of the opacified tissue, reflecting that the opacity is comprised of lung parenchyma that is now collapsed with resulting crowding of the arterial vessels that thereby exhibit much more enhancement of the tissue (Figure 3.18).

Interstitial lung diseases

The term "interstitial lung disease" (ILD) is synonymous with "diffuse parenchymal lung diseases," although the actual pathology may occur in both interstitium and airspace of the lungs. ILDs are a heterogeneous group of diseases that diffusely affect the lungs, resulting in lung damage, but have similar clinical presentation, pathology, and radiographic findings. The etiology of ILD may be related to a broad spectrum of diseases, but principal diseases include collagen vascular disease, environmental exposures, and drugs. If the etiology of ILD cannot be identified, the term "idiopathic interstitial pneumonias" (IIPs) or "idiopathic ILDs" is used.

The classification of ILD is based on the morphologic pattern of histologic findings. However, the actual diagnosis requires a multidisciplinary approach that correlates clinical information, imaging, and histologic features. ILDs associated with diseases such as connective tissue diseases and inhalational exposures can possess identical morphologic patterns, and the features of IIP are considered the prototype for these morphologic alterations. The most common clinical presentations of ILD are shortness of breath and cough.

The diagnostic approach to IIPs has long been subject to confusion because these disorders have been variably categorized according to different clinical, radiologic, and histologic classifications. In 2001, the American Thoracic Society (ATS)/European Respiratory Society (ERS) developed a classification system based on the morphologic patterns on which clinical–radiologic–pathologic diagnosis of IIP is based.

IIP includes seven entities: idiopathic pulmonary fibrosis (IPF), which is characterized by the morphologic pattern of usual interstitial pneumonia (UIP); nonspecific interstitial pneumonia (NSIP); cryptogenic organizing pneumonia (COP); respiratory bronchiolitis-associated ILD (RB-ILD); desquamative interstitial pneumonia (DIP); lymphoid interstitial pneumonia (LIP); and acute interstitial pneumonia (AIP):

- Chest radiographs are the first-line imaging test to evaluate ILD, as it is widely available, fast, and inexpensive. The details of parenchymal and interstitial diseases are generally not clearly definable on chest radiographs.
- HRCT techniques provide excellent imaging resolution and anatomical detail, similar to gross pathologic specimens, and can identify anatomical detail at the level of the secondary pulmonary lobule.
- HRCT plays an important role in the diagnosis of ILD and can visualize disease of the interstitium in great detail, which is not demonstrable on chest radiographs. HRCT can also clarify the pattern of abnormality seen on chest radiographs; evaluate disease severity; predict response to therapy; predict survival; aid the decision of what route to use to obtain histological material among surgical lung biopsy, bronchoscopy, or bronchoalveolar lavage; and guide the appropriate location for biopsy.

HRCT findings of common ILDs include:

1 *UIP*: Predominantly basal and peripheral reticular opacities with honeycombing and traction bronchiectasis.
2 *NSIP*: Basal ground-glass opacities tend to predominate over reticular opacities, with traction bronchiectasis only in advanced disease (Figure 3.19).
3 *COP*: Patchy peripheral or peribronchovascular consolidation.
4 *RB-ILD and DIP*: Smoking-related disease characterized by ground-glass opacities, often in combination with cystic lesions.
5 *AIP*: Diffuse lung consolidation with ground-glass opacities, which usually progress to fibrosis in patients who survive the acute phase of the disease.

The histologic diagnosis is the most important factor to determine survival in patients with suspected IIPs; the median survival rate for patients with a histopathologic diagnosis of UIP has been reported as 78 months, compared with 178 months for NSIP. However, patients with UIP may also be at higher risk for death following surgical biopsy. Fortunately, HRCT features in the diagnosis of UIP have a very high specificity; therefore, in patients who show the characteristic distribution and HRCT pattern of UIP and who have the appropriate clinical features, the diagnosis can be reliably made without lung biopsy. In patients with ILD in whom the clinical and HRCT features are not consistent with UIP or who have an uncertain clinical diagnosis, a surgical lung biopsy is indicated and is most helpful.

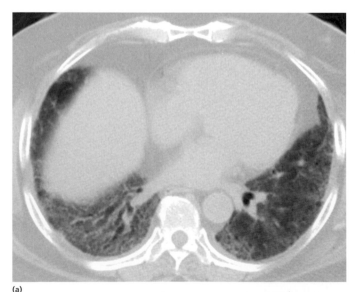
(a)

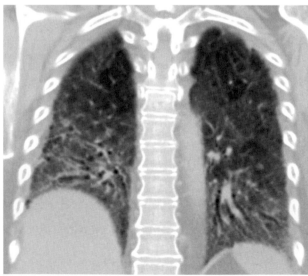
(b)

Figure 3.19 *Nonspecific interstitial pneumonia (NSIP):* axial CT image at lung bases (a) and coronal image (b) in lung window setting show predominantly ground-glass opacities in basal lungs with mild traction bronchiectasis. Note no evidence of honeycombing.

Neoplasm

Mediastinal masses

The mediastinum consists of many structures and is bounded by the right and left pleural spaces laterally, thoracic inlet superiorly, and diaphragm inferiorly. There are differing descriptions of radiological compartmentalization of the mediastinum for the purpose of rendering differential diagnoses. In this chapter, the mediastinum will be divided into three compartments, which can be drawn in outline on the lateral chest radiograph (Figure 3.20).

The anterior mediastinum is the compartment anterior to the heart and great vessels and posterior to the sternum and contains the thymus gland, fat, internal mammary vessels, lymph nodes, and occasionally thyroid gland extending from the neck to the retrosternal region.

The posterior mediastinum is the compartment behind the posterior border of the heart and trachea containing the descending aorta, esophagus, azygos vein, lymph nodes, autonomic ganglia, and thoracic duct.

The middle mediastinum is the compartment between the anterior and posterior mediastinum, containing the heart, pericardium, ascending aorta, aortic arch and its branches, SVC, brachiocephalic vein, pulmonary vessels, trachea and main bronchi, fat, phrenic nerves, left recurrent laryngeal nerve, and lymph nodes. Knowing the contents of each mediastinal compartment facilitates the creation of a differential diagnosis for mediastinal masses. Table 3.1 shows the differential diagnoses of mediastinal masses by compartment location.

The patient with a mediastinal mass may be asymptomatic or may have symptoms caused by mass effect or involvement of adjacent structures including dysphagia, cough, and SVC syndrome:

- Posteroanterior and lateral views of chest radiograph are the initial imaging study to evaluate a mediastinal mass, which is generally observed as creating an abnormal contour of the mediastinum.

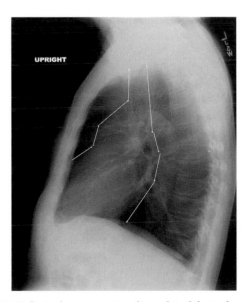

Figure 3.20 *Mediastinal compartments outline on lateral chest radiograph*: the anterior mediastinum is the compartment anterior to the heart and great vessels and posterior to the sternum. The posterior mediastinum is the compartment behind the posterior border of the heart and trachea. The middle mediastinum is the compartment between the anterior and posterior mediastinum.

Table 3.1 Common differential diagnosis of mediastinal masses.

Anterior mediastinal mass
Thyroid
Thymus
Teratoma
Lymphoma
Middle mediastinal mass
Lymph nodes
Benign cysts
Aortic arch aneurysm/vascular
Posterior mediastinal masses
Neurogenic tumor
Descending aortic aneurysm
Extramedullary hematopoiesis

- CT is the most important imaging modality to evaluate a mediastinal mass, because of its high accuracy to localize tumor and high imaging spatial resolution to demonstrate the relationship of the mediastinal mass to adjacent structures.

The most common frequent lesions encountered in the mediastinum are thymoma, neurogenic tumors, and benign cysts, altogether representing 60% of mediastinal masses. Patient's age is an important guide to predict the likelihood of the type of mediastinal tumor. In adults, primary thymic neoplasms, germ cell tumors, and lymphomas are most common, whereas in children, the most common mediastinal tumors are neurogenic tumor, lymphoma, and germ cell tumor.

The combination of location and tissue components of a mediastinal mass is very important to narrow the differential diagnosis. Tissue characterization on CT is based on specific attenuation of the air, calcium, water, and fat. For example, if the mass is in the anterior mediastinum and has fluid attenuation, the differential should include thymic cyst, thymoma, pericardial cyst, and germ cell tumor (Figure 3.21). Components of mediastinal masses are shown in Table 3.2. Vascular lesions (e.g., aortic aneurysm) may present as a mediastinal mass and should be recognized by contrast-enhanced CT to avoid biopsy:

- MRI and CT are equally effective in demonstrating mediastinal lesions, but CT is superior for displaying calcifications within a mass and for demonstrating associated lung abnormality, whereas MRI is superior for showing fluid content in certain solid lesions, like a neurogenic tumor or paraganglionoma.
- MRI may also be useful to differentiate thymic hyperplasia from other thymic tumors in myasthenic patients, showing chemical shift artifact (signal drop) on in-phase and opposed-phase T1-W images in thymic hyperplasia. The high soft tissue contrast resolution of MRI also facilitates characterization and evaluation of tumor extension for neurogenic mediastinal masses.

Pleural tumors

Primary benign tumors of pleura are much less common than metastatic cancers or diffuse malignant mesothelioma. The majority of benign pleural tumors are lipoma and solitary fibrous tumor of pleura. Chest radiographs are the initial imaging modality to evaluate patients with a suspicion of pleural disease. It may not be possible to differentiate benign and malignant disease in many cases. CT plays an important role to evaluate pleural abnormalities and has better sensitivity and specificity to differentiate benign and malignant pleural disease.

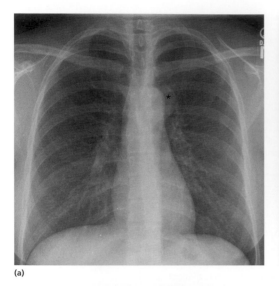

(a)

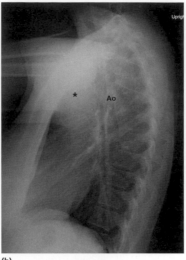

(b)

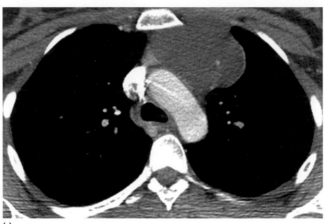

(c)

Figure 3.21 *Anterior mediastinal mass*: (a) PA upright chest radiograph shows an outline of a soft tissue mass (*) over the aortic knob without obscuration of aortic outline, indicative that a mass does not contact to the aortic knob, which locates in posterior mediastinum. (b) Lateral chest radiographs show increased density at the superior part of anterior mediastinum (*), the aortic knob (Ao) is clearly outlined, and a mass locates in the anterior mediastinum. (c) Axial postcontrast image at the level of aortic arch shows a well-defined soft tissue mass at the left anterior mediastinum. The differential diagnoses include thymic cyst, pericardial cyst, and cystic thymoma. The patient underwent surgery and pathology revealed pericardial cyst.

Table 3.2 Components of mediastinal masses.

Cystic
  Thymic cyst
  Bronchogenic cyst
  Duplication cyst
  Necrotic node
  Cystic thymoma
  Lymphoma
  Neurenteric cyst
  Lymphangioma
Fat
  Pericardial fat pad
  Lipoma
  Thymolipoma
  Liposarcoma
  Extramedullary hematopoiesis
Calcifications
  Teratoma
  Vascular lesion
  Thymic lesion
  Calcified wall of cystic lesions

Lipoma

Pleural lipomas are encapsulated fat-containing tumors originating from submesothelial parietal pleura and extend into the subpleural, pleural, and extrapleural space. They are most often discovered incidentally on chest CT obtained for other reasons:

- Definite diagnosis of these tumors based on plain chest radiographs is difficult.

- CT shows a well-circumscribed mass with obtuse angle along the chest wall with homogeneous fat attenuation (−50 to −150 HU). A heterogeneous attenuation greater than −50 HU should be considered suspicious for liposarcoma.

Solitary fibrous tumors of pleura

Solitary fibrous tumors of pleura or localized fibrous tumors of pleura are rare mesenchymal tumors that most commonly affect the pleura. The majority of these tumors are benign and slow growing, but malignant forms may rarely occur. Most patients are older than 40 years at time of initial observation. The average maximum tumor diameter at surgery is approximately 15 cm, and 70% have a maximum diameter greater than or equal to 10 cm. In about half of all patients with small tumors, the tumor is discovered incidentally on radiographs obtained for other reason:

- Radiologically, they are intrathoracic masses of variable sizes. Small lesions usually appear as homogeneous and well-defined masses. Large lesions appear more inhomogeneous.
- A smooth tapering margin at the junction of the mass with the pleural surface is a reliable CT sign of a tumor of pleural origin. Usually, tumors are well-circumscribed extrapulmonary soft tissue mass with an obtuse angle along the chest wall and mild contrast enhancement on CT.
- Rarely tumors may be pedunculated and may change in location based on patient position. Multiplanar CT and MRI are comparable for preoperative assessment.

Excision is curative in the majority of patients.

Malignant mesothelioma

Malignant mesothelioma is the most common primary malignant tumor of the pleural space and arises from mesothelial cells. This tumor is associated with asbestos exposure in up to 80% of patients. The prognosis is poor, with a median survival of 9–17 months after diagnosis. The mean age of patients at diagnosis is about 59–62 years old. Patients usually present insidiously with dyspnea, chest pain, cough, and weight loss:

- The common radiographic findings include a unilateral pleural effusion, a pleural mass, or a diffuse nodular pleural thickening that encase the lung (Figure 3.22). In most cases, plain radiographs show sufficient detail to define the abnormality and determine its extent.
- CT is superior to plain radiography and is able to reveal in greater detail findings such as thickening of the diaphragm, invasion of the chest wall and mediastinum, and detailed contralateral lung evaluation. Concomitant bilateral pleural calcifications and plaques are indicative of previous asbestos exposure and are seen on CT in 15–16% of patients. Contrast-enhanced CT plays a key role in the diagnosis, pretreatment assessment, treatment planning, monitoring, and posttreatment surveillance.

Pleural metastases

Pleural metastasis accounts for the vast majority of pleural neoplasms. The most common primary tumors to result in pleural metastases are adenocarcinoma of the breast, lung, and gastrointestinal tract. Other tumors with a predilection for pleural spread include renal cell carcinoma, melanoma, and thymoma. Pleural effusion is the most common manifestation of pleural metastasis that is usually unilateral, and malignancy is the most common cause of a massive effusion:

- Radiographic and CT manifests as irregular or nodular pleural thickening may be indistinguishable from mesothelioma (Figure 3.23). However, circumferential pleural thickening, fissural involvement, and contraction of the hemithorax are more in favor of mesothelioma.

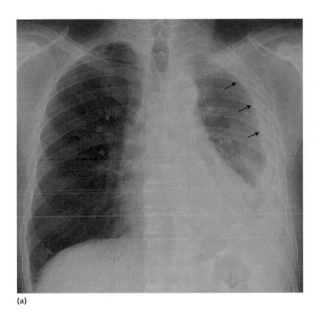

(a)

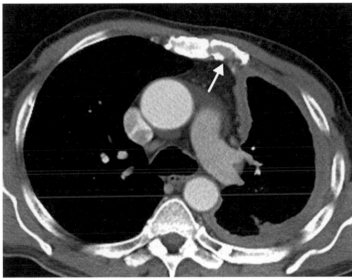

(b)

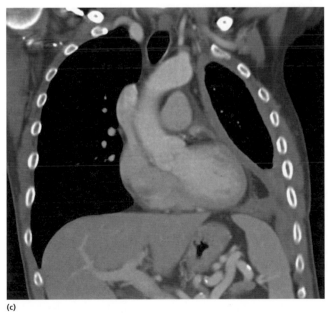

(c)

Figure 3.22 *Malignant mesothelioma*: PA upright chest radiograph (a) shows diffuse left pleural density (arrows) with rather small-sized left hemithorax as compared to the right. Axial (b) and coronal (c) post-IV contrast CT at the level of carina shows diffuse marked thicken left pleura encircling the left hemithorax. Note cortical destruction at the left side of sternum (arrow) adjacent to a tumor.

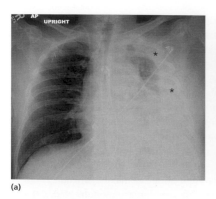
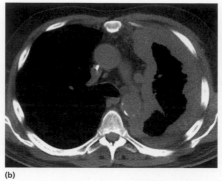
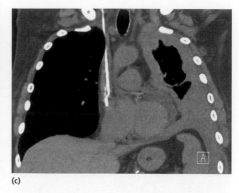

(a) (b) (c)

Figure 3.23 *Lung metastasis*: (a) AP upright chest radiograph shows evidence of left pleural opacity along the left costal margin (*) with obliteration of left hemithorax and left cardiac border. The pleural opacity also extends to the upper and medial part of the left hemithorax. (b) Axial and (c) coronal noncontrast CT of the chest shows diffuse irregular pleural thickening encircling the left hemithorax. Note rather small-sized left hemithorax as compared to the right.

Table 3.3 Recommendations for follow-up and management of nodules smaller than 8 mm detected incidentally at nonscreening CT.

Nodule size (mm)*	Low-risk patient†	High-risk patient‡
≤4	No follow-up needed§	Follow-up CT at 12 mo; if unchanged, no further follow-up¶
>4–6	Follow-up CT at 12 mo; if unchanged, no further follow-up¶	Initial follow-up CT at 6–12 mo and then at 18–24 mo if no change¶
>6–8	Initial follow-up CT at 6–12 mo and then at 18–24 mo if no change	Initial follow-up CT at 3–6 mo and then 9–12 and 24 mo if no change
>8	Follow-up CT at around 3, 9, and 24 mo, dynamic contrast-enhanced CT, PET, and/or biopsy	Same as for low-risk patient

Note: Newly detected indeterminate nodule in persons 35 years of age or older.
mo, months.
*Average of length and width.
†Minimal or absent history of smoking and of other known risk factors.
‡History of smoking or of other known risk factors.
§The risk of malignancy in this category (<1%) is substantially less than that in a baseline CT scan of an asymptomatic smoker.
¶Nonsolid (ground-glass) or partly solid nodules may require longer follow-up to exclude indolent adenocarcinoma.

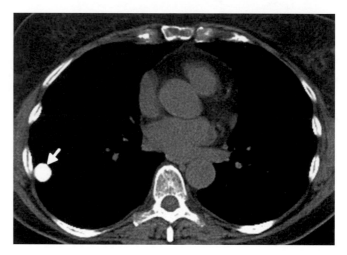

Figure 3.24 *Calcified granuloma*: a noncontrast axial CT at the level of the left atrium shows a round dense calcification of calcified granuloma (arrow) at the periphery of the right lung.

Benign lung tumors

Benign lung nodules are very common findings on chest imaging studies. The frequency of benign lesions stymies the efforts to use imaging tests to screen for lung cancers, because benign lesions are so common; and when lesions are small in size, benign and malignant lesions are difficult to distinguish from each other. The Fleischner society has created an imaging algorithm to evaluate for the solitary pulmonary nodule and is shown in Table 3.3.

Granulomas

Granulomas are very common pulmonary nodules:
- Clues to their benign nature include multiplicity of lesions, central calcification, or diffuse solid calcification (Figure 3.24) or laminated calcification and no change in lesion size over serial investigation. However, not all calcified nodules are benign.
- Pulmonary metastasis from osteogenic sarcoma or chondrosarcoma and carcinoid tumor may calcify, and although rare, primary lung cancer can also calcify. To classify calcification in a benign pulmonary nodule, certain criteria need to be fulfilled. Benign calcification should encompass over 10% of the pulmonary nodule and calcification should be central, diffuse, popcorn type, or laminated.

Hamartomas

Hamartomas are the most common benign lesion occurring in the lung. The components of tumor are tissues that are normally present in the lung including fat, epithelial tissue, fibrous tissue, and cartilage. Lesions typically have a lobular or potato-like morphology:
- On chest radiograph, the lesion is a well-defined, lobulated, round, or oval, and usually solitary pulmonary nodule, usually not greater than 4 cm. About 10–15% of lesions may show varying patterns of calcification on radiograph, but only popcorn calcification is virtually diagnostic.
- CT findings include a well-defined, smooth outline with area of fat attenuation and/or calcification (Figure 3.25). The finding of fat and calcification together is a specific combination for pulmonary hamartoma. Calcification is found in only 10% of lesion less than 2 cm, but 75% for lesions larger than 5 cm.

Lung cancer

Lung cancer remains the leading cause of death in both men and women in the United States, despite that an extensive list of risk factors has been well established and considerable governmental and cancer society efforts have been directed at curbing smoking,

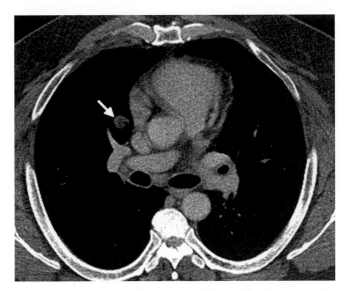

Figure 3.25 *Hamartoma*: axial noncontrast CT at midchest displays in soft tissue window. There is a well-defined pulmonary nodule (arrow) in the right lung adjacent to the right heart border. This nodule has the same attenuation as the subcutaneous fat, consistent with pulmonary hamartoma.

the single most important cause of lung cancer. Active smoking of tobacco causes the majority of cancer cases, but passive smoking (i.e., inhaling smoke from the active smoking of another individual, usually a close family member) also contributes to the lung cancer burden.

Although chest radiography is often the initial imaging study in cancer patients, small cancers are missed in at least 30% of cases, and therefore, plain films have limited reliability to detect early-stage lung cancer. Patients are usually in an advanced stage when the tumor is detected on plain radiographs.

CT can demonstrate smaller lesions and plays an important role in the evaluation and staging of lung cancer. CT has limited sensitivity and specificity to determine nodal metastases, as, on CT, mediastinal nodes are considered abnormal if they exceed 1 cm in short-axis diameter. Therefore, metastases arising in normal-sized nodes can be missed, and enlarged nodes due to hyperplasia can be false-positive.

MRI and FDG positron-emission tomography (PET)/CT for assessment of nodal stage are more sensitive and more accurate than CT and can be considered in selected cases. In particular, PET/CT has achieved an important role for staging lung cancer patients.

On imaging studies, cancers can be categorized as peripheral or central in location. Peripheral lung cancers arise beyond segmental bronchi. Peripheral lung cancers usually present as a solitary pulmonary nodule or mass. Small lesions or early-stage disease may be difficult to detect on plain chest radiographs, as mentioned earlier. Central lung cancers may present with hilar enlargement and consolidation or collapse of peripheral lung due to tumor bronchial obstruction or invasion (Figure 3.18). Hilar enlargement may be due to the tumor itself or lymphadenopathy.

Lung cancer can be divided into two major groups: *small cell lung cancer (SCLC)*, which has generally more rapid growth and early metastases, and *non-small cell lung cancer (NSCLC)*.

SCLC

SCLC accounts for 10–15% of all lung cancers. This type of lung cancer generally is rapidly growing, usually has metastasized at the time of initial presentation, and has a strong association with

tobacco smoking. SCLC is considered nonoperable because it is generally a systemic disease (i.e., widespread) at presentation, and the treatment is radiation and chemotherapy:

- Imaging findings usually are a central lesion and/or hilar enlargement. SCLC is staged as limited or extensive, with limited stage confined to the primary and regional lymph nodes, which can be treated with a single radiation port.
- Standard staging procedures for SCLC include CT scans of the chest and abdomen to evaluate liver and adrenal metastases, bone scan, and MRI of the brain. The brain is a common site of treatment failure; therefore, evaluation of the brain prior to treatment remains mandatory. The utility of whole-body PET imaging has been described and likely improves the accuracy of staging. PET is routinely used in many centers as an additional diagnostic tool, which may change the clinical stage of the disease in a number of patients.

NSCLC

NSCLCs account for about 85% of all lung cancers. There are three different main histologic cell types of NSCLC: adenocarcinoma, squamous cell carcinoma (SCC), and large cell carcinoma (LCC). The staging system of NSCLC is different from SCLC, and the purpose of staging is to determine resectability. The International Association for the Study of Lung Cancer (IASLC) recently announced a major revision of the new seventh edition of TNM staging system for lung cancer. When tumor is restricted to the lungs in stage I and II, surgery or stereotactic radiation is usually considered.

SCC

SCC is the most frequent histological type, found in all age groups and both genders, and accounts for 64% of all lung cancers SCC that is strongly associated with tobacco smoking:

- Imaging findings usually reveal a central lesion, which is commonly cavitary.

Adenocarcinoma

Adenocarcinoma is the most common type of lung cancer in life long nonsmokers. Recently, substantial changes in the pathologic classification of lung adenocarcinoma have been described from the 2011 IASLC/ATS/ERS lung adenocarcinoma classification. The new classification includes categorization of tumors as preinvasive lesions, minimally invasive adenocarcinoma (MIA), invasive adenocarcinoma, and variants of invasive adenocarcinoma. The former mucinous bronchioloalveolar carcinoma and mixed subtype adenocarcinoma are now called invasive mucinous adenocarcinoma. The terms bronchioloalveolar carcinoma and mixed subtype adenocarcinoma have been discontinued. These tumors are usually peripheral in location:

- The radiographic findings of adenocarcinoma correlate with histopathologic subtypes, which include a spectrum of ground-glass and solid opacities on CT. The more solid the composition of the lesion, the more likely the tumor is being invasive (Figure 3.26).

Adenoma *in situ* (AIS) is a preinvasive subtype of adenocarcinoma with a lipidic growth pattern, wherein tumor cells grow along and line the alveolar septa:

- Preinvasive lesions and early-stage cancers are rarely detected on plain chest radiographs. AIS is typically a pure ground-glass nodule less than 3 cm on CT.

AIS patients will have 100% 5-year disease-free survival, if the lesion is completely resected.

The entity of MIA was introduced to define a population of patients with small more solid-appearing tumors than preinvasive

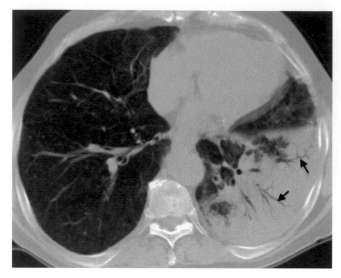

Figure 3.26 *Pulmonary adenocarcinoma (bronchoalveolar carcinoma):* axial CT image in lung window setting at the lower lungs shows consolidation of the left lower lobe with air bronchogram (arrows). Based on radiological findings, airspace pneumonia cannot be differentiated. However, this patient had no fever and the findings were persistent for more than a year (not shown).

lesions, who should have a 100% or near 100% 5-year disease-free survival if the lesion is completely resected:

- On CT, MAI appears as a solid or part-solid nodule with a predominant ground-glass component, with the solid component not greater than 5 mm.

LCC

LCC is the least common type of NSCLC. The histologic morphology in tumor specimens does not have definite criteria of adenocarcinoma or SCC. Imaging findings usually show a large mass in the periphery of the lungs. Imaging findings include:

1 Lung mass or nodule
2 Persistent pulmonary consolidation or collapse
3 Enlarged hilar or mediastinal lymph nodes
4 Adjacent bony destruction, pleural effusion, and pleural thickening
5 Ground-glass nodule or part-solid nodule on CT in early-stage cancer
6 Evidence of distant metastases

Suggested reading

Andreu, J., Caceres, J., Pallisa, E. & Martinez-Rodriguez, M. (2004) Radiological manifestations of pulmonary tuberculosis. *European Journal of Radiology*, **51**, 139–149.

Aquino, S.L., Kee, S.T., Warnock, M.L. & Gamsu, G. (1994) Pulmonary aspergillosis: imaging findings with pathologic correlation. *American Journal of Roentgenology*, **163**, 811–815.

Barst, R.J., McGoon, M., Torbicki, A. *et al.* (2004) Diagnosis and differential assessment of pulmonary arterial hypertension. *Journal of the American College of Cardiology*, **43**, 40S–47S.

Franquet, T., Muller, N.L., Gimenez, A., Guembe, P., de La Torre, J. & Bague, S. (2001) Spectrum of pulmonary aspergillosis: histologic, clinical, and radiologic findings. *Radiographics: A Review Publication of the Radiological Society of North America, Inc*, **21**, 825–837.

George, A., Gupta, R., Bang, R.L. & Ebrahim, M.K. (2003) Radiological manifestation of pulmonary complications in deceased intensive care burn patients. *Burns: Journal of the International Society for Burn Injuries*, **29**, 73–78.

Killeen, K.L., Mirvis, S.E. & Shanmuganathan, K. (1999) Helical CT of diaphragmatic rupture caused by blunt trauma. *American Journal of Roentgenology*, **173**, 1611–1616.

Kim, E.A., Lee, K.S., Primack, S.L. *et al.* (2002) Viral pneumonias in adults: radiologic and pathologic findings. *Radiographics: A Review Publication of the Radiological Society of North America, Inc*, **22**, S137–149.

Laurent, F., Latrabe, V., Lecesne, R. *et al.* (1998) Mediastinal masses: diagnostic approach. *European Radiology*, **8**, 1148–1159.

Lee, H.J., Lee, C.H., Jeong, Y.J. *et al.* (2012) IASLC/ATS/ERS International Multidisciplinary Classification of Lung Adenocarcinoma: novel concepts and radiologic implications. *Journal of Thoracic Imaging*, **27**, 340–353.

MacMahon, H., Austin, J.H., Gamsu, G. *et al.* (2005) Guidelines for management of small pulmonary nodules detected on CT scans: a statement from the Fleischner Society. *Radiology*, **237**, 395–400.

Martinez, S., McAdams, H.P. & Batchu, C.S. (2007) The many faces of pulmonary nontuberculous mycobacterial infection. *American Journal of Roentgenology*, **189**, 177–186.

Metintas, M., Ucgun, I., Elbek, O. *et al.* (2002) Computed tomography features in malignant pleural mesothelioma and other commonly seen pleural diseases. *European Journal of Radiology*, **41**, 1–9.

Mirsadraee, S., Oswal, D., Alizadeh, Y., Caulo, A. & van Beek, E., Jr (2012) The 7th lung cancer TNM classification and staging system: review of the changes and implications. *World Journal of Radiology*, **4**, 128–134.

Mueller-Mang, C., Grosse, C., Schmid, K., Stiebellehner, L. & Bankier, A.A. (2007) What every radiologist should know about idiopathic interstitial pneumonias. *Radiographics: A Review Publication of the Radiological Society of North America, Inc*, **27**, 595–615.

Pena, E., Dennie, C., Veinot, J. & Muniz, S.H. (2012) Pulmonary hypertension: how the radiologist can help. *Radiographics: A Review Publication of the Radiological Society of North America, Inc*, **32**, 9–32.

Salahudeen, H.M., Hoey, E.T., Robertson, R.J. & Darby, M.J. (2009) CT appearances of pleural tumours. *Clinical Radiology*, **64**, 918–930.

Scaglione, M., Pinto, A., Pinto, F., Romano, L., Ragozzino, A. & Grassi, R. (2001) Role of contrast-enhanced helical CT in the evaluation of acute thoracic aortic injuries after blunt chest trauma. *European Radiology*, **11**, 2444–2448.

Simonneau, G., Robbins, I.M., Beghetti, M. *et al.* (2009) Updated clinical classification of pulmonary hypertension. *Journal of the American College of Cardiology*, **54**, S43–54.

Sostman, H.D., Stein, P.D., Gottschalk, A., Matta, F., Hull, R. & Goodman, L. (2008) Acute pulmonary embolism: sensitivity and specificity of ventilation-perfusion scintigraphy in PIOPED II study. *Radiology*, **246**, 941–946.

Stark, D.D., Federle, M.P., Goodman, P.C., Podrasky, A.E. & Webb, W.R. (1983) Differentiating lung abscess and empyema: radiography and computed tomography. *American Journal of Roentgenology*, **141**, 163–167.

Value of the ventilation/perfusion scan in acute pulmonary embolism (1990) Results of the prospective investigation of pulmonary embolism diagnosis (PIOPED). *The Journal of the American Medical Association*, **263**, 2753–2759.

Webb, W.R. (2006) Thin-section CT of the secondary pulmonary lobule: anatomy and the image—the 2004 Fleischner lecture. *Radiology*, **239**, 322–338.

Wittram, C., Maher, M.M., Yoo, A.J., Kalra, M.K., Shepard, J.A. & McLoud, T.C. (2004) CT angiography of pulmonary embolism: diagnostic criteria and causes of misdiagnosis. *Radiographics: A Review Publication of the Radiological Society of North America, Inc*, **24**, 1219–1238.

CHAPTER 4

Cardiac imaging

Nicole T. Tran[1] and J. Larry Klein[2]
[1] Department of Cardiology, University of Oklahoma, Norman, USA
[2] University of North Carolina, Chapel Hill, USA

Introduction

The field of cardiac imaging includes traditional modalities such as echocardiography and coronary angiography, with more recent additions of myocardial perfusion imaging, cardiac computed tomography (CCT), and cardiac magnetic resonance imaging (CMRI). Advances in cardiovascular imaging enable a multimodality, multidisciplinary approach to the evaluation and treatment of cardiac pathophysiology. This chapter reviews the assessment of normal cardiac anatomy and physiology and cardiac pathology using cardiac echocardiography, coronary angiography, myocardial perfusion imaging, CCT, and CMRI.

Cardiac anatomy

Pericardium

The pericardium is formed of two layers: the outer fibrous pericardium and the inner serous pericardium. The inner serous pericardium is also composed of two layers: the parietal pericardium, which is adherent to the outer fibrous pericardium, and the visceral pericardium, which are normally separated from the parietal pericardium by 15–50 ml of serous fluid. The pericardium is best imaged by CCT or CMRI and is normally less than 2 mm in thickness. On echocardiography, the parietal pericardium is the most echogenic structure.

Right atrium

The right atrium has a smooth component formed from the right horn of the embryologic sinus venosus and a trabeculated appendage formed from the primitive atrium. The right atrial appendage is triangular in shape and can be used on CCT or CMRI to help identify the morphologic right atrium. A muscular band called the crista terminalis separates the smooth venous component of the right atrium and the right atrial appendage. The crista terminalis is another identifying characteristic of the morphologic right atrium but can sometimes be mistaken for a right atrial mass.

Left atrium

The left atrium is located beneath the carina, anterior to the esophagus, which facilitates left atrial imaging on transesophageal echocardiography (TEE). Like the right atrium, it is composed of a smooth venous component and a trabeculated appendage. The venous component receives oxygenated blood from four pulmonary veins. The left atrial appendage is long and tubular when compared to the right atrial appendage and can be used to identify the morphologic left atrium on CCT or CMRI.

Interatrial septum

The interatrial septum is formed from the septum primum, the fossa ovalis, and the septum secundum. The septum primum extends from the roof of the atrium caudally, and the cranial portion degenerates to form the ostium secundum. The septum secundum extends to partially cover the ostium secundum and fuses with the septum primum after birth. In 20–25% of adults, the septum primum does not fuse with the septum secundum, resulting in a patent foramen ovale.

Right ventricle

Both the right and left ventricle can be divided into an inlet, an apical portion, a trabecular portion, and an outlet. With normal bulboventricular looping (D-looping), the right ventricle is located anterior and to the right of the left ventricle. It is a thin-walled structure that wraps around the left ventricle and is supplied by the right coronary artery (RCA). On cardiac imaging, the right ventricular free wall is usually less than 3 mm in thickness. The crista supraventricularis is a ridge of muscle separating the tricuspid valve and the pulmonic valve and can be used to differentiate the morphologic right ventricle from the morphologic left ventricle (where the mitral valve and aortic valve are in fibrous continuity).

Critical Observations in Radiology for Medical Students, First Edition. Katherine R. Birchard, Kiran Reddy Busireddy, and Richard C. Semelka.
© 2015 John Wiley & Sons, Ltd. Published 2015 by John Wiley & Sons, Ltd.
Companion website: www.wiley.com/go/birchard

Left ventricle

The left ventricle is thick walled (unlike the right ventricle) and conical in shape. The bileaflet atrioventricular (AV) valve (mitral valve) always enters a morphologic left ventricle. In contrast to the tricuspid valve, the mitral valve does not have a septal attachment. The left ventricular apical trabeculations are fine, and there is normal gradual thinning of the left ventricular apex. There is no moderator band in the left ventricle (which is present in the right ventricle), and the mitral valve is in fibrous continuity with the aortic valve.

Interventricular septum

The interventricular septum is composed of the membranous septum and the muscular septum. The membranous septum forms from the AV endocardial cushions and is located at the base of the heart. The muscular septum forms from fusion of the medial walls of the trabeculated ventricles and extends apically.

AV valves
Tricuspid valve

The tricuspid valve is trileaflet and always enters a morphologic right ventricle. It has anterior, posterior, and septal leaflets, and the septal leaflet attaches to the interventricular septum. The tricuspid valve is more apically displaced than the mitral valve and is separated from the pulmonic valve by the crista supraventricularis. The anterior and posterior papillary muscles are usually larger with a smaller supracristal septal papillary muscle. The moderator band runs from the base of the anterior papillary muscle to the interventricular septum.

Mitral valve

The mitral valve is bileaflet and always enters a morphologic left ventricle. It is composed of two leaflets with some area of overlap. There are two commissures where the leaflets meet. The anterior commissure is lateral and adjacent to the left atrial appendage. The posterior commissure is medial and closer to the tricuspid annulus. The posterior leaflet of the mitral valve is quadrangular in shape and is attached to two thirds of the mitral annulus. The anterior leaflet of the mitral valve is semicircular and attaches to the aortic valve via the intervalvular fibrosa.

Semilunar valves
Pulmonic valve

The pulmonic valve always enters the pulmonic artery. It is separated from the tricuspid valve by the crista supraventricularis. It has three leaflets, which are designated right, left, and posterior.

Aortic valve

The aortic valve always enters the aorta. It is in fibrous continuity with the mitral valve and is composed of three leaflets or cusps. The right coronary cusp gives rise to the RCA. The left coronary cusp gives rise to the left coronary artery (LCA). Normally, no coronary arises from the noncoronary cusp.

Cardiac veins
Coronary sinus

The coronary sinus runs in the AV groove superior to the RCA and enters the right atrium between the inferior vena cava (IVC) and the tricuspid valve. It drains the majority of the myocardium.

Great cardiac vein

The great cardiac vein runs in the left AV groove with the left circumflex (LCX) artery and drains into the coronary sinus. The great cardiac vein is the largest tributary of the coronary sinus. Beneath the left atrial appendage, it forms the base of the triangle of Brocq and Mouchet with the left main coronary artery (LMCA) bifurcation into the left anterior descending (LAD) artery and the LCX artery.

Anterior interventricular vein

The anterior interventricular vein runs in the anterior interventricular groove with the LAD artery and drains into the great cardiac vein. It drains the anterolateral left ventricle (via the diagonal veins) and the anterior two thirds of the interventricular septum.

Middle cardiac vein

The middle cardiac vein or the posterior interventricular vein runs in the posterior interventricular groove with the posterior descending artery (PDA). It drains the remainder of the interventricular septum.

Other cardiac veins

The small cardiac vein runs in the right AV groove and drains into the coronary sinus, the middle cardiac vein, or the right atrium directly. It drains the posterior right atrium and right ventricle and is present 36% of the time.

Coronary arteries
LMCA

The LMCA normally arises from the left sinus of Valsalva in the upper one third of the sinus. Its ostium is usually more cranial than the ostium of the RCA. The LMCA runs beneath the left atrial appendage and bifurcates into the LAD artery and the LCX artery (LCX forming the triangle of Brocq and Mouchet with the great cardiac vein).

LAD artery

The LAD artery runs in the anterior interventricular groove alongside the anterior interventricular vein and supplies the anterior and anterolateral left ventricle and the anterior two thirds of the interventricular septum. 80% of the time, the LAD artery wraps around the apex supplying the inferior wall.

LCX artery

The LCX artery runs in the left AV groove along with the great cardiac vein and supplies the lateral and posterolateral walls of the left ventricle. 80% of the time, the RCA gives rise to the PDA (right dominant circulation).

RCA

The RCA arises from the right sinus of Valsalva, more caudally than the LMCA, and runs in the right AV groove under the right atrial appendage along with the small cardiac vein (if it is present).

The first branch of the RCA is usually the conus branch, which supplies the right ventricular outflow tract. The sinoatrial (SA) nodal artery is generally the second branch off of the RCA. Two thirds of the time, the SA nodal artery arises from the RCA. The remainder of the time, in 15%, the SA nodal artery arises from the LCX artery, and in 10%, both the RCA and the LCX artery supply blood to the SA node.

The RCA then gives off several acute marginal branches, which supply blood to the right ventricle. At the crux of the heart, the RCA bifurcates into the PDA and one or more posterolateral branches. The RCA gives rise to the PDA, which supplies the posterior one third of the interventricular septum, 80% of the time. The PDA runs in the posterior interventricular groove alongside the middle cardiac vein. Just distal to the take-off of the PDA, the RCA gives rise to the AV nodal artery. If the circulation is left dominant, the AV nodal artery arises from the LCX artery.

Echocardiography
Basics
Echocardiography is the primary noninvasive imaging method used to evaluate cardiac structure and function.

Normal views
In the typical echocardiographic exam, the heart is imaged in several standard views: the parasternal long-axis (PLAX) view, the parasternal short-axis (PSAX) view, the right ventricular inflow view, the apical views (four chamber, two chamber, and three chamber), the subcostal view, and the suprasternal view.

PLAX
Approximately 75% of the information available on an echocardiogram can usually be gleaned from the initial PLAX.

PSAX
PSAX cuts are usually obtained at the level of the mitral valve papillary muscles and the left ventricular apex and at the level of the aortic valve.

Right ventricular inflow
The right ventricular inflow view shows the right ventricle, tricuspid valve, and right atrium. The moderator band is seen extending from the base of the anterior papillary muscle to the interventricular septum. Adjacent to the tricuspid annulus, the coronary sinus drains into the right atrium. Inferior to the coronary sinus, the IVC is seen draining into the right atrium. The crista terminalis, which divides the trabeculated anterior portion of the right atrium from the smooth posterior portion of the right atrium, can be seen in this view and is used to identify a morphologic right atrium.

Apical views
In the apical four-chamber (A4C) view, the left ventricular apex is closest to the probe. The left ventricle, mitral valve, left atrium, right ventricle, tricuspid valve, and right atrium can be identified.

Subcostal
In the subcostal view, the right atrium, tricuspid valve, and right ventricle are anterior; the left atrium, mitral valve, and left ventricle are posterior. This is an optimal view for assessing for a pericardial effusion. Color flow Doppler of the interatrial septum can be used to evaluate for an atrial septal defect (ASD) or patent foramen ovale in this view. By rotating the probe, the IVC can be visualized entering the right atrium. The size and respiratory changes of the IVC can be used to estimate central venous pressures in the absence of positive pressure ventilation. The hepatic veins can also be interrogated in this view.

Suprasternal notch
The suprasternal notch view shows the ascending aorta, the aortic arch, the origins of the arch vessels (innominate artery, left common carotid, left subclavian artery), and a portion of the descending aorta.

M-Mode echocardiography
M-mode looks at motion of cardiac structures over time and has higher temporal resolution than standard 2D echocardiography. It can therefore be optimal for chamber measurements, in looking for abnormal septal motion with constriction and for early diastolic collapse in tamponade, and in evaluating the motion of valves over time. 2D echocardiography is used to optimally position the M-mode sampling line.

TEE
TEE involves the insertion of an echo probe into the esophagus, generally under conscious sedation. The overall rate of complications associated with TEE is less than 1%. Indications for TEE include the evaluation of native valvular disease, prosthetic heart valves, cardiac masses, congenital heart disease, atrial fibrillation with inadequate anticoagulation, aortic dissection, endocarditis, and etiology of stroke and to aid in the performance of percutaneous procedures and cardiac surgery. Contraindications include esophageal stricture, mass, or perforation; upper gastrointestinal bleeding; and inability to tolerate conscious sedation.

Stress echocardiography
Stress echocardiography uses either exercise or pharmacologic stress to detect a change in cardiac wall motion from baseline. With coronary stenoses between 50% and 70%, adequate resting coronary blood flow is maintained via autoregulation. With increased myocardial oxygen demand during exercise or via pharmacologic stress, autoregulation is unable to further increase coronary blood and ischemia results. Once a coronary stenosis is greater than 80–90%, autoregulation will be unable to maintain adequate resting blood flow, resulting in resting ischemia. Ischemic myocardium will have abnormal motion and impaired thickening that can be detected on echocardiogram.

Exercise stress echocardiography
Stress modalities include exercise or pharmacologic stress, usually with a combination of dobutamine and atropine. In either protocol, baseline images in the PLAX, PSAX, apical four-chamber, and apical two-chamber views are recorded.

In exercise stress echocardiography, the patient then exercises either by a Bruce treadmill protocol or a supine bicycle. A second set of images is recorded at the target heart rate. Exercise stress echocardiography is most sensitive if images are recorded at maximal stress. This may be a problem with an exercise treadmill protocol where peak images are obtained after exercise. Using a supine bicycle and recording peak images during ongoing exercise increase the sensitivity of the test.

Dobutamine stress echocardiography
Dobutamine is a beta-agonist that increases heart rate and myocardial contractility. In dobutamine stress echocardiography (DSE) protocols, baseline images are obtained, and then a dobutamine infusion is started at 5–10 µg/kg/min. Dobutamine is increased every 3 min in increments of 10 to a maximum of 50 µg/kg/min or until the target heart is reached. If the target heart rate is not reached with dobutamine, 0.25–0.5 mg of atropine (to a total maximum dose of 2.0 mg) can be given. The test should be stopped early for ST elevation, significant hypertension or hypotension, significant chest pain, or any significant arrhythmia. Images are obtained at baseline, low dose dobutamine, target heart rate, and after recovery. Potential complications include premature complexes,

nonsustained ventricular tachycardia, hypotension, hypertension, and rarely myocardial infarction or sustained ventricular arrhythmias.

Myocardial perfusion imaging
Basics

Radionuclide myocardial perfusion imaging uses a radioactive isotope to evaluate myocardial perfusion at stress and at rest. The isotope is taken up into the myocardium proportional to the degree of blood flow. Photons are emitted by the tracer and captured by a gamma camera. The heart is imaged in multiple slices (tomograms) that are displayed in standardized views: short-axis slices from apex to base, vertical long-axis slices from septal to lateral, and horizontal long-axis slices from anterior to inferior.

Each scan also shows a polar plot of the tomograms, which is a 2D representation of the 3D myocardium. To construct the polar plot, each short-axis tomogram is sampled in rays every 3–6° for 360°. The maximum counts at each pixel in the ray are recorded and compared with a composite of normals stratified by age and sex. These quantitative methods add to the visual interpretation of the tomograms.

Stress modalities

If the patient is able to exercise, exercise stress is preferred to pharmacologic stress as it provides additional physiologic data and prognostic information. Exercise can increase coronary blood flow two to three times over resting blood flow.

Coronary vasodilators are the most commonly used pharmacologic stressors in myocardial perfusion imaging and can increase myocardial blood flow by four to five times over baseline. A diseased coronary vessel will already be maximally vasodilated. Administration of a vasodilator will create differential perfusion by increasing blood flow to normal areas. Coronary vasodilators include dipyridamole, adenosine, and regadenoson. Regadenoson (Lexiscan), a derivative of adenosine, is currently the most frequently used coronary vasodilator.

SPECT

Single-photon emission computed tomography or SPECT imaging uses labeled thallium or technetium to image the myocardium.

Thallium-201

Thallium is a monovalent cation, similar to potassium, that is actively taken up into myocytes via the sodium/potassium/ATPase pump. Thallium uptake is proportional to myocardial blood flow. In normal myocardium, there is initial increased uptake of thallium compared to diseased myocardium. With redistribution, thallium diffuses out of normal myocardium more rapidly than ischemic myocardium due to the increased gradient between myocytes and blood.

If thallium-201 is injected at rest, both ischemic myocardium and scar will show decreased perfusion when compared to normal myocardium. After redistribution, the ischemic myocardium will have some uptake of tracer (reversible), whereas the scar will be irreversible.

Technetium (^{99m}Tc)

Technetium (^{99m}Tc) is a lipid soluble cation that passively diffuses into myocytes proportional to blood flow. It is then retained in the mitochondria with minimal redistribution. ^{99m}Tc protocols require two separate (rest/stress) injections. In general, stress images are obtained 15–30 min after exercise stress and 30–60 min after pharmacologic stress to minimize attenuation from tracer uptake in the liver and gut. Ischemic myocardium will have normal ^{99m}Tc uptake at rest but decreased uptake with stress. Lack of ^{99m}Tc uptake both at rest and stress is consistent with scar.

Positron emission tomography

Compared to SPECT imaging, positron emission tomography (PET) has improved spatial and temporal resolution. PET images are displayed in the same format as SPECT images. Tracers used with PET can be divided into perfusion tracers (^{82}Rb-rubidium and ^{13}N-ammonia) and metabolic tracers.

Metabolic tracers are used to evaluate the myocardial cell membrane activity and metabolic activity and to determine the myocardial viability. The main metabolic tracer used is 2-[^{18}F]fluoro-2-deoxyglucose or FDG. After administration, FDG is phosphorylated to FDG-6, trapping it in the myocyte. It is best used in combination with a perfusion tracer (i.e., ^{82}Rb) to evaluate for perfusion/metabolic mismatch. If the myocardium is severely ischemic but viable, there will be a perfusion defect on rest ^{82}Rb imaging, but FDG imaging will show tracer uptake.

Radionuclide ventriculography/angiography

Radionuclide imaging can also be used to assess chamber size, contraction, segmental wall motion, right and left ventricular contractile function, and wall thickness. This is most often done using multiple-gated acquisition (MUGA) scanning with ^{99m}Tc-labeled red blood cells or albumin.

Coronary angiography
Basics

Coronary angiography is the gold standard for evaluation of coronary artery stenoses and coronary anatomy. In adults, selective coronary angiography with engagement of the coronary ostia is performed. Coronary angiography has the advantage of being both a diagnostic and therapeutic modality. It is also better suited to evaluate collateral flow, which is less well characterized on noninvasive imaging. It has superior spatial and temporal resolution when compared to coronary CTA and coronary MRA. However, it is an invasive technique requiring arterial puncture. As with myocardial perfusion imaging and CCT, there is exposure to ionizing radiation. In addition, basic coronary angiography provides a "luminogram" of the coronary vessel, but does not characterize the degree or type of plaque. It tends to underestimate the severity of diffuse disease.

CCT
Basics

CCT is a noninvasive modality that is used to assess coronary artery disease and evaluate for coronary anomalies, cardiac masses, complex congenital heart disease, pulmonary veins prior to atrial fibrillation ablation, coronary veins prior to biventricular pacemaker placement, and other intrathoracic anatomies (acute aortic syndromes, pulmonary emboli, etc.). Currently, the minimum requirements for the performance of CCT include a minimum 16-slice CT scanner (32 detector rows are ideal and a slice thickness of 0.5–1 mm (ideally <0.6 mm) with images spaced at a distance less than the slice thickness). A patient heart rate of less than 60 beats per minute (BPM) is optimal for image quality. Irregular heart rhythms and heart rates greater than 80 BPM are relative contraindications for CCT.

Contrast agents

Contrast timing can be done via three different methods. The least accurate is starting the scan approximately 22–25 s after contrast administration. Alternatively, a bolus tracking method can be used. The contrast is administered and then a region of interest is sampled every several seconds. When that region is greater than 100 HU, the scan is triggered. Finally, a test bolus of 10–20 ml of the contrast can be given to calculate the scan delay.

Gating

CCT scans are done during breath hold to minimize respiratory motion. ECG gating is used to minimize cardiac motion. There is minimal motion of the coronary arteries during diastole and end systole. The majority of CCT scans are done using ECG-based dose modulation.

CMRI
Basics

CMRI is increasingly being used as a noninvasive method to evaluate cardiac anatomy and morphology. In patients without implantable pacemakers/defibrillators, it is an accurate way to assess perfusion and viability. There is increasing data supporting its use in the evaluation of coronary anomalies and proximal coronary artery disease. It is ideal for assessing complex congenital heart disease. Like CCT, CMRI is ECG gated, allowing for imaging during diastole when there is minimal cardiac motion.

Steady-state free precession

Each MR system manufacturer has their own tradename for steady-state free precession (SSFP), but the sequences are all essentially the same (i.e., trueFISP, FIESTA, balanced-FFFE). Cine images are ECG gated and can be obtained either over several cycles, each at a certain percentage of the R–R interval, or during a complete cardiac cycle in real time. There is a high (optimal) signal-to-noise ratio. These images are ideal for assessing cardiac structure, motion, cardiac valves, and blood flow.

Black blood imaging

Black blood imaging can be ideal for evaluating cardiac morphology as the blood suppression keeps bright blood from masking intracardiac structures. There is good differentiation between blood and myocardium and the signal-to-noise ratio is high. Half-Fourier acquisition single-shot turbo spin-echo (HASTE) imaging can reduce imaging time and decrease breath-hold time; however, it decreases the signal-to-noise ratio.

Perfusion imaging

To assess perfusion, gadolinium contrast is administered and then first-pass imaging is obtained. This can be combined with a stress modality (regadenoson, adenosine, and dipyridamole) to obtain functional myocardial perfusion imaging. The signal intensity changes in a linear fashion with the concentration of gadolinium in the myocardium. Normal myocardium will enhance (brighten), and ischemic myocardium will remain dark (hypoenhancing). Perfusion imaging can be combined with coronary MRA to determine the hemodynamic significance of visualized lesions.

Viability imaging (delayed hyperenhancement)

In patients without an ICD in place, CMRI has become the primary method to assess myocardial viability. To evaluate viability, gadolinium contrast is administered. On first pass, infarcted tissue does not enhance with gadolinium. Then, over time, gadolinium diffuses into the interstitium of infarcted myocardium and is not easily washed out due to the low blood flow. Scar (dead, nonviable myocardium) will show delayed hyperenhancement. Infarctions of less than 25% of the myocardium will often improve with revascularization. Transmural infarction greater than 50% of the myocardium is unlikely to regain function with revascularization. Perfusion imaging can be combined with delayed hyperenhancement imaging to identify ischemic, hibernating, but viable myocardium, which will have a perfusion defect but no delayed hyperenhancement. The pattern of delayed hyperenhancement can also be useful in the evaluation of a newly developed cardiomyopathy.

Coronary angiography

Whole-heart imaging during breath hold can be used to evaluate the proximal coronary arteries and to rule out anomalous origins of the coronary arteries. The coronary arteries can also be imaged in targeted oblique views, much like during cardiac catheterization. CMRI appears to be best suited for the evaluation of significant proximal coronary disease.

Congenital heart disease

ASD

An ASD causes an interatrial communication with left to right shunting. It should be considered in patients with right-sided enlargement, a fixed split of S2 on physical exam, and classic EKG findings. There are many types of ASDs. A primum ASD is located at the inferior portion of the atrial septum and forms a partial AV canal defect. Secundum ASDs are the most common form of ASD. Sinus venosus defects are a relatively uncommon form of ASD:

- Transthoracic echocardiography (TTE) is usually the initial imaging modality and should also evaluate the right heart size, function, and pulmonary artery pressures.
- TEE and CMRI can improve imaging quality, and CMRI is the gold standard for the assessment of right ventricular function.
- CMRI and CCT are useful to evaluate for partial anomalous pulmonary venous return associated with a superior sinus venosus defect. There are four types of ASDs.

Ventricular septal defects

A ventricular septal defect (VSD) is the most common congenital heart defect at birth and accounts for 10% of adult congenital heart disease. There are five general types of VSDs: membranous, muscular, supracristal, inlet, and Gerbode defects. Membranous VSDs are the most common type of VSD in North America:

- The initial diagnostic modality of choice is usually TTE, which has an 88–95% detection rate for VSD. It is most sensitive for the detection of VSDs that are at least 5 mm in size. An apical muscular defect can be difficult to detect.
- Echocardiography should also focus on evaluation of pulmonary pressures and for evidence of volume overload of the left heart. The right heart is usually normal in the absence of Eisenmenger's physiology.

Tetralogy of Fallot

Tetralogy of Fallot (TOF) is the most common form of cyanotic congenital heart disease in infants. It is characterized by an overriding aorta, an infundibular or pulmonic stenosis, a right ventricular hypertrophy, and a VSD. The VSD is usually large and unrestrictive with equalization of pressure between the left ventricle and right ventricle. TOF results from anterior and cranial displacement of the aorticopulmonary septum during embryologic development:

- Echocardiography is usually the initial diagnostic modality of choice in the evaluation of TOF. In unrepaired TOF, the degree of infundibular obstruction, the location of the VSD(s), and the right ventricular function should be assessed.
- The PLAX will show the overriding aorta. The right ventricular outflow tract, pulmonic valve, and pulmonary artery can be seen in the PSAX at the level of the aortic valve. The right ventricular hypertrophy and contraction should be assessed in multiple views (PLAX, PSAX, A4C).
- Postrepair, echocardiography can be used to follow the effects of pulmonic regurgitation and evaluate for right ventricular volume overload. If transthoracic echocardiographic imaging is inadequate, TEE or CMRI may be useful.

Aorta

Aortic dissection

The patient with an acute aortic dissection will classically present with acute onset of severe chest pain, which may be described as "sharp" or "tearing." Pain may radiate to the neck and jaw if the arch and arch vessels are involved or to the back if the descending aorta is involved. Patients may have a history of hypertension, a family history of acute aortic syndromes, a history of a connective tissue disorder (i.e., Marfan's syndrome, Ehler's–Danlos syndrome, Loeys–Dietz syndrome), a history of coarctation or a bicuspid aortic valve, or may present post-trauma or as a post-procedural complication. Mortality from aortic dissection is high, at a rate of 1% per hour for the first 48 h with an overall 70% mortality in the first 2 weeks. Aortic dissections can be classified as type A or type B based on whether the ascending aorta is involved (type A involves the ascending aorta and is a surgical emergency) (Figure 4.1a, b).

On TTE, a dissection flap can sometimes be visualized. A linear, mobile, echogenic flap will be visualized in the lumen of the aorta, separating the true lumen from the false lumen. The true lumen is often smaller than the false lumen and expands during systole. The false lumen is often larger and crescentic and decreases in size during systole. It will often have evidence of slow flow with spontaneous echocontrast and possible intraluminal hematoma:

- Concern for acute aortic dissection is one of the indications for TEE. Similar to TTE, a dissection flap will appear as a linear, mobile echogenicity in the lumen of the aorta. Color flow Doppler can confirm systolic flow into the true lumen. Sensitivity and specificity for TEE to detect aortic dissection are both high (>97%).
- Echocardiography can also assess for complications of aortic dissection such as aortic regurgitation, pericardial effusion and tamponade, and wall motion abnormalities from involvement of the coronary ostia. The arch vessels should also be interrogated for involvement in the dissection.
- Both cardiac CT angiography (CTA) and MRA are also highly sensitive and specific for the detection of acute aortic syndromes (see Chapters 3 and 12).

Penetrating atherosclerotic ulcer

A penetrating atherosclerotic ulcer (PAU) is classically seen in older males, with a history of hypertension, tobacco abuse, and other atherosclerotic vascular diseases. Like acute aortic dissection, patients present with acute onset of severe chest pain. The ulcer penetrates through the intima into the media of the aorta. A PAU can lead to aortic dissection, saccular aneurysm, or aortic rupture. It is classified and managed similarly to an acute aortic dissection:

- On echocardiography, a PAU will appear as a localized outpouching of the aortic wall without evidence of a dissection flap. There is often significant associated atherosclerosis. A PAU is most commonly found in the descending thoracic aorta. Further evaluation is by CT or MRI (refer to the Chapters 3 and 12).

Intramural hematoma

An intramural hematoma is a localized collection of blood within the aortic wall without evidence of a dissection flap. It is classified and managed similarly to an aortic dissection, as approximately 10–15% will progress to dissection. Clinical presentation is similar to that of a dissection, with chest pain often correlating to the involved area of the aorta:

- TEE is better than TTE for the diagnosis of intramural hematoma and will show a smooth, circumferential, or crescentic echogenic thickening of the aortic wall.
- Noncontrast CT scan is recommended first to identify the subtle circumferential thickening associated with intramural hematoma. This should be followed by a contrasted CT scan to evaluate for a dissection flap.

Symptomatic aneurysm

Echocardiography remains the initial screening test for thoracic aortic aneurysms.

Genetic conditions

Patients with Marfan's syndrome should have an initial echocardiogram and then a follow-up study 6 months later to evaluate for progression of aortic disease. If there is no rapid enlargement, then patients should have yearly screening echocardiograms.

Patients with Turner's syndrome should have initial imaging of the heart and aorta, which can be repeated every 5–10 years in the absence of symptoms. Patients with bicuspid aortic valves should have evaluation of the aortic root and ascending aorta. In patients with a bicuspid aortic valve, the mid-ascending aorta is most commonly affected.

Thoracic aortic aneurysms

There is a critical risk of rupture once the ascending aorta reaches a diameter greater than 6 cm and the descending aorta a diameter greater than 7 cm. Current indications for surgery include an ascending aortic aneurysm greater than 5.5 cm or between 4.0 and 5.0 cm in size in a patient with connective tissue disease (Marfan's syndrome, Ehler–Danlos syndrome, Loeys–Dietz syndrome) or a bicuspid aortic valve. Surgery is also indicated for symptomatic aneurysms, rapidly expanding aneurysms (increase in size of more than 0.5 cm per year), or mycotic aneurysms.

Abdominal aortic aneurysms

Most abdominal aortic aneurysms (AAA) are infrarenal. The US Preventive Services Task Force (USPSTF) now recommends a one-time screening ultrasound for AAA in men between 65 and 75 years who have ever smoked. Indications for surgical repair include size greater than 5.0–5.5 cm, rapid expansion, symptomatic aneurysms, and contained rupture or rupture.

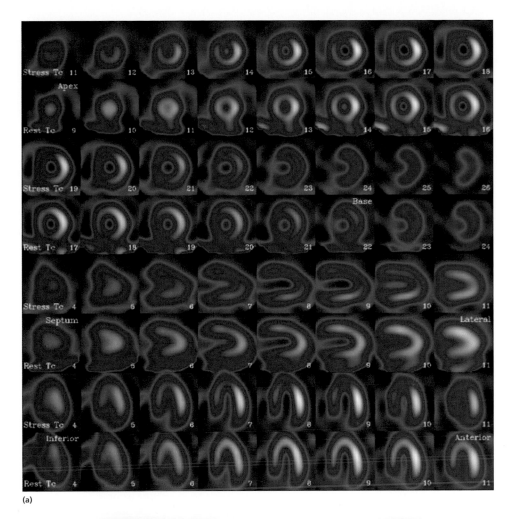

(a)

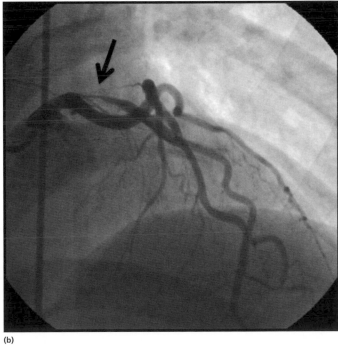

Figure 4.1 Coronary artery disease—
myocardial perfusion imaging. PET
82-rubidium nuclear stress test with a
large, severe, completely reversible
anterior/anteroseptal defect consistent
with ischemia (a). Coronary angiography
(RAO cranial projection) from the same
patient shows a 99% proximal LAD artery
stenosis (arrow) (b).

(b)

Sinus of Valsalva aneurysm

Aneurysmal dilatation of one or more of the sinuses of Valsalva is a relatively uncommon finding of the general population. Often, patients are asymptomatic and this is an incidental imaging diagnosis. They most commonly originate from the right sinus of Valsalva followed by the noncoronary sinus. They can be congenital or acquired from infection (syphilis, endocarditis), connective tissue disease, atherosclerosis, or trauma:

- On TTE, an aneurysm of the right or noncoronary sinus of Valsalva can be seen in the PLAX. A right sinus of Valsalva aneurysm may protrude into the right ventricular outflow tract causing obstruction to flow. This can be detected by color flow Doppler showing a continuous jet from the high-pressure aorta to the low-pressure right ventricle.
- These aneurysms are also readily imaged with CCT or CMRI.

Coronary arteries

Ischemia
TTE

Resting TTE includes evaluation for any regional wall motion abnormalities, which can indicate prior ischemic events or acute-onset severely ischemic myocardium. In the setting of a previous myocardial infarction, the myocardium will often be thinned and akinetic or dyskinetic. This can affect the overall systolic contraction. In areas of previous infarction, aneurysms or pseudoaneurysms may be present.

An aneurysm involves dilatation of all layers (endocardium, myocardium, and pericardium) and often has a wide neck when compared to the base of the aneurysm. A pseudoaneurysm is an area of contained rupture. It does not contain all three layers and the base is often formed by laminated thrombus contained by pericardium.

TTE can also be used to assess for other complications following myocardial infarction including VSDs or papillary muscle dysfunction or rupture.

Stress echocardiography

Stress echocardiography can be used to evaluate for coronary ischemia if there are no baseline wall motion abnormalities and no contraindication to dobutamine or exercise stress. With either stress modality, resting images are compared to images at peak stress. Ischemic myocardium will have decreased myocardial thickening and contraction compared to surrounding normal myocardium.

Myocardial perfusion imaging

Myocardial perfusion imaging, either SPECT or PET, compares myocardial tracer uptake at stress with rest uptake. A defect on stress imaging that is not present at rest is consistent with myocardial ischemia. A defect present at both rest and stress is consistent with myocardial scar. Myocardial perfusion imaging can detect the presence, location, and severity of defects (Figure 4.2a, b).

Thallium myocardial perfusion and FDG PET imaging can also be used to assess myocardial viability. A resting thallium defect that shows tracer uptake on redistribution images is consistent with severely ischemic but viable myocardium. On FDG PET, a defect that is present on the perfusion images but not present on metabolic images has severely impaired blood flow but intact metabolism, consistent with ischemic but viable myocardium.

Coronary calcium score

Coronary calcium score (the Agatston score) using CT describes the presence and extent of calcium in coronary arteries, with the intention of predicting the likelihood of myocardial infarction. The lesion scores ranged from one to four with increasing HU.

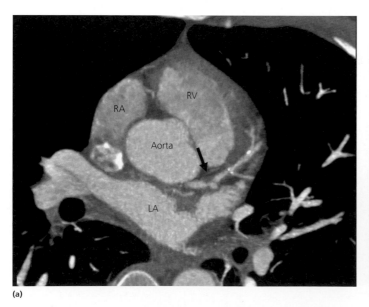

(a)

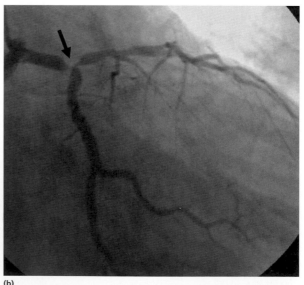

(b)

Figure 4.2 Coronary CT angiography shows greater than 75% obstructing, non-calcified plaque in the distal LMCA and proximal LAD with negative remodeling of the vessel wall (Arrow) (a) RA: Right atrium; RV: Right ventricle; LA: Left atrium. Coronary angiography (RAO caudal projection) from the same patient shows a 99% stenosis involving the distal LMCA, proximal LAD and proximal LCX (Arrow) (b). The patient went for CABG.

Coronary CTA

Currently, 16-slice (or greater) CT scanners possess sufficient temporal and spatial resolution to allow for evaluation of the coronary lumen, the plaque characteristics, the course of anomalous coronary arteries, and the general cardiac and thoracic anatomy. Current coronary CTA has a sensitivity of 80–100% and a specificity of 80–90% for the detection of flow-limiting plaque. It has a high negative predictive value of 98–100% and therefore may be an optimal imaging modality in low-risk patients. The prognostic value of coronary CTA has been validated, and the absence of coronary disease on coronary CTA is associated with a very low cardiac event rate.

Current guidelines recommend CCTA as an option in the evaluation of symptomatic patients with an intermediate pretest probability for coronary artery disease that are unable to exercise, have an equivocal stress test, and have suspected anomalous origins of the coronary arteries and of asymptomatic patients with new heart failure who require evaluation of coronary anatomy (Figure 4.3a, b).

Cardiac MRA

Cardiac MR coronary angiography is acquired during breath hold and using ECG gating in diastole. It can assess the proximal LMCA, LAD artery, and proximal RCA. Oblique imaging is generally better to image the LCX artery and distal RCA. CMRA can generally exclude significant proximal coronary disease.

Some centers are now performing stress CMRI. First-pass perfusion imaging combined with a stress agent has a high sensitivity and specificity for the evaluation of obstructive coronary artery disease (83 and 82%, respectively) (Figure 4.4).

Late gadolinium enhancement (LGE) on CMRI is the most accurate method in the assessment of myocardial scar and viability. LGE of less than 25% of transmural myocardial thickness is predictive of improved function following revascularization. LGE of greater than 50% transmural myocardial thickness is rarely associated with improvement in myocardial function postrevascularization. LGE on CMRI is also an independent predictor of death (Figure 4.5a, b).

Myocardial thickening on CMRI cine imaging, with a change of greater than 2 mm between systole and diastole, is also highly predictive of contractile reserve. It is associated with a sensitivity of 89% and a specificity of 94% for the prediction of myocardial viability.

LGE can be combined with cardiac MR coronary angiography and cardiac MR stress perfusion imaging to identify coronary stenoses, assess the hemodynamic effect of stenoses, and evaluate for viability and the potential benefit of revascularization of stenoses. It therefore has the potential to be the most complete evaluation of coronary disease in suitable patients.

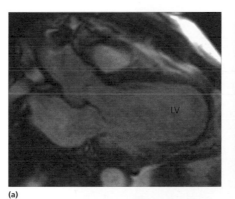 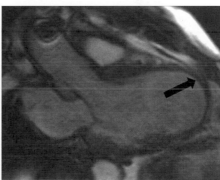

(a)

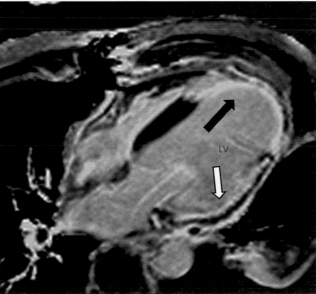

(b)

Figure 4.3 Ischemic cardiomyopathy. Cardiac MRI true FISP cine imaging in diastole (left) and systole (right) shows a dilated left ventricle, severely decreased left ventricular contraction, and a thinned, akinetic apex (arrow) in this patient with severe ischemic cardiomyopathy (a). Late gadolinium enhancement imaging of the same patient shows transmural infarction in the apex (black arrow) and nontransmural infarction of the lateral wall (white arrow). The basal septum is spared (b). LV, left ventricle.

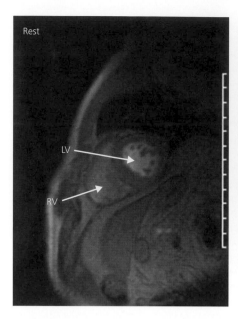
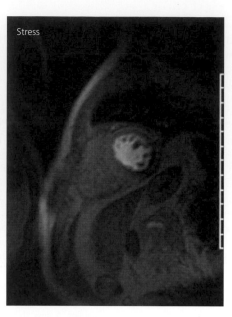

Figure 4.4 Coronary artery disease—stress MRI. Stress MRI shows normal perfusion at rest (left) and inferolateral ischemia with stress (right). RV, right ventricle; LV, left ventricle.

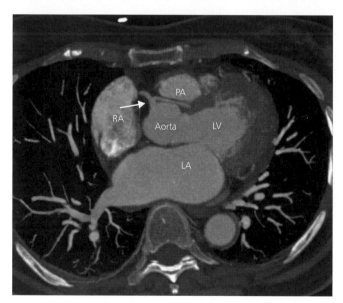

Figure 4.5 Anomalous origin of the coronary arteries. Coronary CT angiography shows a single coronary artery originating from the right coronary cusp with the left coronary artery following an interarterial course between the aorta and pulmonary artery (PA) (arrow). RA, right atrium; LA, left atrium; LV, left ventricle.

Coronary angiography

Coronary angiography remains the gold standard for the assessment of coronary disease and is the only imaging modality that is both diagnostic and therapeutic. Indications for coronary angiography include a high-risk exercise treadmill test (hypotension with exercise or diagnostic ECG changes with poor functional status), new cardiomyopathy, extensive wall motion abnormalities on stress echocardiography, a large perfusion defect on myocardial perfusion imaging, defects in multiple coronary distributions on myocardial perfusion imaging, TID, lung uptake on myocardial perfusion imaging, unstable angina (which is intermediate to high risk), and ST-elevation myocardial infarction.

Anomalous coronary artery from the opposite sinus

A coronary anomaly is defined as a variant of vessel origin or supply and occurs in less than 1% of the population. The majority of these are considered benign. Common anomalous coronary arteries are LCA from the right coronary cusp, an anomalous LCX artery arising from the right coronary cusp, and RCA arising anomalously from the left coronary cusp or the LCA. It is rare to have a coronary artery arise from the noncoronary cusp, but this can occasionally be seen in patients with transposition of the great arteries (TGA) (Figure 4.6):

- The gold standard for evaluation was previously coronary angiography with direct engagement of the anomalous ostium. Currently, coronary CTA and CMRI are increasingly used to identify and characterize anomalies of the coronary circulation.

Anomalous origin of the left coronary artery from the pulmonary artery

Anomalous origin of the left coronary artery from the pulmonary artery or ALPACA (Bland–White–Garland syndrome) is a rare but often fatal coronary anomaly. The LCA arises from the pulmonary artery and the RCA arises normally. Cardiac CTA will show the anomalous origin of the LCA and extensive collateral network.

Myocardial bridging

Normally, the coronary arteries sit on the epicardial surface of the heart. Myocardial bridging occurs when a portion of the coronary artery has an intramyocardial course. This occurs most commonly in the mid-LAD artery and can be seen in up to 5% of patients undergoing coronary angiography. Cardiac CTA can directly visualize the intramyocardial segment.

Coronary artery fistula

Coronary artery fistulae are connections between a coronary artery and a cardiac chamber. Contrast injection will show filling from coronary artery to the affected chamber. Most commonly, fistulae come from the RCA and drain into the right atrium, right ventricle, or pulmonary artery.

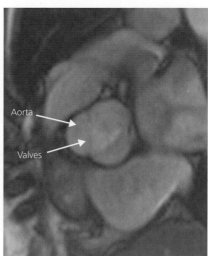

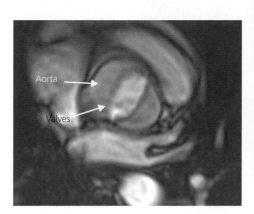

Figure 4.6 Bicuspid aortic valve. Cardiac MRI true FISP cine imaging shows a congenitally malformed bicuspid aortic valve (left) and a normal tricuspid aortic valve (right). RV, right ventricle; LV, left ventricle.

Valvular disease

After a careful history and physical exam, the initial diagnostic modality in the evaluation of valvular heart disease remains echocardiography. Echocardiography allows the clinician to confirm the presence of valvular pathology, assess its severity, and assess the effects of valvular pathology on downstream chambers. Echocardiography can also be used to follow valvular disease over time and determine optimal timing of surgery.

Cardiac catheterization, which previously had been the mainstay in the evaluation of valvular disease, however, is no longer a routine step in the evaluation of valvular pathology.

CMRI is evolving as an alternate noninvasive method to assess valvular pathology. It is not limited by acoustic windows and is not limited by bone or lung interference. Phase-contrast imaging can be used to quantitate flow velocity and volumes similar to Doppler echocardiography. Using this technology, regurgitant volumes and shunt fractions can be quantified.

Stenosis
Mitral

The most common cause of mitral stenosis worldwide remains rheumatic heart disease. Rheumatic heart disease most commonly affects the mitral valve, followed by the mitral and aortic valves, the aortic valve, and then the tricuspid valve (often in concert with rheumatic mitral and aortic disease). Rheumatic heart disease causes thickening of the leaflet tips and fusion of the medial and lateral commissures of the mitral valve:

- The initial diagnostic evaluation for rheumatic mitral stenosis is TTE. On the PLAX view, the posterior mitral leaflet will be relatively fixed. The anterior leaflet tip will be thickened, and there will be doming of the body of the leaflet during diastole, creating the classic "hockey stick" appearance.
- In the PSAX view at the level of the mitral valve, fusion of the medial and lateral commissures is seen, which creates a "fish mouth" appearance.
- The left atrium is usually dilated due to chronic pressure overload. With more significant mitral stenosis, pulmonary hypertension will develop, and right ventricular hypertrophy may be present.
- Continuous wave Doppler echocardiography can be used to assess the mean and peak gradient across the valve. Valve area can be calculated using Doppler parameters or by planimetry of the valve in the PSAX.
- Mitral annular calcification occurs more frequently with age and increasing cardiovascular risk factors; it is associated with increased cardiovascular risk and can be visualized by echocardiography.

Aortic

The most common cause of aortic stenosis is progression of calcific aortic sclerosis. This is related to both age and cardiovascular risk factors. In general, calcific aortic sclerosis will progress to significant aortic stenosis between 70 and 80 years of age. Calcification occurs initially at the base of the leaflets and then progresses inward, steadily limiting flow through the left ventricular outflow tract:

- Echocardiography will show a thickened, calcified valve with limited systolic excursion of leaflets. Gradients can be estimated across the aortic valve using Doppler echocardiography.
- A common cause of aortic stenosis in younger individuals is a congenitally malformed or bicuspid aortic valve. In the PLAX, the coaptation of the aortic cusps may not be midline, and there is often bowing of the leaflets into the left ventricular outflow tract during systole, creating a "dome-like" appearance (Figure 4.7).
- M-mode echocardiography can confirm that the closure line is not midline. A congenitally malformed valve is confirmed in the PSAX at the level of the aortic valve during systole.
- In a bicuspid valve, the line of closure is either more anterior or posterior (creating right and left cusps), and in 70–80%, the right and left coronary cusps will be fused. In 20–30%, the right and noncoronary cusps will be fused. These patients are also at risk for aortopathy and dilatation, generally of the mid-ascending aorta. They should be screened as discussed in the aorta section earlier section "Symptomatic aneurysm".
- In the United States, rheumatic aortic stenosis is less commonly seen. It affects approximately 30% of patients with rheumatic mitral stenosis. Like rheumatic mitral disease, there will be thickening of the leaflet tips, fusion of the commissures, and doming of the leaflets during systole.

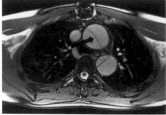 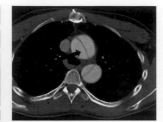

(a)

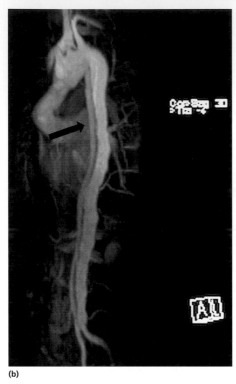

(b)

Figure 4.7 Aortic dissection. Cardiac MRI (left) and cardiac CTA (right) from the same patient show a dissection (arrows) at the level of the aortic arch (a). 3D reconstruction from the same patient shows the dissection (arrow) extending down the descending aorta to the level of the iliac bifurcation (b).

Tricuspid/pulmonic

Tricuspid stenosis is relatively uncommon and if present is often due to rheumatic heart disease. It is usually mild. Rheumatic tricuspid regurgitation is more common than rheumatic tricuspid stenosis. In the majority of these cases, rheumatic mitral and aortic disease will also be present.

Pulmonic stenosis is nearly always associated with congenital heart disease, particularly TOF and congenitally corrected TGA. CMRI can be useful to help distinguish infundibular stenosis from valvular stenosis and supravalavular stenosis.

Regurgitation
Mitral

Causes of mitral regurgitation include dilatation of the left ventricle and mitral annulus in the setting of a dilated cardiomyopathy, degenerative mitral valve disease, rheumatic mitral regurgitation, endocarditis, ischemic mitral regurgitation, and papillary muscle rupture:

• TTE remains the first-line imaging modality for the evaluation of mitral regurgitation. The mitral valve should be assessed for

the cause of regurgitation, the severity of regurgitation, and the downstream effects of regurgitation (progressive left atrial and left ventricular dilatation due to chronic volume overload).

• Using color flow Doppler imaging, physiologic mitral regurgitation can be detected in 70–80% of individuals.

• If the degree of regurgitation is no more than mild, the jet will be central, and there will be no associated valvular abnormalities or downstream effects of mitral regurgitation.

• Patients with dilated cardiomyopathy will have dilatation of the mitral valve annulus with resultant functional mitral regurgitation. Echocardiography will reveal a dilated left ventricle. The mitral valve itself is often normal.

• Degenerative or myxomatous mitral valve disease is a primary disorder of the mitral leaflets and chordae. Leaflets will appear thickened and redundant with increased chordal laxity. Mitral valve prolapse may be present. Mitral valve prolapse is best evaluated in the PLAX on TTE that shows leaflets "sagging" into the left atrium, behind the level of the mitral annulus, during systole. In Marfan's syndrome, the anterior leaflet in particular is redundant and prolapses into the left atrium during systole.

• Rheumatic mitral valve disease is characterized by thickening of leaflet tips and commissural fusion, generally resulting in mitral stenosis. Associated mitral regurgitation occurs when there is associated thickening and shortening of the chordae tendineae.

• Ischemic mitral regurgitation occurs when decreased coronary blood flow leads to papillary muscle dysfunction and rarely papillary muscle rupture. If the papillary muscle becomes ischemic, the leaflet motion of the mitral valve is reduced and the leaflet is tethered during systole. With actual papillary muscle rupture, there is acute severe mitral regurgitation, and the papillary muscle can be seen prolapsing into the left atrium during systole and the left ventricle during diastole.

Aortic

Aortic regurgitation may be secondary to calcific aortic stenosis, rheumatic aortic disease, a congenitally malformed aortic valve, aneurysmal dilatation of the aortic root, endocarditis, or acute aortic dissection. Echocardiography is the initial imaging modality in the evaluation of aortic regurgitation. Aortic regurgitation is rarely physiologic in adults.

Tricuspid/pulmonic

Tricuspid regurgitation can be detected in 80–90% of normal individuals. Pathologic tricuspid regurgitation may be due to annular dilatation in the setting of right heart failure or pulmonary hypertension, rheumatic tricuspid disease (usually associated with rheumatic mitral and aortic disease), carcinoid heart disease, endocarditis, or Ebstein's anomaly:

• Carcinoid heart disease causes thick, shortened, fixed tricuspid leaflets with resultant regurgitation.

• Ebstein's anomaly is characterized by significant apical displacement of the septal leaflet of the tricuspid valve with varying involvement of the posterior leaflet. The anterior leaflet is usually large, dysplastic, and sail-like. The valve is dysfunctional and regurgitant. If the anterior leaflet is also apically displaced, it can cause obstruction of the right ventricular outflow tract.

• Pulmonic regurgitation can be detected in 70–80% of normal individuals. Pathologic pulmonic regurgitation is often the result of congenital heart disease or dilatation of the pulmonic annulus/ pulmonary artery from pulmonary hypertension. Carcinoid syndrome can also affect the pulmonic valve.

Endocarditis

TTE often followed by TEE is the initial imaging modality of choice in the evaluation of possible endocarditis. The study should confirm the presence of a vegetation, assess the size of the vegetation, and evaluate for an associated paravalvular abscess and for any evidence of valvular destruction:

- Vegetations are found on the upstream side of cardiac valves (the atrial side of AV valves and the ventricular side of semilunar valves). They appear as an echogenic, independently mobile structure on the affected valve.
- Right-sided vegetations occur most frequently in intravenous drug users or are associated with the lead of an implantable cardiac device.
- A paravalvular abscess usually affects the annulus adjacent to the infected leaflet and appears as an echolucency in the area of the aortic annulus or an area of increased thickening and echogenicity in the area of the mitral and tricuspid valve annulus.
- If TTE is nondiagnostic, TEE is the next step in the evaluation for endocarditis and is preferred in the evaluation of endocarditis associated with prosthetic heart valves.

Myocardium

Nonischemic cardiomyopathy

On echocardiography, nonischemic cardiomyopathy will usually show global left and sometimes right ventricular dysfunction. There may be increased trabeculation of the left ventricular apex, which should be differentiated from left ventricular noncompaction:

- A normal myocardial perfusion study in a patient with nonischemic cardiomyopathy has a high negative predictive value for the absence of coronary artery disease.
- CMRI may show T2 edema in the acute setting. There may be no LGE, or there may be patchy, linear LGE not in a coronary distribution. This is often seen in the mid-basal septal wall and is independently associated with sudden cardiac death.

Ischemic cardiomyopathy

Ischemic cardiomyopathy is defined based on the presence of two or more epicardial coronary arteries with a greater than 50% luminal stenosis:

- On echocardiography, patients with ischemic cardiomyopathy may have evidence of segmental wall motion abnormalities with areas of myocardial thinning and akinesis/dyskinesis.
- CMRI can be used to evaluate the thickness of scar on LGE imaging to predict whether revascularization is likely to improve myocardial function.

Hypertrophic obstructive cardiomyopathy

- On echocardiography, patients with hypertrophic obstructive cardiomyopathy (HOCM) will have asymmetric septal hypertrophy with a ratio of septal wall thickness to posterior wall thickness of greater than 1.5:1. If the septal wall thickness is greater than 30 mm, it is considered a high-risk feature for the development of ventricular arrhythmias. There will often be systolic anterior motion (SAM) of the mitral valve, subaortic valvular turbulence, early closure of the aortic valve, and posteriorly directed mitral regurgitation. There may be a dynamic left ventricular outflow tract gradient (Figure 4.8a, b).
- CMRI can also be used to evaluate for myocardial fibrosis on LGE. Fibrosis is often related to the degree of hypertrophy, is not in a coronary distribution, and is associated with an increased risk of ventricular arrhythmias.

Sarcoidosis

- On echocardiography, cardiac sarcoidosis can present with segmental wall motion abnormalities not in a coronary distribution (i.e., midseptal) and a pericardial effusion.
- FDG PET can be used to differentiate active versus chronic disease in patients with cardiac sarcoidosis. FDG accumulates in areas of active inflammation. With the transition from acute inflammation to chronic, the granulomas mature and there are fewer macrophages and inflammatory cells present. As a reflection of this, FDG uptake diminishes.
- CMRI will show areas of LGE that are usually midmyocardial or subepicardial and not in a coronary distribution. The basal septum is often involved. The degree of LGE is associated with an increased risk of ventricular arrhythmias and death. T2-weighted MR images may show tissue edema in areas of active inflammation (Figure 4.9).

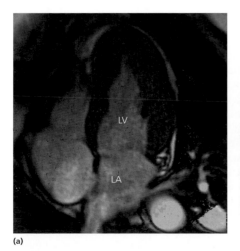
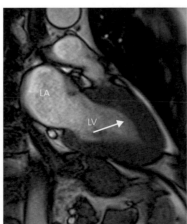
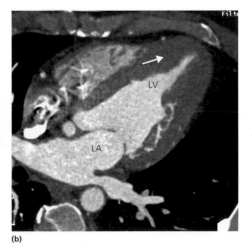

(a) (b)

Figure 4.8 Apical variant hypertrophic cardiomyopathy. Cardiac MRI true FISP cine imaging shows apical variant hypertrophic cardiomyopathy (arrow) with the classic "spade sign" (a). Cardiac CTA shows apical variant hypertrophic cardiomyopathy (arrow) (b). LA, left atrium; LV, left ventricle.

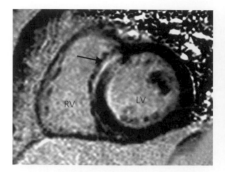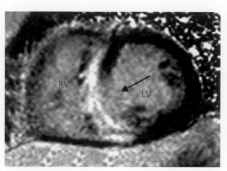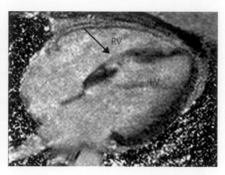

Figure 4.9 Cardiac sarcoidosis. Cardiac MRI in a patient with cardiac sarcoidosis shows midmyocardial hyperenhancement of the basal septum (top) and midseptum (bottom) not corresponding to a coronary distribution (arrows). RV, right ventricle; LV, left ventricle.

Amyloidosis

- On echocardiography, cardiac amyloidosis is classically associated with significant ventricular hypertrophy, often described as having a "speckled" appearance. Surface ECG, however, will show low voltage. Atria are often markedly dilated consistent with underlying restrictive physiology, and there is often a small pericardial effusion.

Hemochromatosis

Hemochromatosis can cause either a dilated or a restrictive cardiomyopathy:

- On CMRI, T2-star-weighted imaging can assess the degree of iron deposition in the myocardium. The degree of iron deposition correlates with worsening of ventricular function.

Chagas disease

Chagas disease is caused by the protozoan *Trypanosoma cruzi* and is mainly seen in Central and South America. If latent infection develops, patients will develop a cardiomyopathy:

- CMRI will show edema on T2-weighted images, consistent with myocarditis, which will evolve into fibrosis that can be seen as areas of LGE.

Arrhythmogenic right ventricular dysplasia

Arrhythmogenic right ventricular dysplasia leads to fibrofatty replacement of the right ventricle and results in arrhythmias and right ventricular failure:

- On echocardiography, there will often be isolated right ventricular dysfunction.
- CMRI can be used to identify fat in the right ventricular free wall on T1-weighted images.

Myocarditis

- With active myocarditis, T2-weighted MR images show high signal corresponding to edema. If myocarditis evolves into fibrosis, LGE will be present in the involved areas.

Takotsubo cardiomyopathy

Takotsubo cardiomyopathy classically occurs in postmenopausal women following a significant emotional stress. ECG can show a variety of abnormalities including ST elevation. Cardiac biomarkers are often elevated:

- Cardiac echocardiography shows basal and midventricular hypercontractility with apical akinesis (the "apical ballooning" syndrome).

- Coronary angiography distinguishes Takotsubo cardiomyopathy from the occlusion of a large, wraparound LAD artery. A ventriculogram at the time of cardiac catheterization will also show apical ballooning as will cine imaging in CMRI.

Endomyocardial disease

Endomyocardial disease is a hypereosinophilic syndrome that can cause a restrictive cardiomyopathy and has two phenotypic variants—Loeffler endocarditis and endomyocardial fibrosis:

- On echocardiography, there will be left ventricular apical thrombus formation and apical obliteration in the absence of apical infarction. Thrombus also forms beneath the posterior leaflet of the mitral valve.

Pericardial disease

Pericarditis

Acute pericarditis is diagnosed with a typical history and ECG. On echocardiography, a pericardial effusion may or may not be present. On CMRI, enhancement of the pericardium can be consistent with either inflammation or fibrosis. Clinical history and diastolic parameters on both echocardiography and CMRI can help to distinguish between the two.

Pericardial effusion

There is normally between 5 and 50 ml of serous fluid between the parietal and visceral pericardial layers. A pericardial effusion can result from acute pericarditis due to infectious etiologies (most commonly viral), uremia, systemic inflammatory diseases, postmyocardial infarction (Dressler's syndrome), malignancy, dissection, or trauma:

- On echocardiography, the subcostal view is often ideal for assessment of a pericardial effusion and is identified between the echogenic parietal pericardium and the visceral pericardium adherent to the myocardium on PLAX.
- A pericardial effusion will track into the oblique pericardial sinus between the aorta and left atrium; this can help to differentiate pericardial fluid from pleural fluid.
- A small pericardial effusion is <0.5 cm in diastole, a moderate effusion is between 0.5 and 2.0 cm, and a large effusion is >2.0 cm. Effusions may be loculated or free-flowing.
- Care should be taken to evaluate for any signs of elevated intrapericardial pressure and tamponade physiology, which include early diastolic collapse of the right ventricle, exaggerated

respiratory variation of left ventricular filling, and a dilated and fixed IVC. With tamponade physiology, there will be a greater than 25% decrease in left ventricular filling at the mitral valve with inspiration. This is the echocardiographic manifestation of a pulsus paradoxus. A dilated and noncompressible IVC indicates elevated right atrial pressure.

Pericardial constriction

Pericardial constriction results from thickening, fibrosis, and adherence of the visceral and parietal pericardium, which limits total cardiac volume and impairs diastolic filling. Given the fixed, inelastic pericardium, nearly all of filling happens in early diastole. Causes of pericardial constriction include idiopathic or viral, postsurgical, postradiation therapy, and postinfection and are associated with connective tissue diseases:

- A pericardial thickness greater than 4 mm on echocardiography is suggestive of constriction. TTE will show exaggerated ventricular interdependence with abnormal septal motion and rapid early diastolic filling with abrupt cessation due to the limits of the rigid pericardium.
- CCT and CMRI permit more accurate measurement of pericardial thickness than TTE and correlate with pericardial thickness measured on TEE. CCT may also show calcification of the pericardium.

Pericardial cyst

A pericardial cyst can be seen on both echocardiography and CMRI. It is an uncomplicated cyst with smooth walls and no internal septae. On CMRI, it will be dark on T1-weighted images and bright on T2-weighted images. It usually contains transudative fluid.

Partial absence of the pericardium

Partial absence of the pericardium is a congenital anomaly associated with sternal defects, ASDs, a patent ductus arteriosus, and anomalies of the great vessels. Pericardium is most often absent over the left heart, and the left atrium or left atrial appendage can herniate through the defect and become strangulated.

Masses/neoplasm

Benign tumors

Myxoma

Myxomas are the most common primary cardiac tumor. Usually, they are single and originate from the fossa ovalis in the interatrial septum. They are most common in the left atrium, followed by the right atrium and rarely the ventricles. They can be either well circumscribed and pedunculated on a stalk or more gelatinous and varied in appearance:

- A myxoma can often be suggested by typical echocardiographic appearance and location.
- Cardiac MRA and coronary angiography may show a tumor blush with contrast administration due to the vascularity of the myxoma. A lipoma can be distinguished from a myxoma on T1-weighted MR images, as lipomas are very bright in signal (and lipomas can be characterized with greater confidence if an additional T1-weighted fat-suppressed sequence is performed that will show loss of signal of the fat).

Rhabdomyoma

Cardiac rhabdomyomas are the most common primary tumor of the heart in children. A rhabdomyoma is a benign tumor of striated muscle and can be associated with tuberous sclerosis where they are often multiple. Rhabdomyomas are most frequently located in the ventricular myocardium. Cardiac rhabdomyomas often regress spontaneously:

- On CMRI, rhabdomyomas will have a signal intensity similar to myocardium on T1-weighted images but will have increased signal intensity on T2-weighted images.

Fibroma

A cardiac fibroma is a benign tumor that occurs most frequently in children. It is the second most common benign cardiac tumor in children after rhabdomyomas. It is usually found in the

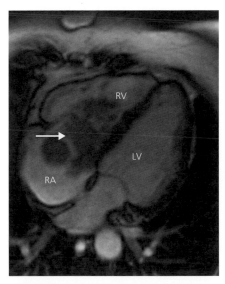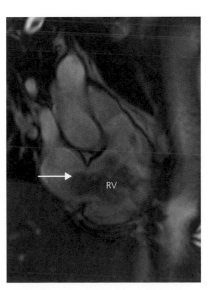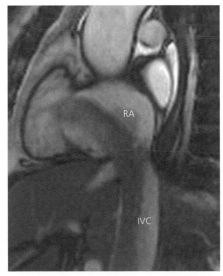

Figure 4.10 Cardiac masses. Cardiac MRI in a patient with a uterine leiomyoma shows a tumor cluster in the right atrium (RA), prolapsing across the tricuspid valve and extending into the right ventricle (RV) (left, middle). Tumor is seen extending up the inferior vena cava (IVC) into the right atrium (right). LV, left ventricle.

interventricular septum or left ventricular free wall. Fibromas can cause conduction abnormalities. They are usually single.

Papillary fibroelastoma

A papillary fibroelastoma is a small, benign, mobile mass found on the downstream side of cardiac valves (the ventricular side of the AV valves or the aortic/pulmonic side of the semilunar valves). This helps to distinguish it from a vegetation. Rarely, it can be associated with systemic embolic events.

Metastatic tumors

Metastatic tumors are more common than primary malignant tumors. They can reach the heart via direct invasion from lung or breast tumors. They can spread to the heart via the lymphatic system like melanoma or lymphoma, or they can reach the heart directly via hematogenous spread. Renal cell carcinoma is the classic example of this and can be seen extending up the IVC into the right atrium. With the exception of renal cell carcinoma, metastatic disease usually affects the pericardium (i.e., melanoma) or epicardium. Associated pericardial effusions are common (Figure 4.10).

Primary malignant tumors

Primary malignant cardiac tumors are much rarer than metastatic tumors. Rarely, angiosarcomas, rhabdomyosarcomas, and fibrosarcomas present in adults.

Suggested reading

Cerqueira, M.D., Weissman, N.J., Dilsizian, V. *et al.* (2002) Standardized myocardial segmentation and nomenclature for tomographic imaging of the heart: a statement for healthcare professionals from the Cardiac Imaging Committee of the Council on Clinical Cardiology of the American Heart Association. *Circulation*, **105**, 539–542.

Dilsizian, V., Bacharach, S.L., Beanland, S.R. *et al.* (2009) PET myocardial perfusion and metabolism clinical imaging. *Journal of Nuclear Cardiology*, **16**, 651.

Ho, V.B. & Reddy, G.P. (2011a) *Cardiovascular Imaging: Embryologic Basis and Segmental Approach to Imaging*. St Louis, MO Elsevier, Saunders.

Ho, V.B. & Reddy, G.P. (2011b) *Cardiovascular Imaging: Coronary Anatomy*. St Louis, MO Elsevier, Saunders.

Jongbloed, M.R.M., Lamb, H.F., Bax, J.J. *et al.* (2005) Noninvasive visualization of the cardiac venous system using multislice computed tomography. *Journal of the American College of Cardiology*, **45**, 749–753.

Kushner, F.G., Hand, M., Smith, S.C., Jr *et al.* (2009) 2009 Focused updates: ACC/AHA guidelines for the management of patients with ST-elevation myocardial infarction and ACC/AHA/SCAI guidelines on percutaneous coronary intervention. *A report of the ACC/AHA Task Force on Practice Guidelines. Journal of the American College of Cardiology*, **54**, 989.

Lang, R.M., Bierig, M., Devereux, R.B. *et al.* (2005) Recommendations for chamber quantification: a report from the American Society of Echocardiography's Guidelines and Standards Committee and the Chamber Quantification Group, developed in conjunction with the European Association of Echocardiography, a branch of the European Society of Cardiology. *Journal of the American Society of Echocardiography*, **18**, 1440–1463.

Mark, D.B. & Lauer, M.S. (2003) Exercise capacity: the prognostic variable that doesn't get enough respect. *Circulation*, **108**, 1534.

Otto, C.M. (2013) *Textbook of Clinical Echocardiography*, 5th edn. Elsevier, Saunders, Philadelphia, PA.

Patel, S. (2008) Normal and anomalous anatomy of the coronary arteries. *Seminars in Roentgenology*, **43**, 100–112.

Pellikka, P.A., Nagueh, D.F., Elhendy, A.A. *et al.* (2007) American society of echocardiography: recommendations for performance, interpretation and application of stress echocardiography. *Journal of the American Society of Echocardiography*, **20**, 1021–1041.

Peterson, G.E. (2003) Brickner E and SC Reimold. *Transesophageal echocardiography: clinical indications and applications. Circulation*, **107**, 2398–2402.

Singh, S. & Goyal, A. (2007) The origin of echocardiography. *Texas Heart Institute Journal*, **4** (34), 431–438.

Wacker, F.J., Brown, K.A., Heller, G.V. *et al.* (2002) American Society of Nuclear Cardiology position statement on radionuclide imaging in patients with suspected acute ischemic syndromes in the emergency department or chest pain center. *Journal of Nuclear Cardiology*, **9**, 246.

CHAPTER 5

Abdominopelvic imaging

Pinakpani Roy[1] and Lauren M.B. Burke[2]

[1]Department of Radiology, University of North Carolina, Chapel Hill, USA

[2]Division of Abdominal Imaging, Department of Radiology, University of North Carolina, Chapel Hill, USA

Normal anatomy and general concepts

Abdominal imaging is an extremely wide and deep field, and therefore, this chapter can provide only an overview of this subject. The goal is to convey the most fundamental and critical ("do not miss") abnormalities that you will encounter in clinical medicine.

The abdomen is roughly divided into four quadrants, right upper quadrant (RUQ), left upper quadrant (LUQ), right lower quadrant (RLQ), and left lower quadrant (LLQ), as well as epigastric and suprapubic regions. Each of these regions contains certain organs and has a finite number of differential diagnoses. From a clarity of diagnosis perspective, it is critical to narrow a patient's symptoms to one (or more) of these regions, which will immensely facilitate the construction of a differential diagnoses, and from there the imaging test that is most appropriate for each region and its constituents (Figure 5.1):

- RUQ
  - Liver
  - Gallbladder
  - Hepatic flexure of colon
  - Duodenum
- LUQ
  - Stomach
  - Spleen
  - Splenic flexure of the colon
  - Pancreas (body and tail)
- RLQ
  - Bowel
    - Distal ileum
    - Cecum
    - Appendix
  - Adnexa/ovary
- LLQ
  - Sigmoid colon
  - Adnexa/ovary
- Epigastric region
  - Pancreas
  - Stomach
  - Esophagus and gastroesophageal (GE) junction
  - Duodenum
- Suprapubic region
  - Urinary bladder
  - Uterus
  - Prostate (Figures 5.2, 5.3, and 5.4)

The abdominal viscera are enclosed within a thin layer of sheetlike tissue called the peritoneum. Any organ that is within this peritoneal cavity is intraperitoneal, while others are extra- or retroperitoneal. The abdominal cavity as a whole contains both the intraperitoneal and retroperitoneal spaces (Figure 5.5).

The small bowel lies within the central abdomen and is composed of (from proximal to distal) the duodenum, jejunum, and ileum.

The large bowel or colon lies peripheral to the small bowel, wrapping around it like a picture frame.

The duodenum has a primarily retroperitoneal location (see section "Small bowel"), as does the ascending colon, descending colon, and rectum. The rest of the small and large bowel is intraperitoneal.

The pancreas has a mainly retroperitoneal location (the tail being the exception), and pancreatic pathology can cause pain that radiates to the back as well as the epigastrium. The duodenum makes a loop, shaped like a C, as it courses through the right hemiabdomen and heads into the retroperitoneum, and the head of the pancreas is surrounded by this C-loop.

The kidneys (and adrenals) are entirely retroperitoneal, and the ureters traverse from the posterior abdomen to the suprapubic region to enter the bladder, coursing through the lower quadrants. As such, pathology within the kidneys typically causes flank pain, whereas ureteral pathology can cause symptoms anywhere along their course.

The two main vessels of the abdomen, the abdominal aorta and inferior vena cava (IVC), are both retroperitoneal structures, lying between the spine and the midline retroperitoneal organs.

With this basic understanding of the general anatomy of the abdomen, it is more evident why pathology within certain organs will cause symptoms that are typically confined to one of the aforementioned regions. This understanding also facilitates choosing

Critical Observations in Radiology for Medical Students, First Edition. Katherine R. Birchard, Kiran Reddy Busireddy, and Richard C. Semelka.

© 2015 John Wiley & Sons, Ltd. Published 2015 by John Wiley & Sons, Ltd.

Companion website: www.wiley.com/go/birchard

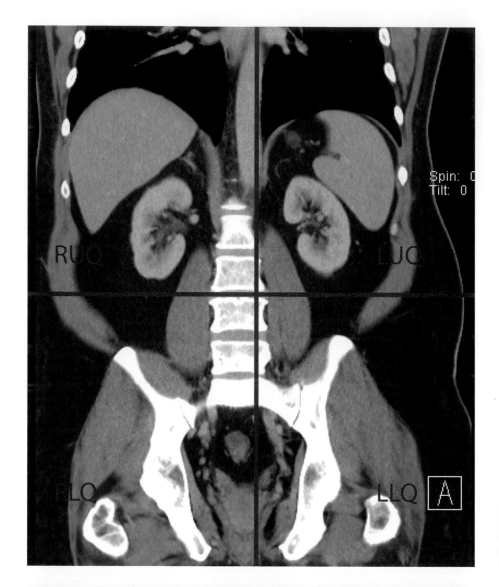

Figure 5.1 Coronal image of the abdomen dividing the abdomen into four quadrants: right upper quadrant (RUQ), left upper quadrant (LUQ), right lower quadrant (RLQ), and left lower quadrant (LLQ).

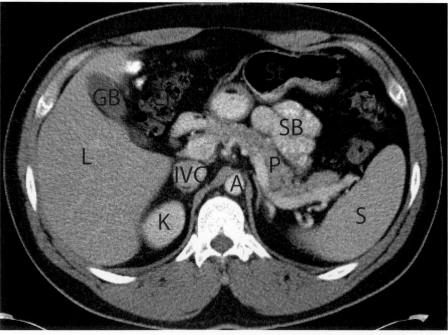

Figure 5.2 Axial contrast-enhanced CT image of the upper abdomen. L, liver; GB, gallbladder; Cn, colon; St, stomach; P, pancreas; S, spleen; SB, small bowel; K, kidney; IVC, inferior vena cava; A, aorta.

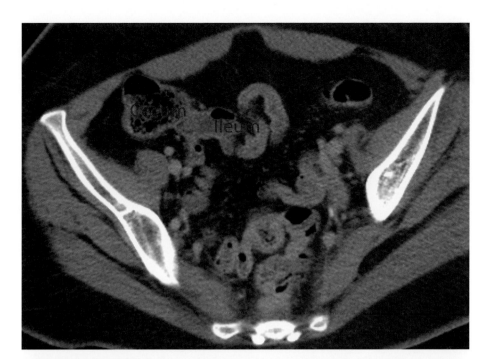

Figure 5.3 Single axial CT image of the right lower quadrant demonstrates the terminal ileum and cecum. The appendix is not included on this single image.

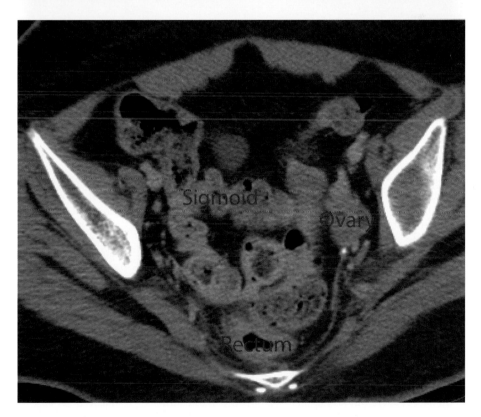

Figure 5.4 Single axial CT image of the pelvis demonstrates the sigmoid, ovary, and rectum.

the appropriate imaging test. Each of the major imaging tests that radiologists employ (plain films, ultrasound (US), computed tomography (CT), nuclear medicine (NM), and magnetic resonance imaging (MRI)) has certain strengths and weaknesses. Different regions of the abdomen and disease processes sought confer certain opportunities and challenges for each of these imaging modalities. Recognizing the primary location of the disease process, and the likely type of disease, permits the selection of the modality that couples the appropriate combination of strengths, offset by its weaknesses, to study the patient. To illustrate this, the words "RUQ pain" raises the consideration of hepatic and/or gallbladder causes first (making US the most appropriate initial test), while seeing "RLQ pain" should trigger the consideration of bowel causes, such as appendicitis or ileitis, or ovarian pathology (CT and US, respectively). MRI can also answer these questions, but due to cost considerations (factored into the weakness formula), this often is used as problem solving for many of the abovementioned examples.

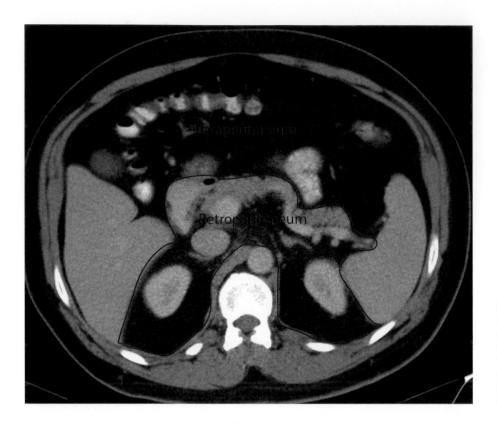

Figure 5.5 Axial contrast-enhanced CT image of the upper abdomen distinguishing the intraperitoneum from the retroperitoneum (outlined in red). The retroperitoneum also includes the ascending and descending colon, not included on this image of the upper abdomen.

Some general concepts in abdominal imaging are as follows and can be thought of as broad rules to evaluating imaging studies:

The first rule is straightforward: air belongs only inside the gastrointestinal (GI) tract (stomach and bowel). Any air not inside the GI tract is abnormal. Bear in mind that abnormal does not necessary mean unexpected. Free intraperitoneal air is expected to be present after an abdominal surgery or air inside the renal collecting system or bladder after instrumentation. However, if there is no history of iatrogenic maneuvers and this rule has been broken, there have been disruption of the GI tract wall (perforated hollow viscus), introduction of air due to a penetrating wound or downward from the thorax, or sequelae of gas-forming infection. Just like outside the body, free air rises and ends up in the highest spots (often termed nondependent), including under the diaphragm in an upright patient or along the liver margin in a supine or laterally positioned patient.

The second rule is that there should be no "free" fluid. Normally, fluid in the abdomen should reside within the bowel, vessels, and certain organs, including but not limited to the gallbladder, renal collecting systems, or uterus. There should be no "free" fluid, which is when the fluid pools or layers inside the abdomen. Unlike free air, free fluid ends up in the most dependent portions of the abdomen. These are the hepatorenal fossa (also called Morrison's pouch), the two paracolic gutters, and the pelvis. In females, the most dependent pelvic space is between the rectum and uterus, called the rectouterine pouch (also called pouch of Douglas or cul-de-sac), whereas in men it is between the rectum and bladder (rectovesical pouch). Free fluid is generally abnormal, with one exception: reproductive age females can have a small amount of physiologic pelvic free fluid. Free fluid is quite nonspecific, but it is a good marker of inflammation or trauma and should serve to heighten suspicion if present.

The third rule is that the plumbing in the body should be free of obstruction and intact. The body, including the abdomen, is full of pipes, which are the bowel, vessels, bile ducts, and renal collecting systems and ureters. Analogous to kinking a garden hose, the portion above the kink expands due to increased pressure, and the hose beyond the kink collapses. The same is observed in the body; whenever there is interruption of proper flow through any of the body's many pipes, there is increased pressure and proximal dilatation, along with distal narrowing or collapse. Therefore, whenever the observation is made of a dilated bowel loop (with narrowed or normal bowel distally), bile duct, vessel, or ureter, interrogate the region of transition where the structure becomes narrowed for a possible cause. It might be an endoluminal object like a ureteral or bile duct stone, bowel obstruction due to an adhesion, or extrinsic compression from a tumor. When the plumbing loses its integrity and becomes disrupted, then the principal contents of those tubes become distributed in surrounding tissues. Among the most dramatic and deadly of these events is disruption of the abdominal aorta, which permits distribution of blood into surrounding tissues at the site of the disruption.

The fourth rule is that the body hates traffic jams, known as stasis. Motility is the preferred state. Therefore, whenever there is stasis due to either obstruction or disruption of normal motility, there are increased risk of infection and associated inflammation.

Taking into consideration these rules, more detail about the normal anatomy and function of specific organs will be discussed.

GI tract

The GI tract is essentially a long tube extending from the mouth to the anus, which includes areas of expansion (the stomach and colon) and a lot of twists and turns. The components include the mouth and oropharynx, esophagus, stomach, small bowel (including the duodenum, jejunum, and ileum), colon, rectum, and anus.

Esophagus

The esophagus is a long tube that connects the pharynx to the stomach, with the pharyngoesophageal sphincter and GE junction being its margins. The main function of the esophagus is to propel food toward the stomach, through synchronized contractions called peristalsis.

The peristaltic contractions can be grouped into three types of waves:

1 Primary: this smooth continuous wave is triggered by swallowing and can push the food bolus to the stomach in about 9 s.
2 Secondary: identical imaging-wise to the primary wave but initiated by a troublesome bolus or esophageal distention.
3 Tertiary: high-frequency contractions that do not propel the food bolus and are seen primarily in esophageal motility disorders.

The lower esophageal sphincter (LES) marks the terminal point of the esophagus and consists of a bundle of smooth muscles that stop the reflux of gastric acid but periodically relax to let food bolus through. Unlike the upper esophageal sphincter, the LES is not under voluntary control.

In broad terms, imaging evaluation of esophageal pathology focuses primarily on the caliber (abnormal dilatation or narrowing) and mucosal appearance (ulcerations or masses; Figure 5.6).

Stomach

The stomach functions as a reservoir that temporarily stores food, liquefies it, and begins the process of protein digestion. It is divided into the cardia, fundus, body, antrum, and pylorus, from proximal

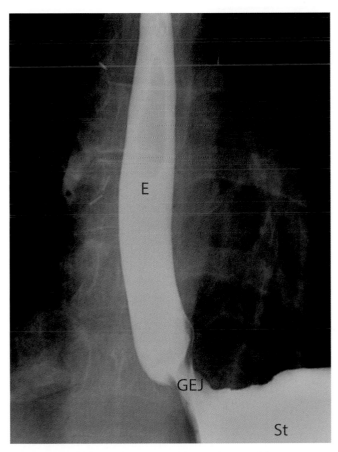

Figure 5.6 Single fluoroscopic image of the esophagus with barium opacifying the esophagus. E, esophagus; GEJ, gastroesophageal junction; St, stomach.

to distal. These separate segments are rather arbitrary and often not distinctly demarcated on imaging, with the exception of the pylorus, which (similar to the distal esophageal sphincter) controls gastric emptying through periodic muscular contractions.

Anatomic imaging evaluation of the stomach focuses primarily on the appearance of the gastric folds (rugae), the presence of ulcers or mass lesions, and the pylorus (in pediatrics). Functional evaluation of the stomach through NM is mainly for the evaluation of gastric emptying (Figure 5.7).

Small bowel

The small bowel (comprised of the duodenum, jejunum, and ileum) is where digestion primarily takes place. The division between the duodenum and jejunum (duodenojejunal junction or DJJ) is important in imaging for evaluation of malrotation, particularly in children. The jejunum–ileum junction is broad and not particularly relevant in imaging.

As discussed previously, the duodenum makes an approximately C-shaped loop (hence the term duodenal C-loop). The ligament of Treitz marks the boundary between the duodenum and jejunum (and suspends it as the initial attachment of the mesentery) and is thus an important anatomic landmark to evaluate the small bowel positioning. At the lower extent, the ileocecal valve is normally situated in the RLQ and forms the junction between the small bowel (upper GI) and colon (lower GI).

The duodenum is split into four parts:

1 First portion, or duodenal bulb—just distal to the gastric pylorus and the only completely intraperitoneal portion of the duodenum.
2 Second portion—the descending or vertical part of the C-loop. The pancreatic head fits into this portion, and it is here that the pancreatic and common bile ducts (CBD) meet and deposit their respective contents (bile and pancreatic enzymes) into the duodenum via the ampulla of Vater. Thus, any mass at the ampulla may cause upstream dilatation of the biliary ductal system as well as the pancreatic duct.
3 Third portion—the horizontal portion of the inferior C-loop.
4 Fourth portion—the transition point from the third portion is where the duodenum is crossed over by the superior mesenteric artery (SMA). The fourth part continues to course horizontally with a slightly superior angulation and to the left before terminating at the ligament of Treitz, which marks the transition to the jejunum. On coronal imaging, the normal DJJ should overlie the left pedicle of the L1 or L2 vertebral body (or further left of it) and should be at least level with the duodenal bulb (if not slightly superior). If the DJJ fails to cross the midline and lies inferior to the bulb, intestinal malrotation should be considered.

Unlike the duodenum, the jejunum and ileum do not have anatomically clear divisions. The most distal small bowel, or terminal ileum, is clinically important as it is the commonly involved bowel site in inflammatory bowel disease such as Crohn's disease (discussed later on in this chapter). The ileum connects to the cecum via the ileocecal valve, typically located in the RLQ.

Colon

From proximal to distal, the colon is comprised of the cecum (with appendix), ascending (or right) colon, transverse colon, descending (or left) colon, sigmoid colon, rectum, and anus. Due to their proximity to the respective organs, the flexed junction between the ascending and transverse colons is called the hepatic flexure, and the flexed junction between the transverse and descending colons is called the splenic flexure.

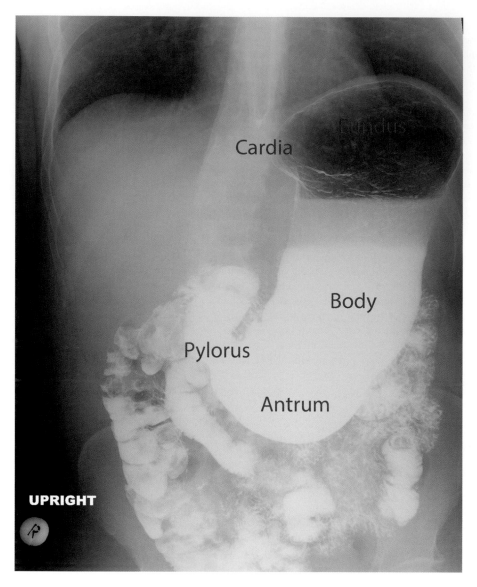

Cardia

Fundus

Body

Pylorus

Antrum

UPRIGHT

Figure 5.7 Single fluoroscopic image demonstrates the anatomy of the stomach (cardia, fundus, body, antrum, and pylorus). Small bowel and colon are partially opacified.

The appendix is a vestigial organ arising from the cecum and clinically significant mainly for appendicitis, which will be discussed later in the section.

Liver, pancreas, gallbladder, and biliary system

The liver is the major solid organ in the RUQ, with the gallbladder tucked inferiorly. The liver is supplied by both the hepatic arterial system (arising from the abdominal aorta, usually the celiac artery) and the portal venous system (which drains blood from the bowel and spleen). The latter provides the majority of hepatic blood supply. The hepatic venous system (consisting of the right, middle, and left hepatic veins) drains blood from the liver to the IVC.

In terms of segmentation, functional anatomy is more relevant in imaging than traditional gross anatomy. Functionally speaking, the liver is divided into the right and left lobes via Cantlie's line inferiorly (drawn from the gallbladder fossa to the IVC) and the middle hepatic vein superiorly. The fossa for ligamentum teres divides the functional left hepatic lobes into medial and lateral segments.

The bile produced by the liver is taken downstream via the right and left hepatic bile ducts, which combine to form the common hepatic duct. This bile is then either stored in the gallbladder (which connects to the common hepatic duct via the cystic duct) or supplied to the duodenum (via the CBD; Figure 5.8).

The pancreas is a primarily retroperitoneal organ, which has a close relationship with the duodenum. The exocrine pancreas generates digestive enzymes, which are supplied to the duodenum via the pancreatic duct. As discussed previously, the CBD and pancreatic duct deposit their respective contents into the duodenum via the ampulla of Vater.

Genitourinary system

The kidneys are paired and bean-shaped (with the bean slightly flattened in the anteroposterior (AP) direction), mainly craniocaudally oriented structures in the retroperitoneum. The adrenals are paired, conical structures closely apposed to the superior aspect of the kidneys. The kidneys and adrenals are housed within the renal or Gerota's fascia, which acts as a structural barrier to spread of disease to and from the renal space.

Each kidney may have one or more renal arteries supplying it, with multiple renal arteries not uncommon. Renal veins are almost always solitary. The distance the right renal vein courses to enter the IVC is short, whereas the left renal vein must cross the aorta to reach the IVC.

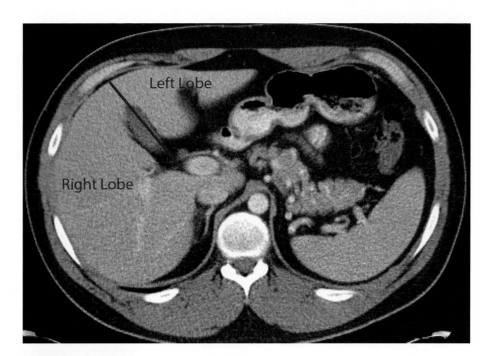

Figure 5.8 Axial contrast-enhanced CT image of the upper abdomen demonstrates both right and left hepatic lobes.

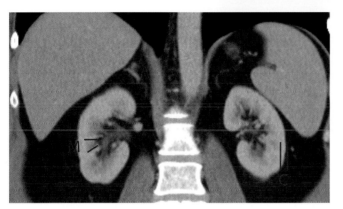

Figure 5.9 Coronal contrast-enhanced CT image of the kidneys. A, adrenal gland, the inverted Y-shaped organ just superior to the kidney; M, medulla of the kidney; C, the cortex of the kidney.

Most often, the vein crosses anteriorly, but posterior crossing is not rare, and circumaortic renal vein is the least common pattern. One anatomic observation that has clinical significance is that the right gonadal/testicular vein drains directly into the IVC, whereas the left gonadal vein drains into the left renal vein. Because of its more circuitous course, left-sided varicocele is more common and may indicate obstructive pathology of the left renal vein (due to mass lesion or thrombus).

The renal parenchyma consists of the cortex and medulla. The renal collecting system is composed of renal calyces, which combine to form the infundibula that then combine to form the renal pelvis. The renal pelvis extends to the ureter (at the ureteropelvic junction or UPJ), and the ureter courses down to connect with the bladder (at the ureterovesicular junction or UVJ; Figure 5.9).

In the female pelvis, the anatomy from anterior to posterior consists of the urinary bladder, uterus (and adnexa), and rectum. The inferior portion of the uterus is the cervix, which communicates with the vagina.

In the male pelvis, the prostate wraps around the proximal urethra (which is why benign prostatic hyperplasia results in bladder outlet obstruction).

Imaging modalities

Plain radiography

Plain radiography is an inexpensive, effective, and popular modality for identification of acute findings such as free air and bowel obstruction. The ability of plain radiography to identify bowel pathology mainly depends on the presence of the extremes of density—air or calcification. As such, it remains a common modality for identification of acute findings such as pneumoperitoneum and bowel obstruction and (to a lesser extent) nephrolithiasis. Due to the silhouette sign, plain radiography is not a preferred modality for evaluation of most solid organs.

Digital fluoroscopy

This is a subset of plain radiography, in which real-time images are obtained. In abdominal fluoroscopy, enteric contrast (water soluble or barium) is used to distend the viscus in question for optimal evaluation.

The use of fluoroscopy in abdominal imaging is limited mainly to evaluation of the GI tract. Opacifying the bowel lumen with barium or water-soluble contrast allows for functional evaluation (esophageal motility, transit time to the colon) as well as bowel wall abnormalities (e.g., mucosal irregularity, ulcers, or stricture).

Fluoroscopy can also be used to opacify the ureters, bladder, and urethra to evaluate for potential filling defects (stones, masses, blood clot) or extravasation in the setting of trauma. While there are still cases where fluoroscopy is helpful, multiphase CT has largely taken over evaluation of the bowel and genitourinary (GU) system (Figures 5.10 and 5.11).

CT

The advent of CT has revolutionized abdominal imaging, as it allows rapid cross-sectional evaluation with great spatial resolution. CT is considered the preferred modality in most of abdominal imaging, with the exception of the liver (where MRI is preferred) and biliary and pelvic pathology (where US and/or MRI is preferred; as a rule, US for simpler and MRI for more complex diseases). It is essential in the evaluation of abdominal trauma and much vascular

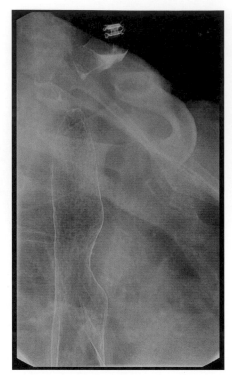

Figure 5.10 Esophagitis—Single image from a double contrast esophogram demonstrates innumerable tiny plaque-like lesions throughout the esophageal mucosa, with associated edema.

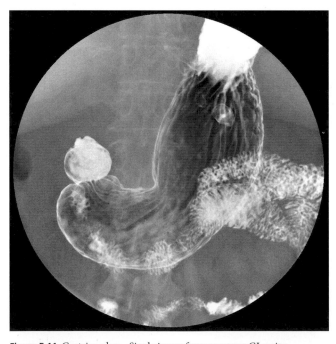

Figure 5.11 Gastric polyp—Single image from an upper GI series demonstrates two polyps in the proximal stomach, with the smaller showing a ring shadow.

pathology and is also used for many abdominal interventions, such as biopsies, ablations, and drainage procedures.

The main drawback of CT imaging remains the risk associated with ionizing radiation, although iterative reconstruction techniques used in modern scanners have allowed for a significant decrease in overall radiation dose while maintaining image quality. It also has lesser intrinsic soft tissue contrast resolution than MRI.

CT is quite dependent on intravenous (IV) contrast for optimal detection of lesions, which limits its utility in patients in whom iodinated contrast is contraindicated (renal disease, anaphylaxis).

MRI

MRI, unlike CT, offers superb soft tissue contrast even without the use of IC contrast, which is extremely helpful in cases of renal insufficiency. The ability of MR to differentiate between different tissue types is instrumental in detection of abdominal solid organ lesions, especially in the liver, the pancreas, and the female pelvis. In addition, the ability to create specialized sequences (such as fat suppressed or in and opposed phase) makes MRI very versatile. MRI also provides the ability to image in any anatomic plane, without the risks associated with ionizing radiation. Drawbacks include longer imaging times and cost.

Gadolinium-based IV contrast agents are considered safe to use in most patients, short of patients with advanced renal disease.

MRI can be (and is being increasingly) used to evaluate most abdominal pathology, including but not limited to evaluation of solid organ lesions (mainly the liver, pancreas, and kidneys), biliary pathology (via magnetic resonance cholangiopancreatography or MRCP), pelvic disease (uterine and ovarian lesions, prostate pathology), and bowel (MR enterography).

US

US imaging is obtained via the use of pulsed sound waves and analysis of the resulting echo. In abdominal imaging, US is valued for its portability, speed, economy, and ability to generate real-time plane-independent images with vascular information (through Doppler imaging). For these reasons, US is heavily relied upon for guidance during image-guided biopsies.

However, US is very user dependent and can therefore lack the precision and reproducibility of other imaging modalities. In addition, it is very dependent on good acoustic windows, and the presence of ample subcutaneous fat or bowel gas can severely impede its utility.

US is mainly used for evaluation of the biliary system (primarily gallbladder and biliary tree) and GU system (kidneys, bladder, and female pelvis). US is also used as a first-line, rapid bedside imaging modality in abdominal trauma (focused assessment with sonography for trauma or FAST).

NM

NM imaging in the abdomen is mainly used as a problem-solving modality. The basic method of diagnostic nuclear imaging involves tagging a physiologically active compound with a radioactive molecule and then mapping its distribution. In therapeutic nuclear imaging or radiotherapy, the radioactive molecule is a particulate emitter, which can deliver targeted radiotherapy to a desired organ while minimizing dose to "bystander" tissues.

In abdominal imaging, NM is mainly used for oncologic diagnosis and staging through positron emission tomography (PET). The combination of PET with either CT or MRI enables the combination of functional and anatomic imaging, and this has achieved importance for oncology imaging. NM can also be used to diagnose gastroparesis and equivocal cases of acute cholecystitis (through cholescintigraphy or hepatobiliary iminodiacetic acid (HIDA) scan) or for renal evaluation (mercaptoacetyltriglycine (MAG)-3, diethylene triamine pentacaetic acid (DTPA), or dimercaptosuccinic acid (DMSA) scans).

Critical observations

In this section, a brief overview is given of the most serious disease processes to recognize in abdominal imaging. This should be considered: the things that "absolutely cannot be missed" survey.

Pneumoperitoneum

Free air in the abdomen is a key finding that must be recognized. Assuming the absence of iatrogenic causes, perforation of a hollow viscus or perforating injury to the abdominal wall is the most likely cause.

This finding should be sought after on any chest and abdominal radiograph. Upright radiographs are preferred, as the observation of air under the diaphragm establishes the diagnosis. If upright images are not possible, a left lateral decubitus position can be used, as the air can be visualized between the lateral margin of the right liver and the abdominal wall. One red herring is interposition of the hepatic flexure of the colon between the liver and diaphragm, creating the false impression of free air (Chilaiditi sign). Gastric air is quite commonly observed in the LUQ and must not be mistaken for free air.

On supine images, free air can be detected through increased prominence of the bowel wall, due to air being present both within and outside the bowel (Rigler's sign).

A large volume of free air can show up as a central lucency, as the midabdomen is the highest location in a supine patient (football sign).

CT is vastly superior to plain films to make the diagnosis of free air, where even a small amount of free air can be detected (typically anterior to the liver margin). So if there is uncertainty about free air

and the patient is physically unwell, CT is indicated. For more information about this topic, refer to the recommended reading [1] (Figures 5.12 and 5.13).

Pneumatosis intestinalis and portal venous gas

Pneumatosis intestinalis is intramural bowel gas, within the bowel wall itself. In the symptomatic patient, this can be secondary to serious pathology such as underlying bowel ischemia and necrosis due to mesenteric ischemia (discussed later in this section). However, this is nonspecific and can also be an incidental finding (seen with COPD, certain medications such as steroids, or indwelling jejunostomy tubes).

On radiographs, pneumatosis appears as curvilinear or linear gas tracking along the bowel wall, often with associated bowel wall thickening.

CT is a much more sensitive, and the best, test to make this diagnosis, and contrast-enhanced (both IV and oral) CT also enables detection of possible underlying causes such as arterial or venous thrombosis or a strangulated hernia. For more information about this topic, refer to the recommended reading [2].

Portal venous gas is the next extension after pneumatosis due to bowel ischemia and necrosis, as the intramural gas is taken via the mesenteric veins and emptied into the portal venous system. This is a serious finding and usually portends a grave prognosis.

A possible mimic of portal venous gas is gas within the hepatic biliary system, or pneumobilia. In contrast to portal venous gas, pneumobilia is usually due to benign or iatrogenic causes (endoscopic retrograde cholangiopancreatography (ERCP), placement of a biliary stent, gastrojejunostomy, etc.) but can be seen with severe cholangitis.

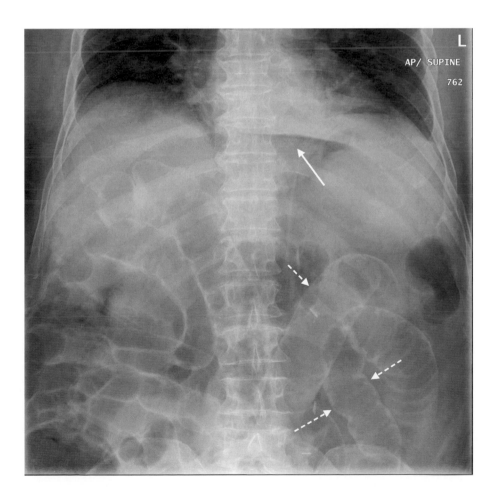

Figure 5.12 Free air – AP supine radiograph of the abdomen demonstrating free intraperitoneal air or pneumoperitoneum. Note the air lining the undersurface of the diaphragm inferior to the heart (solid arrow). Also note the increased conspicuity of the bowel wall (dashed arrows) due to presence of air both inside and outside the bowel lumen (Rigler sign).

A critical observation on imaging is that portal venous gas is usually located peripherally within the liver, whereas pneumobilia is more central (within the main biliary ducts; Figure 5.14).

Bowel obstruction

Bowel obstruction is one of the most common bowel pathologies, with small bowel obstruction (SBO) being significantly more common than large bowel obstruction. Typical causes include adhesions from prior surgeries, incarcerated hernias, bowel mass lesions,

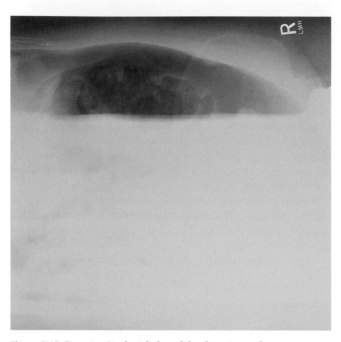

Figure 5.13 Free air—Single right lateral decubitus image demonstrates free intraperitoneal air outside the bowel lumen, rising to the most antidependent position. Also note the air–fluid level within the abdomen due to layering of ascitic fluid.

or abnormal twisting of the bowel (volvulus or closed loop). The severity of bowel obstruction ranges from simple luminal obstruction to closed-loop obstruction, where a loop of bowel twists upon itself and becomes ischemic. If uncorrected, the ischemia can progress to frank necrosis. Unlike arterial-occlusive mesenteric ischemia, where buildup of lactic acid from bowel death can be detected by lab testing of circulating venous blood, a high-grade closed-loop obstruction creates loss of both arterial inflow and venous outflow, with the venous outflow obstruction preventing lactic acid to enter into the systemic circulation. This renders clinical detection difficult and makes imaging diagnosis all the more important.

Imaging findings

As described earlier, a bowel obstruction creates dilatation of the loops proximal to the point of obstruction, while the distal loops are of normal caliber (early) or decompressed (late). This differential bowel dilatation or presence of a transition point is key, because diffusely dilated bowel can represent adynamic ileus (lack of bowel motility) as opposed to obstruction.

Plain radiographs are commonly diagnostic of bowel obstruction, as they show dilated loops of bowel with presence of air–fluid levels that indicate loss of normal peristalsis. However, if all the loops are fluid filled, this observation may not be apparent.

Cross-sectional imaging such as CT is typically performed to determinate the cause of obstruction, presence of vascular compromise, and better localization of the transition zone and to determine if the patient has findings that require an operation.

A closed-loop obstruction will usually appear as a dilated C- or U-shaped loop of bowel. Additional findings concerning for bowel ischemia may be seen in severe cases of obstruction. This will be discussed in detail later.

In terms of maximal normal bowel caliber, the following are some good numbers to keep in mind:
- Small bowel: 3 cm
- Large bowel (except cecum): 6 cm
- Cecum: 9 cm

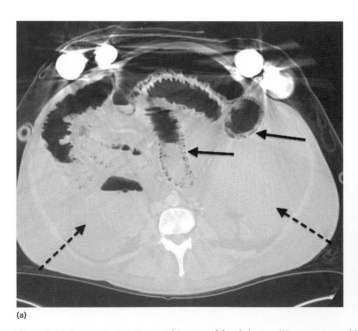

(a)

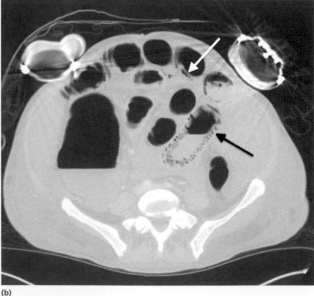

(b)

Figure 5.14 Pneumatosis – Two axial images of the abdomen (Figures 14 a and b) in lung windows demonstrate air interdigitating within the bowel wall (arrows). Also note the presence of ascites (14a, dashed arrows) with the central positioning of the bowel loops.

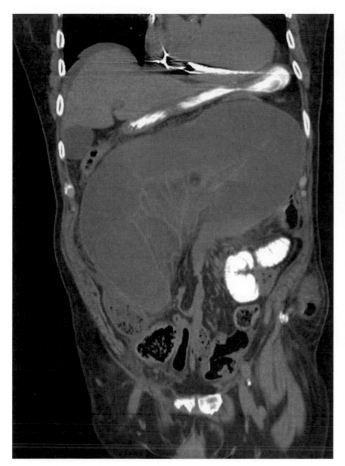

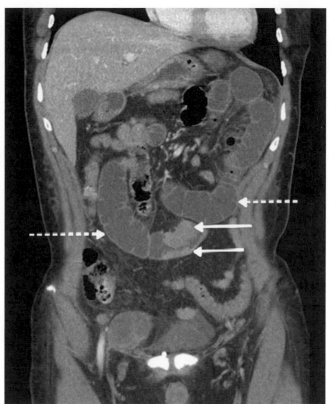

Figure 5.16 Small bowel obstruction secondary to lymphoma – Single coronal image of the abdomen demonstrating enhancing soft tissue within the small bowel lumen (solid arrows), with dilation of the proximal small bowel (dashed arrows).

Figure 5.15 Closed-loop obstruction—Single coronal image of the abdomen demonstrates an inverted U-shaped loop of dilated small bowel. Notice that the proximal and distal segments of the dilated bowel point toward the same location, which is the site of the twisting or obstruction. Oral contrast is noted in the left lower quadrant small bowel, which is not dilated as it is not part of the closed loop.

For more information about this topic, refer to the recommended reading [3] (Figures 5.15, 5.16, and 5.17).

Intra-abdominal infection

There are many different forms of intra-abdominal infections, and they will be discussed in more detail in the dedicated infection/inflammation section later in this chapter.

However, one important concept is to evaluate for the progression of infection, recognizing the spectrum from fat stranding to abscess formation.

Normally, intra-abdominal fat should have the same appearance as subcutaneous fat, with little to no fluid interdigitating within this fat. On US, fat should have a hyperechogenic appearance, and on CT, it should be homogeneously hypoattenuating. On MRI, fat should be hyperintense on non-fat-suppressed T1-weighted images and relatively hyperintense on non-fat-suppressed T2-weighted images. Fat signal is minimized (hypointense) on fat-suppressed MRI sequences.

As the inflammatory response develops, there is increase in free fluid—which seeps into the mesenteric fat. This transitions the appearance of fat toward that of fluid on each modality—on US, the fat demonstrates infiltrating hypoechoic strands; on CT, infiltrative hyperattenuating fluid is seen throughout the fat; and

on MRI, the signal of fluid is introduced into fat on the various sequences.

In the setting of worsening inflammation, the amount of free fluid increases, and on imaging, the appearance goes from ill-defined "stranding" to frank free fluid. If this process continues unabated and if there is active bacterial infection, the relatively transudative fluid can become organized. This is termed loculation. A loculated fluid collection is a poor sign, since it represents the progression to an abscess, reflecting complex fluid collection or frank pus surrounded by a rind of soft tissue. Generally, antibiotics alone cannot fully treat an abscess, and one important method of more definitive treatment entails percutaneous drainage. Many untreated intra-abdominal infectious processes can give rise to abscesses; two of the most common causes are perforated viscus with spillage of bowel contents and bacteria into the peritoneal cavity and secondary to surgery. The presence of gas in a loculated fluid collection is always an adverse sign (unless the air has been introduced by needle aspiration or open surgery), as it indicates either formation of an abscess or a fistula (communicating tract) with the bowel.

Mesenteric ischemia

The arterial supply to the bowel is provided by the SMA and inferior mesenteric artery (IMA) (and partially via the celiac artery), which arise off the abdominal aorta. The venous drainage is similarly via the superior mesenteric vein (SMV) and inferior mesenteric vein (IMV). The IMV drains into the splenic vein, while the SMV

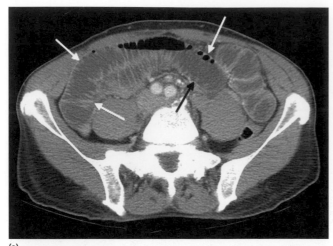

(a)

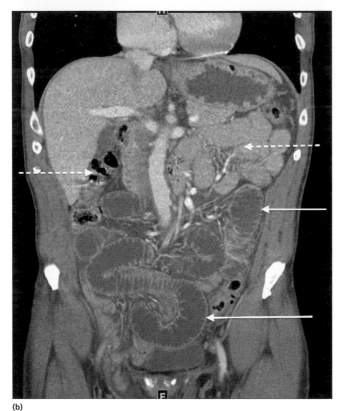

(b)

Figure 5.17 Small bowel obstruction – Axial and coronal contrast enhanced images of the abdomen and pelvis demonstrate long-segment small bowel dilatation (solid arrows, figures 17a and 17b). Decompressed small and large bowel loops are noted on the coronal image (Figure 17b, dashed arrows), indicating this is a likely a small bowel obstruction (although the exact point of obstruction is not seen on these images).

connects with the splenic vein to form the portal vein, which then drains to the liver.

Both arterial and venous vascular flows can be interrupted, and the result is mesenteric ischemia due to either poor inflow of oxygen-rich blood or poor outflow of venous blood.

Arterial interruption is usually caused by embolic disease, due to dislodging of unstable atherosclerotic plaque or embolic event from the heart (e.g., atrial fibrillation), or from atherosclerotic wall thickening.

Venous thrombosis usually arises from a local cause and typically involves the SMV and portal vein.

Imaging findings

Mesenteric ischemia typically results in bowel wall edema, which translates to thickened bowel wall on imaging. This bowel wall thickening can be seen on radiographs, but CT is the preferred modality.

There is also accompanying mesenteric edema, which presents as stranding of mesenteric fat on CT. In more advanced cases, this stranding can actually coalesce to form free fluid in the mesentery, which should raise concern for ischemic bowel (especially in cases of strangulated hernia or obstruction).

On MRI, there is increased T2 signal due to the edema and fluid.

There is often dilatation of the affected bowel due to loss of normal intestinal tone and peristalsis, leading to adynamic ileus.

An additional finding is decreased attenuation/enhancement due to edema and decreased perfusion, which generally requires IV contrast to be observed.

Contrast-enhanced arterial and venous-phase CT and MRI are preferred for direct visualization of the vascular obstruction. This typically takes the form of a filling defect in the vessel or severe narrowing of the arterial caliber due to atherosclerotic plaque or calcification. For more information about this topic, refer to the recommended reading [4] (Figure 5.18).

Testicular or ovarian torsion

The testicular blood supply is provided through the spermatic cord. If the testicle twists on the spermatic cord, this can result in obstruction of the testicular blood supply. Venous outflow is obstructed first, followed by arterial inflow. The severity of the ischemia depends on the degree of twisting (which can range from 180° to 720°). Time is of the utmost importance, as torsion lasting more than 6h usually means the testicle is not salvageable.

The ovary can also experience torsion, with a similar pattern of venous obstruction first, followed by arterial inflow obstruction. The ovary is usually enlarged and heterogeneous in echogenicity reflecting the ischemic damage. In some cases, torsion can be intermittent with intermittent preservation of flow. Alternatively, in a small number of cases, arterial and venous flow can be preserved in the setting of ovarian torsion. In these cases, secondary findings and clinical suspicion are helpful in diagnosis.

US is by far the best modality for evaluation of possible testicular or ovarian torsion. It is quick, easy, and dynamic and offers easy comparison between the two sides. MRI may be of value as a second-line test for ovarian torsion, if uncertainty persists.

Imaging findings in both testicular and ovarian torsions are analogous. These include:

- Enlargement of the affected testicle or ovary due to obstruction of venous outflow. This is the most common finding.
- Free fluid in the pelvis (in case of ovarian torsion) or scrotum (hydrocele, usually reactive and simple).
- Reduced or absent blood flow on Doppler US:
  - Associated "whirlpool" appearance of the twisted vasculature may also be present.
  - As stated earlier, remember that arterial flow may still persist in cases of intermittent torsion.
- Horizontal orientation and superior position of the affected testis compared to the contralateral side. The superior positioning is due to shortening of the pedicle as it twists.
- Large ovarian masses may predispose the patient to torsion.

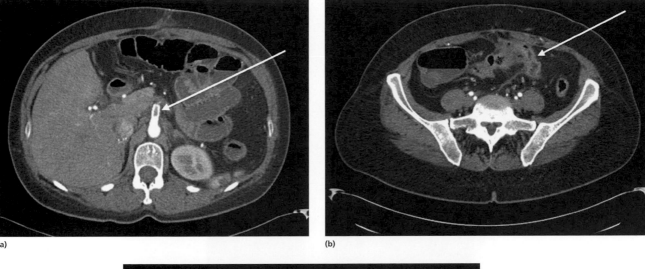

(a)

(b)

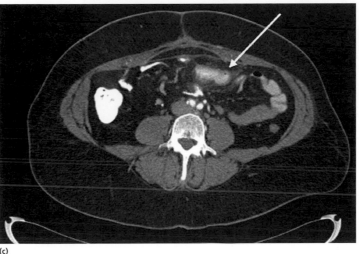

(c)

Figure 5.18 Mesenteric ischemia—Axial arterial-phase contrast images demonstrate hypoattenuating filling defect in the superior mesenteric artery (arrow) (a) and segmental bowel wall thickening and associated mesenteric stranding that reflects bowel ischemia (b and c).

For more information about this topic, refer to the recommended reading [5] (Figure 5.19).

Congenital/genetic disease

A great variety of congenital/genetic diseases possess abdominal features or components. Five of the more common entities will be described.

Hemochromatosis

This is a disorder of iron storage. The primary form (also known as hereditary or genetic hemochromatosis (GH)) results from increased and unregulated iron uptake in the bowel, with direct tissue deposition of this excessively absorbed iron. Iron is deposited in greatest amounts into the liver, pancreas, and myocardium. The secondary form is iatrogenic and seen most often in patients who have received repeated blood transfusions (transfusional siderosis). In transfusional siderosis, iron deposition is primarily in the reticuloendothelial system organs (liver, spleen, and bone marrow). Transfusional siderosis is not of genetic origin and relates purely to the amount and frequency of blood transfusions, but it is critical to distinguish this usually harmless process from GH, which, if left untreated, is progressive and fatal. The direct tissue deposition in GH causes dysfunction of the organs affected, including cirrhosis in the liver (with a relatively high incidence of developing hepatocellular carcinoma (HCC)), chronic pancreatitis in the pancreas, and myocardial dysfunction (which historically was one of the most common causes of death, in addition to HCC), and skin changes (the so-called bronze diabetes). Treatment involves repeated phlebotomy and occasionally iron chelation.

Although biopsy is the definitive method of diagnosis, MRI has become an important means of diagnosis in recent years. MR may in fact be the first diagnostic tool that alerts the clinician to the underlying disease process of GH.

Findings on MRI include markedly decreased intensity on T2-weighted imaging. Specialized sequences (R2-MRI) can quantify the iron deposition in the liver and are being used as an alternative to biopsy.

Horseshoe kidney

This results from fusion of the inferior poles of the kidneys, which prevents the normal superior migration of the kidneys as the conjoined portion gets trapped at the level of the IMA. Associated issues include other GU defects and abnormal drainage (resulting

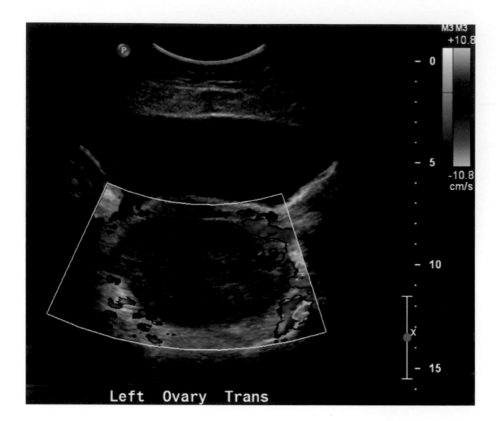

Figure 5.19 Ovarian torsion—Single transverse pelvic ultrasound image with color Doppler demonstrates an enlarged left ovary with small peripheral follicles and no internal vascular flow.

in hydronephrosis, which in turn increases risk of infection, urolithiasis, and transitional cell carcinoma (TCC)).

Polycystic kidney disease

This genetically inherited disorder comes in two forms. The autosomal recessive polycystic kidney disease (ARPCKD) variety is a rare disease of infancy and childhood that causes fetal or early childhood death. Those that survive require renal transplants before the age of 20.

The autosomal dominant polycystic kidney disease (ADPCKD) variety is one of the most common genetic disorders and will be discussed in more detail.

Imaging findings include:
- Enlarged kidneys with innumerable cysts. Many of the cysts appear simple (imperceptible walls, hypoattenuating on CT and T1 hypointense/T2 hyperintense on MRI), but an important feature of ADPCKD is that a fair number of cysts contain blood, which shows increased density on CT and T1 hyperintensity on MRI.
- Over time, the normal renal parenchyma atrophies, with concomitant development of renal impairment and eventual failure. The kidneys generally are massively enlarged, filled with innumerable cysts by the time the patient is 40 years of age.
- Innumerable cysts are often noted in the liver and less prominently within the pancreas, spleen, and ovaries.
- Some may demonstrate intracranial aneurysms, and a screening CT or MR angiogram is often performed (Figure 5.20).

Refer to the selected reading for more information about additional cystic renal diseases, including von Hippel–Lindau (VHL) [6].

Intestinal malrotation

Normal bowel anatomy is the result of coordinated rotation of the midgut during the embryonic period. Abnormal rotation (either

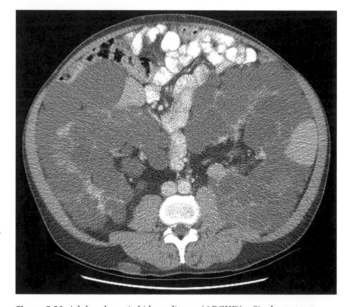

Figure 5.20 Adult polycystic kidney disease (APCKD)—Single contrast-enhanced axial image at the level of the kidneys demonstrates severe atrophy of the kidneys, with innumerable renal cysts bilaterally replacing nearly the entire renal parenchyma. Innumerable splenic and liver cysts are also noted.

lack of rotation or hyperrotation) results in abnormal intestinal positioning and development of the mesentery. Findings include:
- Displacement of the small bowel, mainly jejunum, to the right side of the abdomen. This is diagnosed by the abnormal rightward position of the DJJ on planar and cross-sectional imaging and by the abnormal position of the SMA to the right of the SMV on cross-sectional imaging.

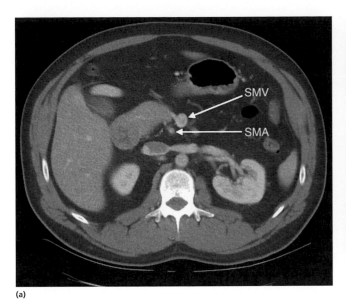 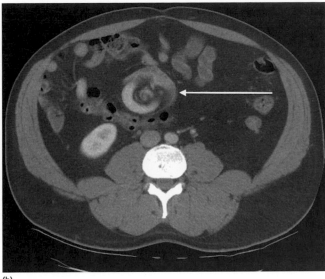

(a) (b)

Figure 5.21 Malrotation—Single contrast-enhanced axial image of the abdomen (a) demonstrates reversal of the normal position of the superior mesenteric artery (SMA) and superior mesenteric vein (SMV) (arrows) (SMV normally lies to the right of the SMA), indicating malrotation. Second axial image (b) demonstrates the swirling of the mesentery (arrow), another finding seen in malrotation.

- Displacement of the cecum to the epigastric or LUQ region.
- Abnormally narrow mesenteric root, which predisposes the patient to midgut volvulus. Acute midgut volvulus is a pediatric surgical emergency that is discussed in more detail in the pediatrics chapter, while chronic midgut volvulus can cause unexplained periodic abdominal pain and symptoms of obstruction in adults for years before being diagnosed (Figure 5.21).

Situs inversus and heterotaxy

This is a group of congenital diseases that involve "mirror image" or abnormal positioning of thoracoabdominal organs across the left–right axis. These include:

- Situs inversus:
  - Heart, stomach, and spleen positioned on the right
  - Liver positioned on the left
- Isolated dextrocardia:
  - Only the heart is positioned abnormally (abdominal organs are normal).
  - Increased association with congenital heart disease.
- Heterotaxy is a collection of heterogeneous disorders that include:
  - Location of the heart and stomach on opposite sides, with a spectrum of cardiac malformations
  - Asplenia
  - Large, midline liver
  - IVC interruption with abnormal continuation of the azygos vein

Trauma/emergency

A wide variety of traumatic injuries may occur throughout the abdomen, and the ability to recognize the specific features of different organ injury is imperative.

US is used in the emergency setting for evaluation of free intra-abdominal fluid via the FAST. During this study, the surgeon or emergency physician uses US to assess the areas most likely to contain free fluid or blood. These locations include the following (the first three have been discussed previously in this chapter):

- Hepatorenal fossa or Morrison's pouch
- Perisplenic space
- Pelvis
- Pericardial sac

The presence of blood in these locations necessitates more urgent action, such as taking the patient to the operating room. In many major trauma centers, the availability of rapid CT obviates the FAST exam.

Because of the critical nature of these observations, specific detail of individual findings in the trauma setting will be described.

Organ injury

Injury to visceral organs is a common finding in serious trauma cases, most commonly seen in high-speed motor vehicle collisions (MVC), although penetrating injuries such as gunshot wounds (GSW) or blunt force traumas are also a cause.

For all organs, one of the key findings is the presence of active contrast extravasation. This means that there is an active vascular injury that has not clotted and the blood (along with the IV contrast) is actively extravasating. This is a serious finding and often necessitates either operative intervention or less invasive interventional radiology catheter-based transarterial embolization of the bleeding vessel.

Below are some of the most common types of injuries. In terms of acute traumatic imaging findings, CT will be focused upon, since it is the most commonly used, and the best, modality to evaluate major trauma:

- Laceration: This typically is a tear in the visceral organ. On CT, this takes the form of a linear hypoattenuation through the tissue. It is important to notice whether a laceration traverses through an important vascular structure such as the intrahepatic portal veins.
- Contusion: This is a bruise within the tissue that takes the form of an irregular or rounded focus of hypoattenuation. More often seen with blunt trauma.
- Subcapsular hematoma: Solid abdominal organs such as the liver and kidneys have a capsule. Occasionally, a hematoma forms along

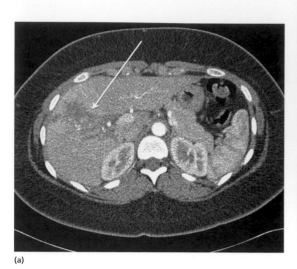
(a)

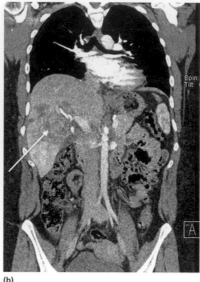
(b)

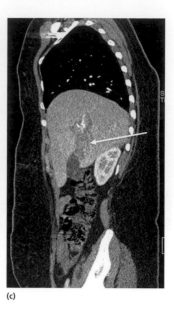
(c)

Figure 5.22 Liver laceration—Axial (a), coronal (b), and sagittal (c) contrast-enhanced CT images demonstrate a grade IV–V laceration involving the right hepatic lobe (arrows), with associated contusion of the parenchyma.

the surface of the organ but still within the capsule. This expanding hematoma can exert extrinsic compression on the organ, deforming the normal contours. In the kidneys, a large hematoma can compress the renal parenchyma sufficiently to cause renal ischemia, if not treated in a timely fashion.

- Pseudoaneurysm: Injury to the arterial structures can cause a tear in the intimal and medial layers of the vessel wall and create a false aneurysm, with the bleeding contained within only a thin adventitial layer. These can rupture and result in life-threatening hemorrhage either at the time of the injury or at a later date. These take the form of a globular contrast "bubble" or "blush" and can sometimes be quite subtle (Figure 5.22).

A few other points regarding abdominal trauma are:

- The spleen is the most commonly injured visceral organ. Pay special attention to the spleen if there are left lower rib fractures. Splenic pseudoaneurysms are a relatively common complication and require timely treatment to prevent life-threatening hemorrhage.
- "Handlebar" or "seat belt"-type injuries: the midabdomen takes the brunt of the force, resulting in pancreatic, left hepatic lobe, and duodenal trauma. Pancreatic lacerations can be subtle, and a high degree of suspicion should be maintained if there is relevant clinical history to indicate this type of injury.
- Subcutaneous soft tissue injuries: These take the form of amorphous foci of stranding in the subcutaneous fat and serve as valuable markers of possible intra-abdominal injuries directly in line with them. Frequently, a "seat belt" sign is seen within the anterior subcutaneous tissues; localized, horizontal fat stranding in the anterior subcutaneous tissues where the seat belt lies across the abdomen.
- Bowel injury can be difficult to diagnose and is discussed in the following.

For more information about this topic, refer to the recommended reading [7].

Ruptured viscus

A ruptured viscus is a major finding that involves urgent operative management. Findings on imaging include:

- Free air
- Bowel wall thickening

- Adjacent mesenteric fat stranding or frank free fluid
- Focally decreased bowel wall enhancement

In cases of penetrating trauma, a very high level of suspicion regarding bowel injury should be maintained (especially in cases of GSW) as bowel injury requires emergent operative repair. If the initial scan (done without oral contrast) is negative and the patient is clinically stable, a repeat study with oral contrast may be warranted to definitively rule out bowel injury.

Urinary bladder rupture

Rupture or perforation of the urinary bladder is an important finding and is associated with pelvic fractures. If there is suspicion of bladder injury (irregularity of the bladder wall, pelvic fractures, or moderate volume pelvic free fluid), a delayed phase scan (20 min to 1 h, allowing time for the kidneys to excrete contrast into the bladder) or a CT cystogram (the study conducted after instilling contrast directly into the bladder through an existing Foley catheter) should be performed. There are two types of bladder rupture, and classification is important as it impacts care:

- Intraperitoneal rupture: If the dome of the bladder ruptures, the result is urine extravasation within the peritoneal cavity. This necessitates surgical correction due to the high risk of complications. On CT, this takes the appearance of a collapsed superior bladder with free intraperitoneal fluid, usually surrounding/abutting loops of bowel.
- Extra- or retroperitoneal bladder rupture: If the base of the bladder is injured, the urine extravasates into the extraperitoneal space. This has a unique CT appearance that is often termed the "molar tooth" sign. This is usually managed nonsurgically.

For more information about this topic, refer to the recommended reading [8] (Figure 5.23).

Infection/inflammation

The concept of stasis leading to pathology has been described in the "Normal anatomy and general concepts" section, and this is a common underlying theme for the various types of intra-abdominal infections, which will be described in this section.

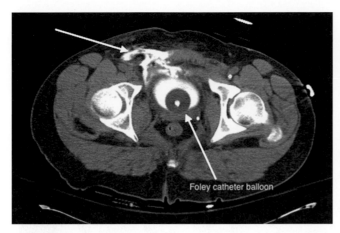

Figure 5.23 Extraperitoneal bladder rupture—Single axial image from a CT cystogram demonstrates anterior pelvic extraperitoneal extravasation of contrast/urine from a ruptured bladder (arrow). Foley catheter is noted within the bladder (arrow).

Appendicitis

The appendix is a blind-ending tubular structure arising from the cecum.

In the normal state, the ostium of the appendix needs to be patent; and if it becomes occluded, due to lymphoid hyperplasia, a fecalith/appendicolith, or inspissated stool, this is sufficient to cause stasis, inflammation, and bacterial superinfection in the blind-ending tube distally. The appendix is typically located in the RLQ but can have a variable position depending on the mobility of the cecum.

Plain radiography is often the first imaging test, but is generally not helpful in either identifying or ruling out this process. In complicated appendicitis (with perforation), free air may be seen on an upright abdominal radiograph.

CT has become the imaging modality of choice for evaluation of suspected acute appendicitis. In children, US is used most often (described in the chapter on pediatric radiology), and MRI may be approximately equivalent to CT in all subjects. MRI is used in pregnant patients due to the lack of ionizing radiation. Relevant imaging findings of uncomplicated acute appendicitis on both CT and MRI include:

- Dilatation of the appendix caliber, usually over 7 mm
- Wall thickening
- Periappendiceal fat stranding or small-volume frank free fluid (increased T2 signal on MRI)

In roughly 25% of patients with untreated acute appendicitis, this progresses, leading to perforation and abscess formation. Clinically, this can present as a sudden transient resolution of the severe RLQ pain, followed by signs of peritonitis (guarding and rebound). In those cases, the imaging findings include the aforementioned, plus:

- Free air.
- Larger volume free fluid. This fluid can organize and form an abscess.

For more information about this topic, refer to the recommended reading [9] (Figure 5.24).

Cholecystitis

Gallstones are common, seen in approximately 15–20% of the population. Of these, roughly 80% are asymptomatic. In the remaining 20%, the stones can obstruct the cystic or bile ducts. If the obstruction is transient, then the result is periodic colicky pain. However, continued obstruction of the cystic duct leads to stasis of

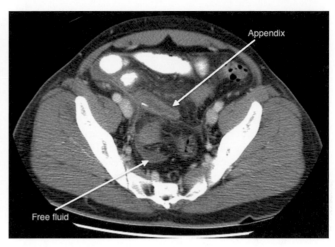

Figure 5.24 Appendicitis—Single axial contrast-enhanced image of the lower abdomen demonstrates a dilated blind-ending viscus with wall thickening and mesenteric stranding (arrow). Small-volume-dependent free fluid is also noted in the pelvis (arrow).

the bile within the gallbladder, which in turn leads to inflammation secondary to the existing bile salts and bacterial overgrowth, thereby causing acute cholecystitis.

Imaging is essential in differentiating acute cholecystitis from other causes of RUQ pain (including hepatitis, peptic ulcer disease, etc.), which is imperative so the correct patient management is performed. Acute cholecystitis is managed surgically, whereas the other causes of RUQ pain are managed medically.

Calculous cholecystitis, or cholecystitis related to the presence of gallstones, is common and will be described in the following. Acalculous cholecystitis is a relatively rare entity that involves inflammation of the gallbladder in the absence of stones, typically noted in critically sick patients who are often bed bound in an ICU setting (burn patients, patients on total parenteral nutrition (TPN)).

Imaging findings

US is the best first test in cases of RUQ due to its low cost, speed, negligible side effects, and high sensitivity and specificity in diagnosing cholelithiasis and acute cholecystitis. Relevant US findings include:

- Gallstones—rounded echogenic foci with posterior shadowing within the gallbladder. Most gallstones are mobile (move with change in patient position), but stones stuck in the gallbladder neck, cystic duct, or biliary ducts (choledocholithiasis) are not.
- Sludge—ill-defined, hyperechoic, layering material without posterior shadowing within the gallbladder.
- Gallbladder wall thickening—normal gallbladder wall thickness is under 3 mm. With inflammation, the wall becomes thickened and edematous. Gas within the gallbladder wall is a critical finding, since this indicates emphysematous cholecystitis (which has a high mortality rate).
- Pericholecystic fluid—the inflammatory process gives rise to free fluid, which localizes around the gallbladder. In gallbladder perforation secondary to untreated infection, free bile can result in a similar appearance. If gas is noted in a pericholecystic fluid collection, this is diagnostic of an abscess.
- Positive sonographic Murphy sign—focal tenderness when US transducer is pressed down over the gallbladder. The ability to create this clinical test with an imaging method is somewhat unique to US.

- The presence of septations within the gallbladder lumen suggests the presence of gangrenous cholecystitis.
- It is important to look at the continuity of the gallbladder wall for signs of possible perforation.

MRI is as sensitive and specific as US, and all of the above findings (with the exception of the sonographic Murphy sign) can be accurately established. Due to the relative speed and low expense of US, MRI is typically reserved for complicated or equivocal cases or when CBD stones are suspected. MRI enables accurate visualization of the complete biliary and pancreatic ductal system via MRCP. This noninvasive alternative to ERCP is excellent for the detection of choledocholithiasis and associated complications.

While findings of acute cholecystitis can occasionally be made on CT, CT is inferior to US or MRI for detection of biliary pathology and is mainly used to rule out alternative pathology once the initial RUQ US is negative.

NM

Hepatobiliary scintigraphy scan is a functional study that examines for cystic and CBD patency. This test is rarely used nowadays, but there are occasionally settings where it may be employed. Technetium-labeled HIDA is used, and the study is often called an HIDA scan. The combination compound is quickly taken up by the liver after injection. It is then incorporated into the bile and excreted into the gallbladder (via the cystic duct) and duodenum (via the CBD). Failure of gallbladder visualization after 4 h usually means the cystic duct is blocked, indicative of acute cholecystitis. Similarly, failure to visualize tracer activity in the small bowel indicates blockage of the CBD. Of note, patients who have been without food or drink for prolonged times can have false-positive examinations.

Morphine can be used to enhance the specificity of this test, as it causes contraction of the sphincter of Oddi and preferentially causes the bile to enter the gallbladder.

For more information about this topic, refer to the recommended reading [10].

In patients with acute cholecystitis who are poor surgical candidates, image-guided percutaneous decompression with cholecystostomy tube placement is a common treatment option. This is discussed in more detail in Chapter 12 (Figures 5.25, 5.26, and 5.27).

Pancreatitis

Pancreatitis is divided into acute and chronic types. Acute pancreatitis refers to recent onset pancreatic inflammation. Chronic pancreatitis is the result of long-term inflammation that affects the normal functioning of the pancreas, which often experiences periods of intermittent acute inflammation. Although chronic pancreatitis can be the result of damage accrued after repeated bouts of acute pancreatitis, often, it is a progressive chronic disease process in isolation and in this setting may be genetic in origin. The underlying problem of pancreatitis is disruption of the pancreatic tissue and autolysis of the pancreatic and peripancreatic tissues by the pancreatic enzymes (unlike the liver and kidneys, the pancreas does not have a capsule). The two most common causes of acute pancreatitis are gallstones (due to stone impaction within the distal biliary system, where obstruction of the pancreatic duct then may occur, and stasis of pancreatic enzyme secretion) and alcohol. Autoimmune pancreatitis is becoming an increasingly more commonly recognized cause of acute pancreatitis. Iatrogenic causes (secondary to ERCP) and trauma are less common causes.

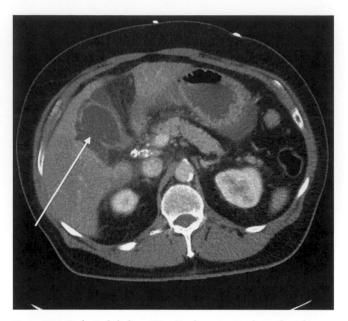

Figure 5.25 Perforated cholecystitis—Single contrast-enhanced axial image of the abdomen demonstrates mucosal enhancement of the thickened gallbladder wall. There is break in the gallbladder wall (arrow), with associated pericholecystic free fluid/bile.

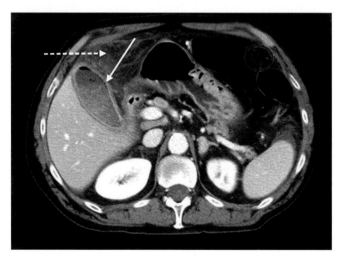

Figure 5.26 Gangrenous cholecystitis – Single contrast enhanced axial image of the abdomen demonstrates wall thickening and mucosal enhancement of the gallbladder wall, with a tiny locules of intramural air (solid arrow). Prominent pericholecystic mesenteric stranding is also noted (dashed arrow); compare this stranding to normal low attenuation fat in the left upper quadrant (circle).

Acute pancreatitis imaging

Acute pancreatitis is primarily a clinical diagnosis. Imaging should be reserved for equivocal cases or to rule out complications of pancreatitis (discussed in the following). However, in daily practice, imaging is often performed at presentation. CT is typically the most frequently used modality, but MRI is more sensitive and specific for this diagnosis and should be used in a variety of complex cases.

Findings of uncomplicated pancreatitis include:

- Pancreatic enlargement (can be focal or diffuse).
- Relative signal change due to edema:
  - Hypoattenuation on CT
  - High signal on T2 and variable signal intensity and enhancement on T1-weighted MRI

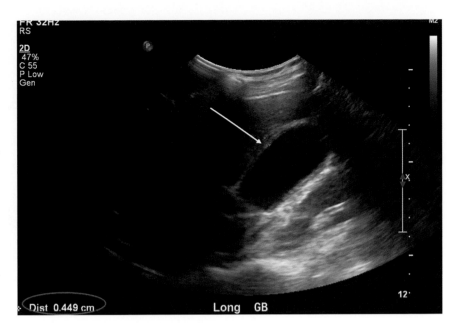

Figure 5.27 Chronic acalculous cholecystitis—Single longitudinal ultrasound image of the gallbladder demonstrates wall thickening (arrow), but no gallstones or sludge. Note that the measured thickness (bottom left of image) exceeds 3 mm.

- Stranding of the peripancreatic fat.
- Frank peripancreatic fluid.
- Obstructing gallstone may be seen in the biliary tree on MRCP images (usually only if the stone is calcified, which is rare with biliary stones, can the stone be seen on CT).

Complications of acute pancreatitis and their imaging findings are:
- Pancreatic necrosis
  ◦ Most important complication given the high mortality rate.
  ◦ Decreased or absent enhancement on CT and T1-weighted MRI images. This can be focal or diffuse.
  ◦ Can progress to emphysematous necrosis, which requires surgical debridement.
- Organized or loculated peripancreatic fluid collections
  ◦ Most common complication.
  ◦ Acutely, these are just organized fluid collections that can resolve with time.
  ◦ When they persist beyond approximately 6 weeks, they often will develop a fibrous capsule and are then termed pseudocysts. Pseudocysts may require percutaneous drainage if large and not spontaneously resolving.
- Pseudoaneurysms
  ◦ Hyperattenuating rounded foci associated with arteries, typically the splenic arterial branches and the gastroduodenal artery
  ◦ On IV contrast administration, demonstrate attenuation similar to arteries
  ◦ Usually require endovascular or surgical repair
- Venous thrombosis
  ◦ Filling defects on contrast-enhanced examinations, typically involving the splenic vein or SMV

For more information about this topic, refer to the recommended reading [11] (Figure 5.28).

Chronic pancreatitis imaging
Unlike acute pancreatitis, this is an imaging-guided diagnosis as symptoms can be vague and lab studies may be equivocal or negative. Chronic pancreatitis involves partial or total loss of the normal exocrine and endocrine function of the pancreas due to chronic inflammation, most commonly secondary to alcoholism, although genetic causes are not uncommon.

Imaging findings on CT and MRI include:
- Multifocal pancreatic calcifications, usually along the pancreatic duct. CT is better at delineating calcifications than MRI.
- Fibrosis, which is often the precursor to calcification, is better recognized on MRI. MRI therefore may be better able to recognize chronic pancreatitis earlier in the course of disease. This may be important in the emergency room setting, as noncalcified chronic pancreatitis is a not uncommon cause of longstanding persistent or intermittent nagging midabdominal pain.
- Atrophy of the pancreatic tissue with pancreatic ductal dilatation:
  ◦ It is important to rule out an underlying pancreatic mass, although clear differentiation is sometimes not possible on imaging alone and biopsy is required. Generally, changes secondary to chronic pancreatitis are diffuse, whereas a pancreatic mass typically causes atrophy and ductal enlargement downstream to the mass.
- Thrombosis of the splenic vein, with formation of varices.

Colitis/enteritis
Colitis is inflammation of the colon/large bowel, while enteritis is inflammation of the small bowel. The bowel involvement can be focal or diffuse, although the former is more common. In terms of pathophysiology, the three most common causes of bowel inflammation are infectious, autoimmune, and ischemic. General features of bowel inflammation will be described, with specific imaging findings that suggest each of the aforementioned causes.

The findings of enteritis are similar to that of colitis, but we will focus on the latter since it is more common.

Plain radiography is useful mainly for ruling out the critical findings of free air, focal bowel dilatation or ileus due to inflammation-mediated loss of peristalsis, and bowel mucosal thickening that occurs with colitis (so-called "thumbprinting" sign). Cross-sectional imaging is generally essential in patients suspected of colitis due to its increased sensitivity and specificity. CT is most commonly used due to its speed and relatively low cost, while MRI is gaining popularity for evaluation of inflammatory bowel disease, especially Crohn's disease in young adults.

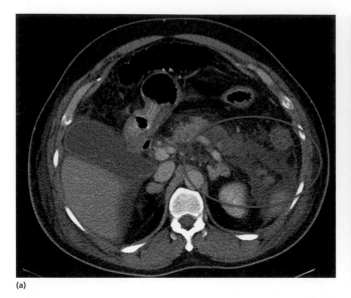

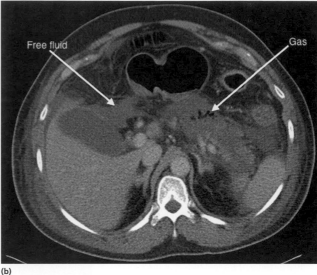

(a) **(b)**

Figure 5.28 Necrotizing pancreatitis—Contrast-enhanced axial CT images of the abdomen demonstrate lack of enhancement of the enlarged pancreatic body and tail, with peripancreatic fat stranding and free fluid (a). Trace gas is also noted within the inflamed, necrotic pancreas (arrow) (b).

The relevant imaging findings of colitis/enteritis include:
- Bowel wall thickening and low attenuation due to inflammation and edema:
  - Focal or diffuse
- Increased mucosal enhancement:
  - The combination of enhancing mucosa and markedly thickened bowel wall is called the "accordion" sign.
- Pericolic fat stranding, which can progress to frank free fluid.
- Findings specific to ischemic colitis are described in the "Mesenteric ischemia" section.
- In inflammatory bowel disease and progressive cases of enterocolitis, breakdown of the bowel wall can result in abnormal connections (fistulas) between bowel loops or between bowel and adjacent structures (urinary bladder, vagina).
- Chronic inflammation in Crohn's or ulcerative colitis (UC) can result in mural fibrosis and focal narrowing (strictures) of the bowel lumen, resulting in functional obstruction.
- Long-standing UC can result in loss of colonic haustration, with a featureless or "lead-pipe" appearance of the colon.

Location is an important consideration and depends on the underlying etiology:
- *Infectious*
  - Clostridium difficile is a type of ischemic colitis that typically affects the entire colon, and the rectum is almost always involved.
  - *Yersinia* enterocolitis and typhoid fever/salmonellosis almost always involve the (distal) ileum. The ascending colon is involved preferentially.
- *Ischemic colitis*
  - The splenic flexure and rectosigmoid junction are watershed regions (where two vascular territories meet, blood supply is often more tenuous) and are affected first and most severely in cases of reduced vascular flow.
- *Inflammatory bowel disease*
  - Crohn's disease can affect the entire GI tract, anywhere from the mouth to the anus. However, the terminal ileum is almost always affected (usually the ileocolic region, which includes the cecum). The involvement of the bowel is discontinuous in many cases resulting in "skip" lesions.

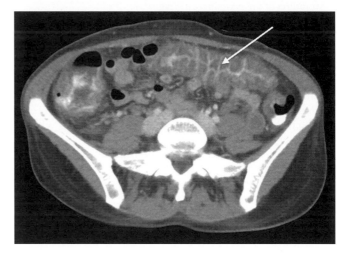

Figure 5.29 Pseudomembranous colitis—Single contrast-enhanced axial image of the lower abdomen demonstrates marked long-segment wall thickening of the colon, with near obliteration of the lumen. Note the linear enteric contrast (arrow) interdigitating between the markedly thickened colonic haustral folds ("accordion sign").

  - UC affects the colon with contiguous involvement from the rectum backward through the colon. Uncommonly, in the setting of complete or pancolitis, a patulous ileocecal valve allows for "backwash" ileitis. Long-standing pancolitis also can result in foreshortened and almost smooth surface to the colon giving a "lead-pipe" appearance. Unlike with Crohn's, focal interspersed areas of sparing are not observed, with the exception that the rectum may appear less involved if the patient has been receiving steroid enemas.

For more information about this topic, refer to the recommended reading [12] (Figures 5.29 and 5.30).

Diverticulitis

Diverticulitis is a specific form of colitis in which the inflammation begins in tiny outpouchings called diverticula. Over half of adults over the age of 60 have diverticula, and the presence of diverticula

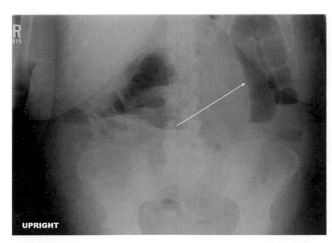

Figure 5.30 "Lead-pipe" colon—Single upright abdominal radiograph demonstrates loss of haustral folds in the distal transverse colon (arrow), consistent with long-standing inflammation secondary to ulcerative colitis.

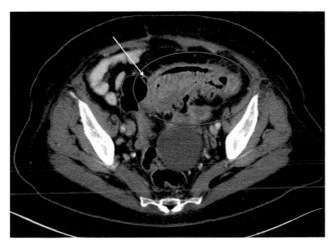

Figure 5.31 Diverticulitis—Single contrast-enhanced axial image of the lower abdomen demonstrates wall thickening, mucosal enhancement, and pericolonic fat stranding involving a focal segment of the sigmoid colon. Background of colonic diverticulosis is also present (arrow).

without superimposed inflammation is called diverticulosis. Not uncommonly, there is luminal obstruction of one or more of these diverticula, which results in stasis, inflammation, and bacterial superinfection that results in diverticulitis (not unlike the pathophysiology of appendicitis discussed earlier).

The presence of associated diverticula and usually focal involvement of the colon suggest the diagnosis. Surrounding stranding, often radiating from diverticula, and small adjacent fluid collections are observed. Longer segment involvement can occur.

Like appendicitis, untreated or severe diverticulitis can result in colonic perforation and abscess formation. Another complication is the formation of fistulous connections between the colon and other structures, most commonly between the sigmoid colon and urinary bladder. Uncomplicated diverticulitis can be managed medically. Abscesses require percutaneous image-guided drainage, whereas severe diverticulitis may occasionally require surgical resection of the affected colon after initial antibiotic therapy. Delay in surgery following institution of antibiotics is often essential as tissue that is severely inflamed has a tendency to break down when sutured, which can result in severe patient complications (Figure 5.31).

Urolithiasis and pyelonephritis

Urolithiasis is the presence of stones within the urinary tract and is seen in up to 10–15% of the population. The vast majority of urolithiasis refers to stones within the renal parenchyma or renal collecting system, and nephrolithiasis is therefore used interchangeably.

Most renal stones contain calcium and are well visualized on CT as high-density foci of calcium, due to CT's high sensitivity to calcification. Non-contrast-enhanced CT is preferred for detection of urolithiasis, as IV contrast can mask small stones. Of note, stones associated with antiretroviral medications (such as indinavir) are radiolucent and cannot be detected by CT.

US is less sensitive than CT, and plain radiography is even less sensitive. On US, stones appear as hyperechogenic foci with posterior acoustic shadowing and twinkle artifact on Doppler imaging. As calcium is dark on MRI, MRI performs well at stone detection only if the stone results in substantial ureteral obstruction.

Once stones enter the ureter, the resulting severity of symptoms (flank pain, hematuria) often but not invariably depends on the size of the stone, as much of the appreciation of pain reflects the extent of mural spasm. Stones less than 5 mm may pass spontaneously, while larger stones can cause obstruction of the involved ureter and renal collecting system, resulting in dilatation of the ureter (hydroureter) and the renal collecting system and calyces (hydronephrosis). The location of the obstruction is usually at the junction between the ureter and bladder (UVJ), the narrowest portion of the system.

Another complication of obstructive uropathy-related stasis is pyelonephritis, which is inflammation of the renal parenchyma (+/− bacterial superinfection). Pyelonephritis can be caused by an ascending urinary tract infection or infection of the bloodstream. Symptoms include fever and exquisite tenderness to palpation over the affected kidney (costovertebral angle tenderness). These symptoms plus pyuria establish the clinical diagnosis of pyelonephritis. Imaging may be obtained to rule out underlying stone disease or complications such as abscess formation, particularly in patients who do not respond to antibiotic therapy.

CT and MRI are the preferred modalities for diagnosing pyelonephritis, as US is quite insensitive. The imaging findings are typically unilateral and include:

- Asymmetric wedge-shaped or globular areas of renal cortical hypoattenuation on CT and increased T2 signal on MRI.
- The same areas demonstrate decreased contrast enhancement on both CT and MRI.
- Perinephric fat stranding on CT and increased signal within the perinephric fat on T2-weighted MRI.
- Enlargement of the affected kidney, with distortion of normal cortical contour due to inflammatory swelling.
- Perinephric or intrarenal abscesses may be seen in severe cases.

For more information about this topic, refer to the recommended reading [13] (Figures 5.32 and 5.33).

Cirrhosis

Cirrhosis is the end point of hepatocellular injury, resulting in the combination of fibrosis and nodular hepatocellular regeneration. The causes are many, including but not limited to alcoholism and chronic hepatitis from either viral or autoimmune causes. Although imaging is not entirely sensitive in the primary diagnosis of cirrhosis, there are several associated conditions and complications where imaging is useful. MRI is by far the best imaging modality for evaluation of cirrhosis, although US is used in low-risk patients.

The classic morphologic appearance of a cirrhotic liver involves atrophy of the posterior right lobe, hypertrophy of the caudate lobe

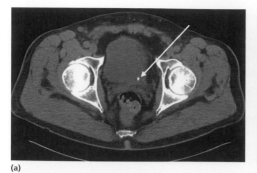

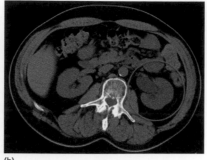

Figure 5.32 Obstructive uropathy—Two unenhanced axial CT images demonstrate a single stone in the left ureterovesicular junction (arrow) (a), with associated ureteral obstruction evidenced by the ipsilateral hydronephrosis (b).

(a)   (b)

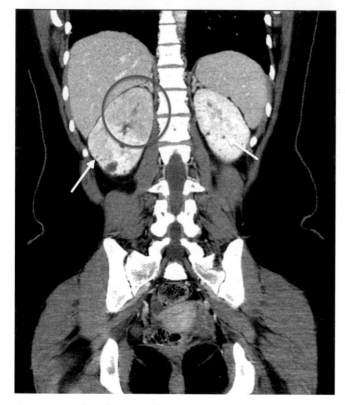

Figure 5.33 Pyelonephritis—Single contrast-enhanced coronal image of the abdomen demonstrates enlargement of the right kidney, with ipsilateral striated nephrogram of the upper pole (oval). Numerous nonenhancing renal cysts are seen bilaterally (arrow).

and left lateral segment, and a nodular contour of the liver. The hepatic parenchyma may demonstrate a heterogeneous appearance (due to underlying fibrosis).

The complications of cirrhosis include:
- Portal hypertension: cirrhosis increased resistance within the portal venous system. These findings are also well evaluated on Doppler US, and include:
  ○ Enlargement of the portal vein, SMV, and splenic vein
  ○ Sluggish portal venous flow and possible thrombosis
  ○ Formation of venous collaterals (varices)
  ○ Splenomegaly
  ○ Ascites
- Hepatic lesions: regenerative nodules, dysplastic nodules, and HCC (the latter is discussed in more detail in the "Neoplasm" section).

- Fibrotic and/or fatty change of the hepatic parenchyma (Figure 5.34).

For more information about this topic, refer to the recommended reading [14].

Orchitis/epididymitis

Orchitis and epididymitis are inflammation of the testicle and epididymis, respectively. Occasionally, these entities can be seen together, which is referred to as "epididymo-orchitis." Inflammation is usually caused by infection (such as gonorrhea or chlamydia).

US is the test of choice for imaging orchitis and epididymitis. Classic imaging features include:
- Asymmetric enlargement and increased hypoechogenicity of the affected testicle or epididymis, secondary to edema.
- Asymmetric increased vascularity.
- Presence of a reactive or complex hydrocele.
- Scrotal wall edema.
- If findings are focal, follow-up imaging is necessary to differentiate findings from neoplastic conditions such as leukemia or lymphoma (Figure 5.35).

Inflammatory conditions of the female pelvis

Pelvic inflammatory disease (PID) is inflammation of the upper female genital tract, usually secondary to underlying infection (most commonly gonorrhea or chlamydia). PID is most prevalent in young, sexually active females. Imaging findings are usually bilateral and consist of soft tissue stranding within the pelvic soft tissues usually with a soft tissue mass-like lesion, thickening of the uterosacral ligaments, dilatation of the fallopian tubes, and potentially abscess formation. If the abscess surrounds the ovary, the diagnosis of a tubo-ovarian abscess is made.

Image findings do not always correlate with the severity of the clinical picture; findings can be subtle in the setting of severe pelvic pain. In general, US is often used to establish the diagnosis. More comprehensive evaluation is obtainable with MRI, which may be indicated in more complicated cases.

For more information about this broad topic, refer to the recommended reading [15].

Neoplasm

Imaging plays an essential role in the diagnosis and management of abdominal neoplasms. Contrast-enhanced CT is often used, with MRI being more important in hepatic, biliary, and pancreatic malignancies. In addition to anatomic imaging, functional imaging with PET plays a role in initial diagnosis, staging, and surveillance.

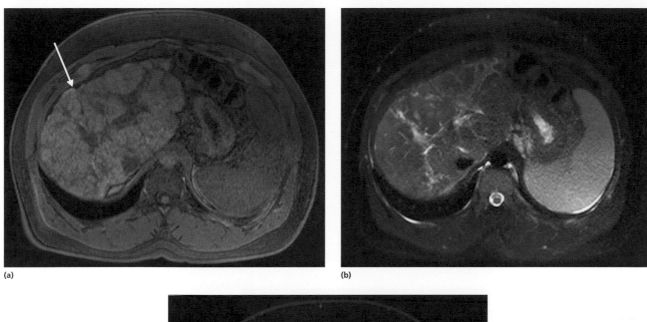

(a)

(b)

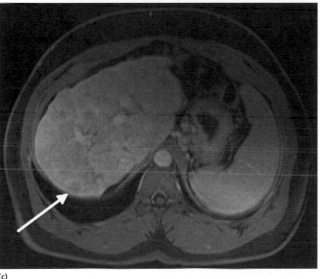

(c)

Figure 5.34 Cirrhosis—Multiple axial MR images demonstrate a nodular liver (a, T1-weighted image with fat saturation) with bands of high T2 signal throughout the liver parenchyma (b, T2-weighted image), suggestive of hepatic fibrosis. There is heterogeneous contrast enhancement on the postcontrast T1-weighted image (c) with a washout lesion that is suspicious for a hepatocellular carcinoma focus (arrow).

Liver

Metastases to the liver and HCC are the two most important and common malignant diseases of the liver. Cholangiocarcinoma is the second most common primary malignant lesion in the liver. These will be described in this section.

Liver metastasis [16]

Liver metastases are far more common than primary hepatic malignancy. The most common primary tumors metastatic to the liver originate from the GI tract, lung, and breast .

Imaging findings of liver metastasis are:

- The hepatic arterial dominant phase of dynamic serial gadolinium-enhanced MR images is particularly important for lesion detection and characterization in patients with known hypervascular primary tumors.
- Generally, hepatic metastases are moderately high in signal intensity on T2-weighted imaging and moderately low in signal intensity on precontrast T1-weighted imaging. The ring enhancement

pattern on early-phase images is the most characteristic appearance of liver metastases.

HCC

HCC is the most common primary visceral malignancy worldwide, accounting for almost 90% of primary liver malignancies. This is mainly due to the high prevalence of (primarily hepatitis-induced) cirrhosis. As discussed previously, cirrhosis leads to formation of hepatic lesions. The histology of these lesions occurs on a spectrum, and the nodules most often advance histologically stepwise from more benign to frankly malignant, with regenerative nodules on the benign end and HCC on the malignant end. In patients with cirrhosis, close imaging surveillance is performed, as early detection of HCC improves survival.

On MR, HCC has a variable appearance on T1-weighted imaging and demonstrates isointensity to mild hyperintensity on T2-weighted imaging.

The main imaging features of HCC are arterial hyperenhancement, early washout of contrast, and late capsular enhancement. This

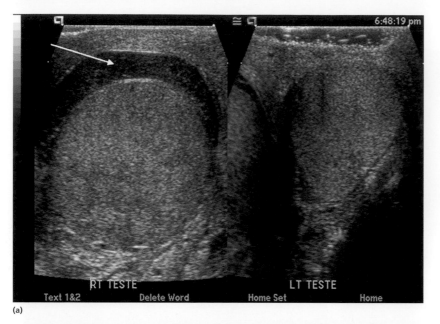

(a)

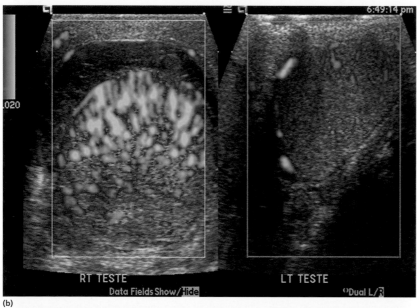

(b)

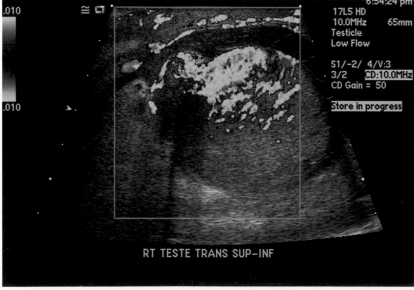

(c)

Figure 5.35 Epididymo-orchitis—Multiple ultrasound images of the testes demonstrate asymmetric enlargement of the right testicle (a and b) with associated hyperemia of both the right testicle (b) and epididymis (c) relative to the normal left side. Small complex right hydrocele is also present (a, arrow).

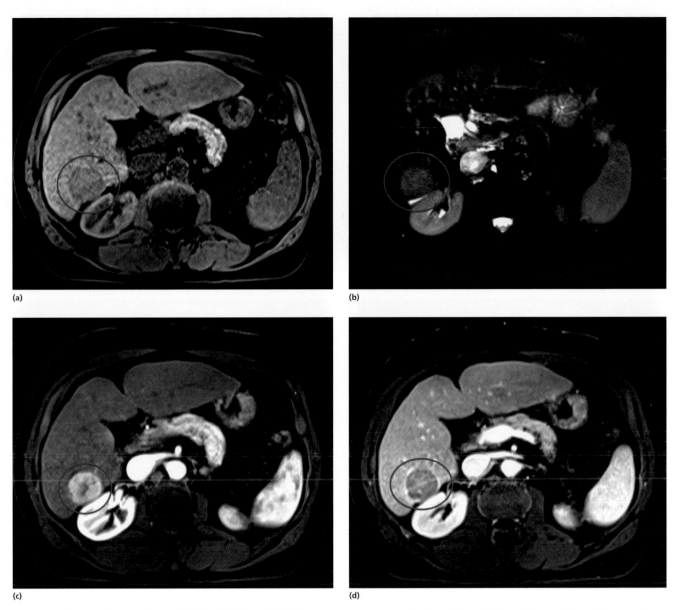

(a)

(b)

(c)

(d)

Figure 5.36 Hepatocellular carcinoma (HCC)—Multiple axial MR images demonstrate a mass in the right hepatic lobe. The mass is hypointense on the precontrast T1-weighted image (a) and slightly hyperintense on the T2-weighted image (b). It also demonstrated early enhancement on the arterial-phase postcontrast T1 image (c), followed by washout with persistent peripheral enhancement on the portal venous-phase postcontrast T1 image (d).

pattern is seen on both contrast-enhanced CT and MR. However, MR is preferred due to its superior soft tissue contrast and ability to differentiate HCC from regenerative and dysplastic nodules.

HCC can invade the portal vein, with tumor thrombus visible on cross-sectional and US imaging.

For more information about this topic, refer to the recommended reading [17] (Figure 5.36).

Cholangiocarcinoma

Cholangiocarcinoma is adenocarcinoma of the biliary ductal epithelium and typically takes the form of an infiltrative periductal mass at the hepatic hilum (Klatskin tumor). Less commonly, intrahepatic cholangiocarcinomas present as a solid mass.

Like other hepatic lesions, MRI is the preferred modality for evaluation of cholangiocarcinoma as it allows good visualization of both the parenchyma and the ductal system (via MRCP).

Imaging features of this lesion include:

- Infiltrative mass with progressive delayed contrast enhancement
- Generally peripheral hyperintensity and central hypointensity on T2-weighted imaging
- Occasionally causes overlying retraction of the hepatic capsule
- Enhancing soft tissue along the biliary ductal system (for infiltrative ductal-type tumors)
- Regional lymph node metastases
- Vascular encasement
- No washout or late capsule formation (Figures 5.37 and 5.38)

Kidney
Renal cell carcinoma

Renal cell carcinoma (RCC) is the most common renal malignancy, accounting for approximately 80% of cases. This tumor arises from the renal cortex. If diagnosed early, surgery can be curative, as more

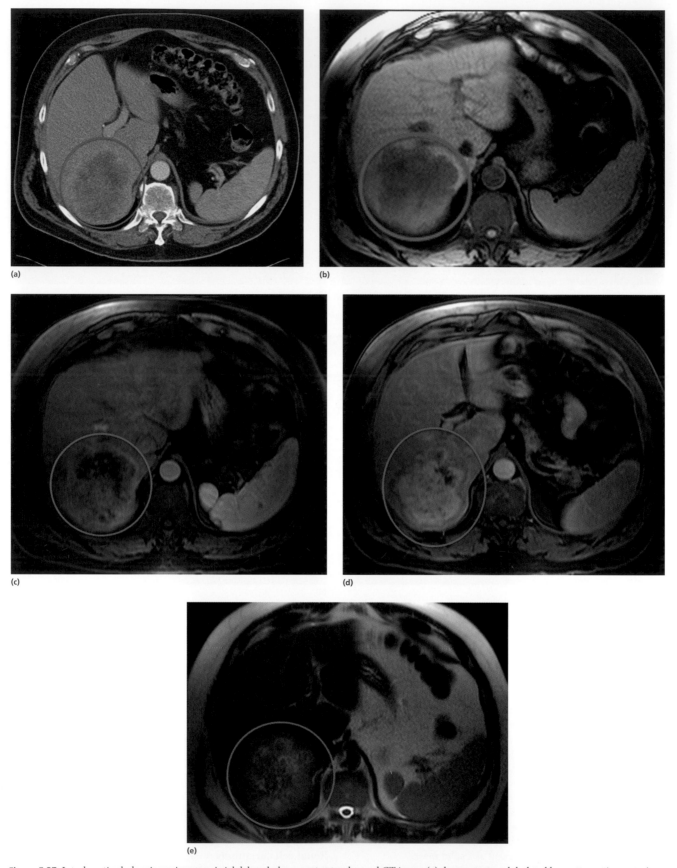

Figure 5.37 Intrahepatic cholangiocarcinoma—Axial delayed phase contrast-enhanced CT image (a) demonstrates a lobulated hypoattenuating mass in the posterior right hepatic lobe. On precontrast T1-weighted MR image (b), the mass is hypointense. On arterial-phase postcontrast T1-weighted MR image (c), the mass shows heterogeneous enhancement, followed by persistent enhancement relative to the liver parenchyma on the portal venous phase (d) due to its fibrous stroma. On T2-weighted MR image (e), the mass demonstrates peripheral hyperintensity (viable tumoral tissue) and central hypointensity (fibrosis).

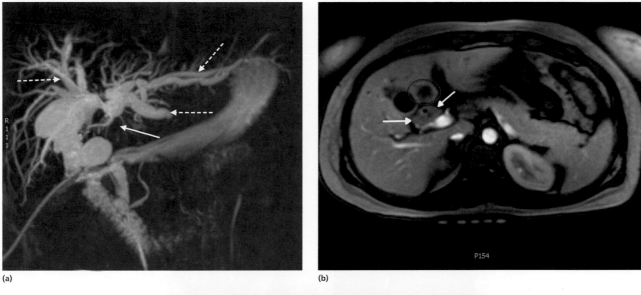

(a)

(b)

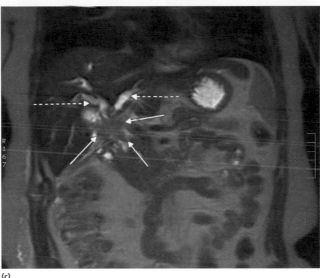

(c)

Figure 5.38 Klatskin tumor – Coronal Maximum Intensity Projection (MIP) image (38a) from a Magnetic resonance cholangiopancreatograph (MRCP) sequence demonstrates marked intrahepatic biliary dilatation (dashed arrows) with high-grade narrowing of the superior aspect of the common bile duct (soild arrow). This narrowing is secondary to the presence of cholangiocarcinoma ("Klatskin tumor") arising at the confluence of the right and left biliary systems. Axial post-contrast arterial phase MRI T1-weighted image (38b) demonstrates circumferential mass-like thickening of the common bile duct (arrows), again compatible with Klatskin tumor. Additionally, there is a poorly enhancing low signal intensity mass in segment IV of the liver (circle), adjacent to the gallbladder fossa, likely metastatic disease. Coronal MRI T2-weighted image (38c) demonstrates an irregular mass (with slightly increased T2 signal intensity) arising from the confluence of the right and left biliary systems (arrows). Marked intrahepatic ductal dilatation is again noted (dashed arrows).

advanced disease carries a poor prognosis. As tumors can be clinically silent until they have reached a large size, imaging is a vital component in initial diagnosis and surveillance of this disease. Contrast-enhanced CT or MRI is the preferred modality for evaluation of renal masses. RCC has the following imaging features:

- Typically exophytic soft tissue lesion arising from the renal cortex.
- Heterogeneous mass with enhancement on contrast-enhanced images. Larger lesions often demonstrate internal necrosis and hemorrhage.
- Noncontrast appearance can be variable on CT and of similar intensity to renal tissue.
- Invasion of the renal vein with enhancing tumor thrombus is not uncommon.
- Although the vast majority of renal cysts are benign, a small percentage can represent cystic RCC. There are several features

(septations, calcification, complex/proteinaceous contents) that suggest that a cystic lesion requires further follow-up [18].

For more information about this topic, refer to the recommended reading [19] (Figure 5.39).

TCC, also known as urothelial carcinoma

TCC is a malignancy arising from the renal collecting system, ureters, and bladder. Although the vast majority of these (90%) arise from the bladder, synchronous and/or metachronous lesions in the upper urinary tracts are not uncommon, and imaging evaluation of the upper tracts accompanies cystographic evaluation of the bladder.

The primary imaging modality for evaluation of TCC is the multiphasic contrast-enhanced CT. The excretory phase, where the contrast is within the renal collecting system and bladder, is most important as TCC appears as a filling defect and often accompanied

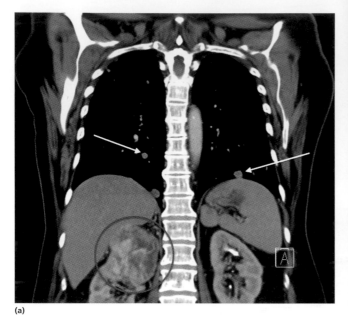

(a)

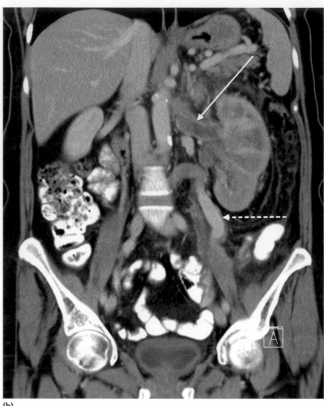

(b)

Figure 5.39 Renal cell carcinoma (RCC)—Single contrast-enhanced coronal image of the abdomen demonstrates a heterogeneous mass arising from the upper pole of the right kidney (a), with multiple lung metastases (arrows). Coronal contrast-enhanced CT image from a different patient (b) shows an enlarged edematous left kidney with infiltrative tumor, with a large poorly enhancing filling defect in the ipsilateral renal vein (solid arrow) that represents tumor thrombus. Also note prominent dilatation of the left gonadal vein (broken arrow) due to obstruction of the left renal vein.

by proximal dilatation of the system. MRI can perform in a comparable fashion, although with MRI emphasis is placed on directly visualizing enhancing tumor to establish the diagnosis (Figure 5.40).

Pancreatic

Pancreatic adenocarcinoma is the most common pancreatic malignancy and carries a very poor prognosis due to the high rate of local peripancreatic tissue and vascular invasion and metastases at the time of diagnosis.

Imaging findings include:
- Irregular, heterogeneous mass with decreased enhancement compared to the normal pancreatic tissue.
- Compared to normal pancreas, the mass is hypodense on CT, T1 hypointense on MR, and hypoechoic on US.
- Pancreatic duct dilatation and tissue atrophy distal to the lesion.
- Local invasion/encasement of the SMA/SMV and mesenteric root is common and precludes surgical cure.
- Distant metastases to the liver and regional lymph nodes are most common.

For more information about this topic, refer to the recommended reading [20].

Islet cell tumors of the pancreas are rare. They are clinically interesting because of their unregulated secretion of hormones. Insulinoma and gastrinoma are the two most common typed tumors. Many of these tumors however go untyped. MRI is the best method to detect these tumors; many are hypervascular (in contrast to pancreatic cancer, which is hypovascular) and show

moderately high signal on T2 and moderately low signal on fat-suppressed T1-weighted images.

Ovarian

Although ovarian cancer is the fifth most common malignancy in women, it is a disproportionately higher cause of mortality, primarily because of its advanced stage at the time of initial diagnosis.

Imaging plays an important role in all phases of this disease—initial diagnosis, staging, assessment of treatment response, and surveillance. US is often used as the initial modality for characterization an ovarian mass, but CT and MRI are used for staging and response assessment, as they provide more overall topographic display of the entire abdomen and pelvis. There are several different subtypes of ovarian cancer, with the epithelial tumors (serous, mucinous, and endometrioid) comprising approximately 80% and germ cell tumors making up most of the remainder.

Imaging findings include:
- Heterogeneous unilateral or bilateral adnexal lesions ranging from cystic with septations to almost completely soft tissue density.
- Peritoneal metastatic disease and carcinomatosis take the form of enhancing soft tissue nodules and are an important finding, portending a poor prognosis. These lesions often involve the omentum and peritoneal surfaces of the liver and paracolic gutters.
- Ascites (Figure 5.41).

For further details regarding ovarian cancer, refer to the article by Jung et al. [21].

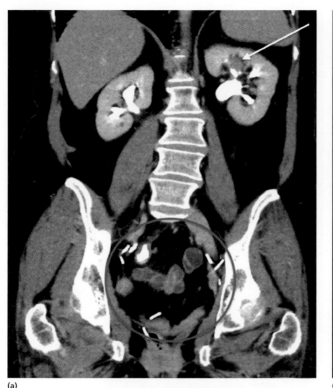
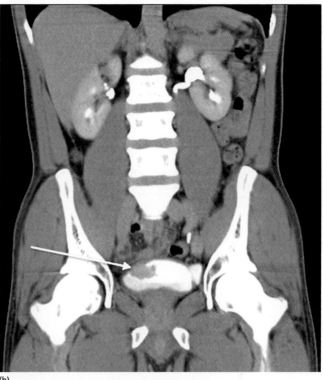

(a)

(b)

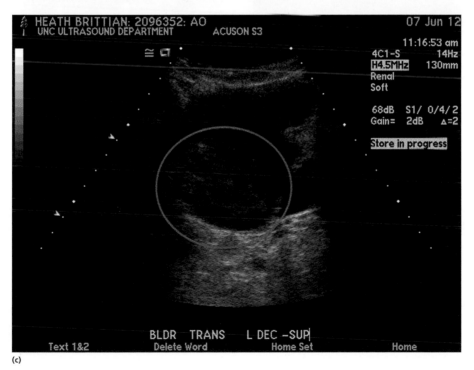

(c)

Figure 5.40 Transitional cell carcinoma (TCC)—Single contrast-enhanced excretory-phase coronal image of the abdomen (a) demonstrates a focal filling defect in the left upper pole calyx (arrow), consistent with TCC. Also note pelvic surgical clips (oval) from resection of the urinary bladder (site of primary disease). Coronal excretory-phase CT image from a different patient (b) demonstrates an irregular soft tissue mass arising from the urinary bladder wall (arrow), which was found to be TCC of the bladder. Ultrasound correlate (c) from this patient shows the same finding.

Lymphoma

Lymphoma is a hematologic malignancy that arises from lymphocytes. It presents as a solid lymphoid tumor and can arise from lymph nodes or lymphoid tissue within any tissue (including the spleen, bone marrow).

In the abdomen, lymphoma typically takes the form of mesenteric or retroperitoneal nodal masses. In contrast to benign causes of retroperitoneal soft tissue formation, lymphoma typically pushes the aorta and IVC anteriorly and away from the spine. In addition, due to the tumor having a soft consistency, it molds to the available

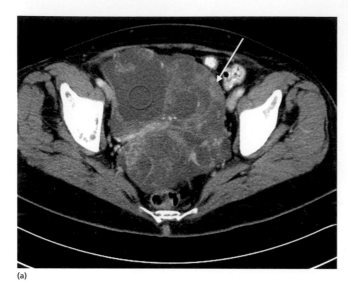

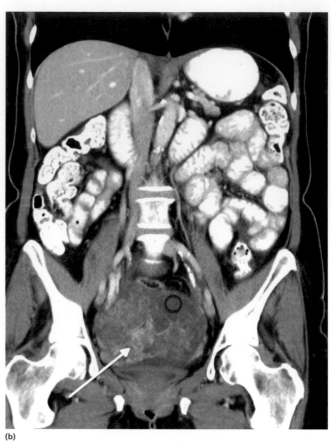

(a)

(b)

Figure 5.41 Ovarian cancer – Contrast-enhanced axial (41a) and coronal (41b) images of the pelvis demonstrate a large, heterogeneously enhancing complex pelvic mass with cystic (circle) and solid (arrow) components.

anatomic space and does not typically cause extrinsic compression or obstruction. This neoplasm also rarely undergoes central necrosis in the untreated state, even when the tumor is large. This also serves as an important distinguishing imaging feature.

PET is extremely (90–95%) sensitive for lymphoma, routinely finding disease in nodes that are not enlarged by CT size criteria (Figure 5.42).

Malignancies of the GI tract

Imaging evaluation of GI tract malignancies (esophageal, gastric, and colon cancer) is typically limited to staging, assessment of treatment response, and detection of metastatic disease both at initial presentation and in the setting of surveillance for recurrent distant disease. Assessment of the primary lesion is often best done through direct visualization with endoscopy, as it is more sensitive at detection and allows obtainment of tissue sample for definitive histologic diagnosis.

Gastric cancer

Gastric cancer typically affects males twice as often as females and is usually diagnosed in the seventh decade of life. While most gastric cancers are sporadic (predisposing conditions include *Helicobacter pylori* infection, pernicious anemia, adenomatous polyps, and dietary nitrates), a small percentage of cases are familial.

The most common form of gastric cancer is adenocarcinoma, which accounts for over 95% of gastric tumors. These tumors can be exophytic or polypoid, ulcerated with an erosive crater, or infiltrative. The infiltrative form leads to thickening and rigidity of the

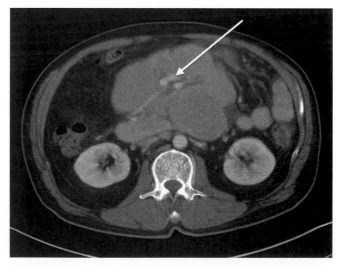

Figure 5.42 Lymphoma—Single contrast-enhanced axial CT image at the level of the kidneys demonstrates a confluent enhancing soft tissue mass in the mesentery that encircles the mesenteric vessels (arrow) but does not compress them. Lymphoma is a "soft" tumor and rarely causes obstruction, even as it grows and encircles vessels and bowel loops.

stomach wall and is commonly called "linitis plastica" ("leather bottle" stomach). Similar to other tumors, prognosis is dependent on the stage of tumor at presentation, but prognosis of gastric adenocarcinoma tends to be poor with a 5-year survival less than 20%.

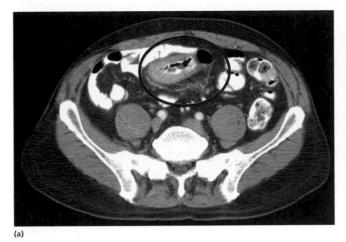
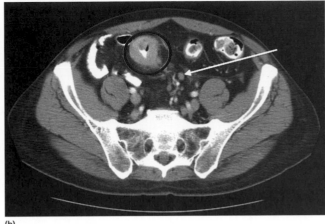

(a)   **(b)**

Figure 5.43 Colon cancer—Axial contrast-enhanced CT images (a and b) demonstrate focal wall thickening and luminal narrowing at the descending colon–sigmoid junction (circle). Multiple prominent mesenteric lymph nodes are also seen (arrow).

Colon cancer

Adenocarcinoma of the colon is the most common GI tract malignancy (following lung and breast cancer in frequency) and the second most common cancer in adults. Imaging is used for detection of local and distant lymph nodes and detection of metastatic disease, which most often develops in the liver, lungs, and bone.

Colon cancer typically arises from tubular and villous adenomas. The former is pedunculated (arises from a stalk), while the latter is usually sessile (with a broad base). Size is a crucial risk factor, and polyps under 1 cm have a minimal risk of harboring malignancy. Although fluoroscopy remains a viable option for colon cancer screening, direct visualization of the colon via colonoscopy has become the more popular method of screening as it allows an instant biopsy of any suspicious lesions. More recently, virtual colonoscopy or CT colonography has emerged as another viable option for screening in low-risk individuals (in whom the chance of a lesion is very low). Conditions that predispose to the development of colon cancer include familial adenomatous polyposis, Gardner syndrome, Lynch syndrome, UC, and Crohn's colitis.

Aside from colonography, CT remains the preferred modality for staging and surveillance of recurrent or metastatic disease in colon cancer. In cases of rectal cancer, MRI is the preferred modality due to its superior performance in the pelvis.

Imaging findings of colon cancer are not specific, but include:

- Circumferential, irregularly marginated, often asymmetric colonic wall thickening with luminal narrowing ("apple-core lesion").
- Affects a short segment of the colon, which can help in distinguishing it from inflammatory causes.
- Nodal and peritoneal metastases. A cluster of local nodes is a suspicious finding (see Figure 5.43).
- Liver is the most common solid organ of metastases.

References

1 Levine, M.S., Scheiner, J.D., Rubesin, S.E. *et al.* (1991) Diagnosis of pneumoperitoneum on supine abdominal radiographs. *American Journal of Roentgenology*, **156**, 731–735.

2 Ho, L.M., Paulson, E.K. & Thompson, W.M. (2007) Pneumatosis intestinalis in the adult: benign to life-threatening causes. *American Journal of Roentgenology*, **188**, 1604–1613.

3 Silva, A.C., Pimenta, M. & Guimarães, L.S. (2009) Small bowel obstruction: what to look for. *Radiographics*, **29**, 423–439.

4 Furukawa, A., Kanasaki, S., Kono, N. *et al.* (2009) CT diagnosis of acute mesenteric ischemia from various causes. *American Journal of Roentgenology*, **192**, 408–416.

5 Chang, H.C., Bhatt, S. & Dogra, V.S. (2008) Pearls and pitfalls in diagnosis of ovarian torsion. *Radiographics*, **28**, 1355–1368.

6 Katabathina, V.S., Kota, G., Dasyam, A.K. *et al.* (2010) Adult renal cystic disease: a genetic, biological, and developmental primer. *Radiographics*, **30**, 1509–1523.

7 Soto, J.A. & Anderson, S.W. (2012) Multidetector CT of blunt abdominal trauma. *Radiology*, **265**, 678–693.

8 Vaccaro, J.P. & Brody, J.M. (2000) CT cystography in the evaluation of major bladder trauma. *Radiographics*, **20**, 1373–1381.

9 Birnbaum, B.A. & Wilson, S.R. (2000) Appendicitis at the millennium. *Radiology*, **215**, 337–348.

10 Hanbidge, A.E., Buckler, P.M., O'Malley, M.E. *et al.* (2004) From the RSNA refresher courses: imaging evaluation for acute pain in the right upper quadrant. *Radiographics*, **24**, 1117–1135.

11 Thoeni, R.F. (2012) The revised Atlanta classification of acute pancreatitis: its importance for the radiologist and its effect on treatment. *Radiology*, **262**, 751–764.

12 Thoeni, R.F. & Cello, J.P. (2006) CT imaging of colitis. *Radiology*, **240**, 623–638.

13 Craig, W.D., Wagner, B.J. & Travis, M.D. (2008) Pyelonephritis: radiologic-pathologic review. *Radiographics*, **28**, 255–277 quiz 327–8.

14 Gupta, A.A., Kim, D.C., Krinsky, G.A. *et al.* (2004) CT and MRI of cirrhosis and its mimics. *American Journal of Roentgenology*, **183**, 1595–1601.

15 Bennett, G.L., Slywotzky, C.M. & Giovanniello, G. (2002) Gynecologic causes of acute pelvic pain: spectrum of CT findings. *Radiographics*, **22**, 785–801.

16 Semelka, R.C. (2010) *Abdominal-pelvic MRI*. Wiley-Blackwell, Hoboken, NJ.

17 Hussain, S.M., Zondervan, P.E., IJzermans, J.N.M. *et al.* (2002) Benign versus malignant hepatic nodules: MR imaging findings with pathologic correlation. *Radiographics*, **22**, 1023–1036 discussion 1037–9.

18 Israel, G.M. & Bosniak, M.A. (2005) How I do it: evaluating renal masses. *Radiology*, **236**, 441–450.

19 Ng, C.S., Wood, C.G., Silverman, P.M. *et al.* (2008) Renal cell carcinoma: diagnosis, staging, and surveillance. *American Journal of Roentgenology*, **191**, 1220–1232.

20 Tamm, E.P., Balachandran, A., Bhosale, P.R. *et al.* (2012) Imaging of pancreatic adenocarcinoma: update on staging/resectability. *Radiologic Clinics of North America*, **50**, 407–428.

21 Jung, S.E., Lee, J.M., Rha, S.E. *et al.* (2002) CT and MR imaging of ovarian tumors with emphasis on differential diagnosis. *Radiographics*, **22**, 1305–1325.

CHAPTER 6

Brain imaging

Joana N. Ramalho[1,2] and Mauricio Castillo[2]

[1]Department of Neuroradiology, Centro Hospitalar de Lisboa Central, Lisboa, Portugal
[2]Department of Radiology, University of North Carolina, Chapel Hill, USA

Introduction

The three main components of the brain are the cerebrum, the cerebellum, and the brainstem. The cerebrum is divided into a right and a left hemisphere by the interhemispheric fissure and is composed of paired frontal, parietal, temporal, and occipital lobes. Basal ganglia (mainly the caudate nucleus, putamen, and globus pallidus) and thalami are deep gray matter structures located off the midline. The cerebellum is located under the cerebrum, and the brainstem is the final pathway between cerebral structures and the spinal cord.

The brain and spinal cord are covered and protected by three layers of meninges: dura, arachnoid, and pia mater. The dura mater is a strong, thick membrane that closely lines the inside of the skull. Its two layers, periosteal and meningeal, are fused and separate only to form venous sinuses and dural folds (such as the tentorium). The dura contains larger blood vessels that split into capillaries in the pia mater. The main dural folds are the falx cerebri, a sickle-shaped structure that separates the cerebral hemispheres, and the tentorium cerebelli, a crescent-shaped structure that separates the occipital and temporal lobes from the cerebellum. Two other dural folds are the falx cerebelli, a vertical infolding that lies inferior to the tentorium cerebelli separating the cerebellar hemispheres, and the diaphragma sella, which covers the pituitary gland and sella turcica. Normally, the dura mater is attached to the skull or to the bones of the vertebral canal. When the dura mater and the bone separate through injury or illness, the space between them is the epidural space. The arachnoid is a thin, weblike membrane that covers the entire central nervous system (CNS). The virtual space between the dura and arachnoid membranes is the subdural space. The pia mater is the meningeal envelope that firmly adheres to the surface of the brain and spinal cord, following the brain's contours (gyri and sulci). The pia mater is pierced by blood vessels to the brain and spinal cord, and its capillaries nourish the brain. The space that normally exists between the arachnoid and pia is the subarachnoid space, which is filled with cerebrospinal fluid (CSF). The arachnoid and pia mater together are sometimes called the leptomeninges or literally thin meninges.

The ventricular system includes the two lateral ventricles that communicate with a third ventricle through the foramina of Monro, the third ventricle that communicates with the fourth ventricle through the cerebral aqueduct, and the fourth ventricle that communicates with the subarachnoid space through the two lateral foramina of Luschka and the single midline foramen of Magendie. The fourth ventricle is continuous with the spinal cord central canal. The third ventricle has two anterior and two posterior protrusions: the supraoptic and the infundibular recesses and the suprapineal and the pineal recesses, respectively.

The CSF is produced mostly by cells of the choroid plexus of the lateral, third, and fourth ventricles. The CSF leaves the ventricular system through the foramina of Luschka and Magendie, flows over the hemispheres within the subarachnoid space, and is absorbed by the arachnoid granulations at the superior sagittal sinus.

The intracranial circulation can be divided into anterior and posterior circulations, on the basis of supply from the internal carotid artery (ICA) and vertebral artery, respectively. At the base of the brain, the anterior and posterior systems form a circle of communicating arteries known as the circle of Willis.

The circle of Willis is formed when the ICA enters the cranial cavity bilaterally and divides into the anterior cerebral artery (ACA) and middle cerebral artery (MCA). An anterior communicating (ACOM) artery bridges the ACAs. Posteriorly, the basilar artery, formed by the left and right vertebral arteries, branches into the left and right posterior cerebral arteries (PCAs), forming the posterior circulation. The PCAs complete the circle of Willis by joining the internal carotid system anteriorly via the posterior communicating (PCOM) arteries. These communications allow equalization of blood flow between the two sides of the brain and permit collateral circulation. A complete circle of Willis is present in about 60–70% of individuals, although well-developed communications between its parts are identified in less than half of the population.

Three vessels supply the cerebellum: the superior cerebellar artery (a branch of the distal basilar artery), the anterior inferior cerebellar artery (a branch of the proximal basilar artery), and the

Critical Observations in Radiology for Medical Students, First Edition. Katherine R. Birchard, Kiran Reddy Busireddy, and Richard C. Semelka.
© 2015 John Wiley & Sons, Ltd. Published 2015 by John Wiley & Sons, Ltd.
Companion website: www.wiley.com/go/birchard

posterior inferior cerebellar artery (a branch of the distal vertebral artery). Perforating arteries from the vertebrobasilar system also supply the brainstem.

The veins of the brain have no muscle in their thin walls and possess no valves. They emerge from the brain and lie in the subarachnoid space; they pierce the arachnoid and the meningeal layer of the dura and drain into the venous sinuses.

There are three main systems for venous drainage of the brain: superficial supratentorial veins, deep cerebral veins, and infratentorial veins. The superficial system comprises the sagittal sinus and cortical veins, which drain the surfaces of both cerebral hemispheres. The deep system consists of the transverse, straight, and sigmoid sinuses along with deeper cortical veins. Both of these systems mostly drain into internal jugular veins. The entire deep venous system is drained by internal cerebral and basal veins, which join to form the vein of Galen that drains into the straight sinus. Though variations in the superficial cerebral venous system are a rule, the anatomic configuration of the deep venous system can be used as landmarks. The infratentorial veins (veins of the posterior fossa) are variable in their course, and angiographic diagnosis of their occlusions is difficult.

Imaging modalities

Among all the imaging techniques available for brain evaluation choosing the best option for a given clinical situation may be a challenge. From a practical point of view, conventional radiography is not used except when documenting fractures for medical/legal reasons. Nuclear medicine studies are useful in specific diseases, such as refractory epilepsy, movement disorders, and dementia in which positron emission tomography (PET)/computed tomography (CT) plays an important role. Ultrasound is useful as the first imaging technique in infants through the still open fontanelles and thin skull bones and also has a role in evaluation of the cervical carotid arteries and intracranial circulation. Catheter digital subtraction angiography is performed in acute setting stenosis, occlusions, or vascular lesions. It is also useful in vascular malformations, aneurysm, and vascular tumors for defining their architecture and for embolization.

The best imaging neuroimaging techniques are CT and magnetic resonance imaging (MRI). As a general rule in brain imaging, CT is performed for acute neurologic illness and MRI for more chronic and subacute conditions or to clarify questionable findings on CT. Nevertheless, CT is the modality of choice for bone evaluation regardless the clinical situation and also plays a role in specific clinical scenarios, including seriously ill patients as those who need assisted ventilation, those who cannot hold still, and patients in whom MRI is contraindicated. Radiation risks of CT and risk of nephrogenic systemic fibrosis (NSF) due to administration of MRI contrast (gadolinium) should not modify the imaging approach for acute neurological syndromes, since the benefits usually exceed the risks.

A standard brain CT consists of axial images processed with brain and bone windows. In certain clinical conditions, such as tumors or abscesses, iodinated contrast may be administered to highlight the lesions. CT angiography (CTA) is used to visualize blood vessels by injecting a large and compact bolus of iodinated contrast intravenously and performing fast and timed image acquisitions. It is an increasingly used technique for acute stroke and aneurysm diagnosis, characterization, and treatment planning. CT perfusion (CTP) measures cerebral perfusion by determining different blood hemodynamic properties including cerebral blood flow (CBF), volume, and time-based parameters. It relies on the first pass of a bolus of contrast during which the brain is imaged sequentially. In clinical practice, CTP is mostly used in acute stroke patients.

A standard brain MRI protocol includes T1- and T2-weighted sequences, diffusion-weighted imaging (DWI), and fluid-attenuated inversion recovery (FLAIR) complemented by T1-WI after gadolinium administration. DWI allows mapping the molecular motion of water in tissues. It takes advantage of the fact that intracellular water molecules have a limited movement compared to extracellular ones. Acute ischemic tissue shows restricted diffusion, seen as bright lesions on DWI with low signal on apparent diffusion coefficient (ADC) maps. This change reflects cytotoxic edema and precedes changes in T2 or FLAIR images making DWI essential in early detection of stroke. DWI is also helpful for tumor, trauma, and infection evaluation. Diffusion of water has also been exploited to map white matter tracts using diffusion tensor imaging (DTI), a technique that relies on the fact that within elongated cell processes such as axons, water diffuses more freely along their longitudinal axis than sideways allowing mathematical reconstructions of white matter tracts (tractography).

Susceptibility-weighted images (SWI) are particularly useful for assessment of hemorrhage and of the veins, while magnetic resonance angiography (MRA) is routinely used for arterial visualization.

MR perfusion imaging refers to several recently developed techniques used to noninvasively measure cerebral perfusion. As in CTP, it is possible to assess various hemodynamic parameters such as cerebral blood volume (CBV), CBF, mean transit time (MTT), and time to peak (TTP). MRI perfusion imaging is particularly useful in cerebrovascular diseases and brain tumors.

Proton magnetic resonance spectroscopy (MRS) is a technique that studies brain metabolites. In practice, three normal metabolites are recognized in brain tissue: choline (Cho), which is a marker of cellular turnover; N-acetyl-aspartate (NAA), which is only found in neurons and therefore is a marker of neuronal density and viability; and creatine (Cr), which is a marker of cellular energetics. Decreased NAA indicates loss or damage to neurons, which results from many types of insults. Increased Cho indicates increase in cell production or membrane breakdown, which can suggest neoplasia and infection or demyelination, respectively. Lactate and lipids are markers of anaerobic metabolism and necrosis, respectively.

Functional magnetic resonance imaging (fMRI) is a procedure that measures brain activity by detecting changes in blood oxygenation and relies on the fact that CBF and neuronal activation are coupled. When an area of the brain is used, its blood flow increases resulting in differences in oxygenation between arterial and venous blood. Reliable localization of motor, visual, auditory, and language areas assists in planning surgery, particularly in tumors or epilepsy. However, the main role of fMRI remains in neurobehavioral and neurophysiological research.

MR and CT permeability are promising techniques that are employed to characterize the functional integrity of the blood–brain barrier (BBB) via estimation of microvascular permeability parameters. However, these techniques still await further clinical validations.

Appearance of normal brain study

CT and MRI scans of the normal brain are shown in Figure 6.1. On CT, the cerebral white matter appears less dense than the gray matter because the white matter contains fat in myelin sheaths.

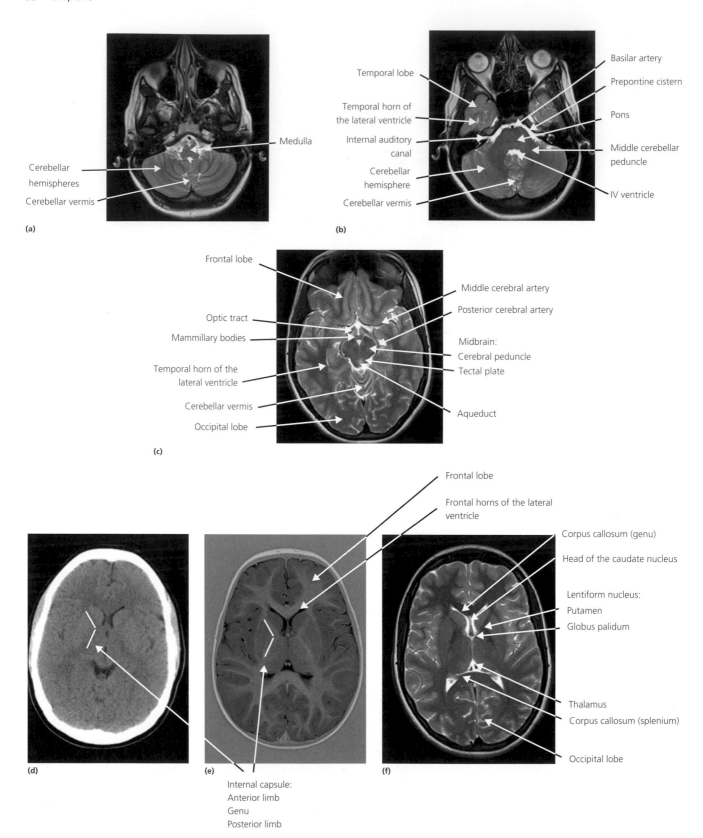

Figure 6.1 CT and MRI scans of the normal brain. Axial T2-WI at the level of the medulla (a), pons (b), and midbrain (c). Axial CT (d), T1-WI (e), and T2-WI (f) at the level of the basal ganglia. Midsagittal T1-WI (g) and coronal T2-WI (h). Sagittal (i) and coronal (j) maximum intensity projection (MIP) image reconstructions from CT angiography and 3D time-of-flight (TOF) MR angiography (k) show the normal course of the common carotid artery (CCA), internal carotid artery (ICA), external carotid artery (ECA), and vertebral arteries (VA). 3D TOF MR angiography (l) of the circle of Willis. (ACA, anterior cerebral artery; ACOM, anterior communicating artery; MCA, middle cerebral artery; PCA, posterior cerebral artery; PCOM, posterior communicating artery; BA, basilar artery) Sagittal (m) and coronal (n) MR venography.

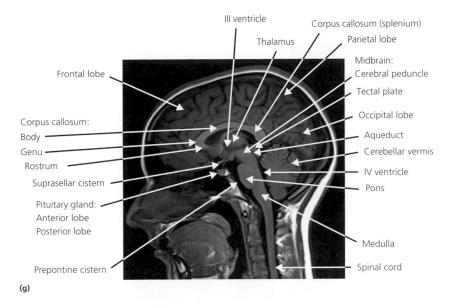

III ventricle
Thalamus
Corpus callosum (splenium)
Parietal lobe
Midbrain:
Cerebral peduncle
Tectal plate
Occipital lobe
Aqueduct
Cerebellar vermis
IV ventricle
Pons
Medulla
Spinal cord

Frontal lobe
Corpus callosum:
Body
Genu
Rostrum
Suprasellar cistern
Pituitary gland:
Anterior lobe
Posterior lobe
Prepontine cistern

(g)

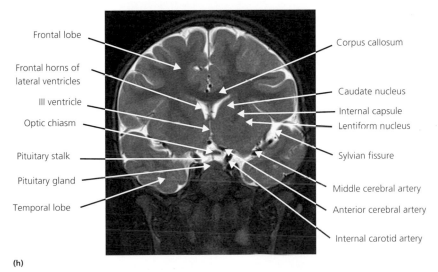

Frontal lobe
Frontal horns of lateral ventricles
III ventricle
Optic chiasm
Pituitary stalk
Pituitary gland
Temporal lobe

Corpus callosum
Caudate nucleus
Internal capsule
Lentiform nucleus
Sylvian fissure
Middle cerebral artery
Anterior cerebral artery
Internal carotid artery

(h)

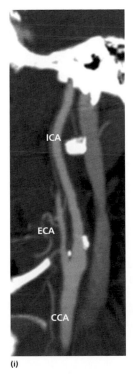

(i)

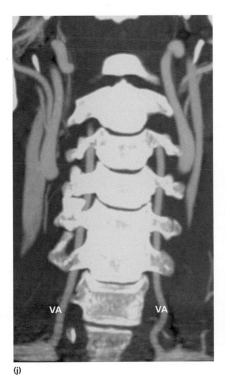

(j)

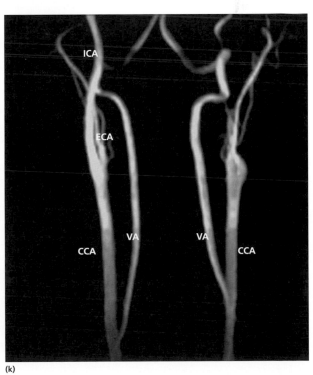

(k)

Figure 6.1 (*Continued*)

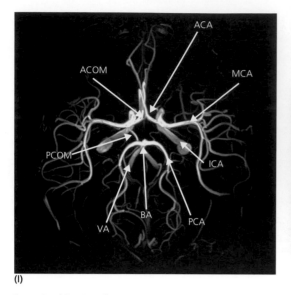

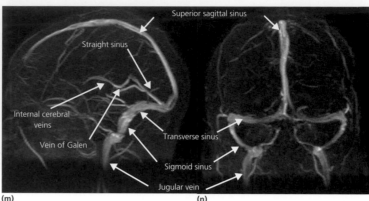

Figure 6.1 (*Continued*)

CSF in the ventricles and subarachnoid spaces appears hypodense, and air and fat are even more hypodense, while bones and calcifications are hyperdense. On CT, the density between different structures remains the same despite the imaging window used. Iodinated contrast agents increase the density of blood inside vessels and vascular structures such as venous sinus so these are hyperdense on postcontrast scans.

MRI is more complicated since the signals of structures vary according to the sequence used. On T1-WI, CSF is hypointense, the white matter is slightly hyperintense compared to the gray matter, and fat-containing structures are strongly hyperintense. Conversely, on T2-WI, CSF has high signal intensity, the white matter is hypointense compared to the gray matter, and fat-containing structures are relatively hypointense. In a simplistic way, most of the brain lesions are hypointense on T1-WI and hyperintense on T2-WI. If an abnormality is hyperintense on T1-WI and hypointense on T2-WI, hemorrhage and fat are probably present. Gadolinium is a paramagnetic substance used as an MRI contrast agent, which shortens T1 and, to a much lesser degree, T2 relaxation time, causing a high T1 signal and low T2 signal in enhancing structures. Postcontrast T1-WI is the most common sequence acquired after gadolinium administration.

Pathological contrast enhancement is due to a breakdown in the BBB or angiogenesis as occurs in tumors, infections, and inflammations. Normal enhancement after contrast administration is seen in structures without BBB, namely, pituitary and pineal glands and the choroid plexi.

The midline of the brain should be in the midline of the skull, and both sides of the brain should look very much alike. Shifts of midline structures or brain asymmetry represent pathologic processes. The sulci pattern should be symmetric, and the interhemispheric fissure should be visualized. The sulci extend out to the inner table of the skull, except in older patients where atrophy occurs and the CSF-containing spaces are widened. The basal cisterns are symmetric and of CSF density/intensity. Some asymmetry of the ventricular system may be normal or may reflect the patient's position in the scanner.

The anatomy of the midline brain is complex and the structures are not duplicated, so the principle of symmetry cannot be applied to its interpretation. On sagittal images, there are three areas that must always be studied: the sella and suprasellar regions, the pineal region, and the craniocervical junction. MRI is the modality of choice for evaluating the sellar, parasellar, and suprasellar regions and the pineal region. Regarding the sellar region, on coronal sections, the pituitary gland is the main structure and rests in a small, midline bony cavity in the sphenoid bone known as sella turcica. The pituitary stalk is a vertically oriented structure, which connects the pituitary gland to the hypothalamus and is thinner at its bottom and thicker superiorly. Another major structure in the suprasellar cistern is the optic chiasm, an extension of the brain where the optic nerves cross. Further cephalic lies the hypothalamus. Anatomically, the hypothalamus forms the lateral walls and floor of the third ventricle. Slightly off the midline are the cavernous sinus and the ICAs. The ICAs have a complex anatomic course passing through the skull base and through the cavernous sinus and then bifurcate into the ACAs and MCAs. The tip of the basilar artery and the PCAs lies at the level of the suprasellar cistern. The pineal gland is adjacent to the dorsal midbrain, which covers the aqueduct of Sylvius. The gland lies superior to the midbrain tectum (quadrigeminal plate).

The craniocervical junction is easily imaged by CT or MRI with axial, coronal, and sagittal views. CT is better for bone evaluation, while MRI is superior for soft tissue assessment. The sharp inferior edge of the bony clivus marks the anterior border of the foramen magnum, known as the basion, and its posterior limit known as the opisthion is the cortical margin of the occipital bone. The cerebellar tonsils should project no more than 5 mm below a line drawn between basion and opisthion. The only structures visualized at the foramen magnum level should be the cervical medullary junction and small portion of cerebellar tonsils.

Critical observations

Mass lesions

The term "mass" is used to mean a space-occupying structure. Because the skull is rigid, a mass lesion results on mass effect upon the brain and displaces the normal cerebral structures away from it. The midline structures may be shifted contralateral to a mass, the sulci adjacent maybe effaced, and the ipsilateral ventricles compressed. Conversely, atrophy is recognized by widening of the ipsilateral sulci or enlargement of the ventricles.

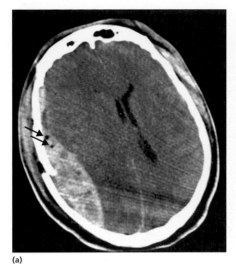
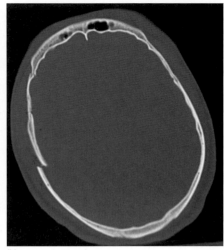

(a) **(b)**

Figure 6.2 Epidural acute hematoma. Axial CT (brain window) (a) shows the characteristic biconvex extra-axial hyperdense collection with mass effect. Note the intracranial pneumocephalus (arrows), an indirect sign of fracture. The bone window (b) shows an underlying depressed fracture.

Brain herniations are secondary to mass effect and can be divided as:

- Subfalcine herniation—the cingulate gyrus is displaced across the midline under the falx cerebri also called "midline herniation."
- Uncal herniation—the medial aspect of the temporal lobe is displaced medially over the free margin of the tentorium.
- Transtentorial herniation—the brain herniates either downward or upward through the tentorial incisura.
- Tonsillar herniation (also called downward cerebellar herniation)—the cerebellar tonsils are displaced downward through the foramen magnum.
- External herniation—the brain herniates through a skull defect.

Trauma

Extracerebral hematomas produce devastating neurologic symptoms that may be completely reversed if treated early.

Epidural hematomas are usually arterial in origin and often result from a skull fracture that disrupts the middle meningeal artery. Epidural hematomas may also occur without fracture, particularly in children. Patients usually present with neurologic deterioration after a lucid interval:

- CT shows a well-defined, high-attenuation, biconvex extra-axial collection that usually does not cross cranial sutures where the periosteal layer of the dura is firmly attached (Figure 6.2).

Subdural hematomas are typically venous in origin and result from stretching or tearing of the cortical veins as they transverse the subdural space:

- CT shows a crescent-shaped, extra-axial, high-attenuation collections typically located along the convexity. Subdural hematomas can also be seen along the fax and tentorium. Because the falx and tentorium are dural folds, a subdural collection does not traverse these structures (Figure 6.3).

Stroke

The management of **acute ischemic stroke** remains challenging due to the limited time window in which the diagnosis has to be made and therapy administered. Intravenous recombinant tissue plasminogen activator (rtPA) within 4.5 h, intra-arterial thrombolysis within 6 h, and mechanical thrombectomy within 8 h of stroke onset are the only treatments currently approved by the US Food and Drug Administration for acute stroke (Figure 6.4):

- CT may be normal or nearly normal.
- Early signs of acute stroke include loss of gray/white matter distinction, low attenuation in the basal ganglia, and poor definition of the cortex in the insula.
- A hyperdense artery, most commonly the MCA, suggests that it contains clot and needs further evaluation by CTA.

MRI is more time consuming and less available than CT but has significantly higher sensitivity and specificity in the diagnosis of acute ischemic infarction, particularly using DWI:

- Diffusion restriction may be seen within minutes following the onset of ischemia.

Ischemic lesions involving a single hemisphere are likely to be caused by a lesion within the carotid circulation ipsilateral to the lesion. However, if those lesions affect both hemispheres, they may represent border zone infarcts resulting from global hypoperfusion or be a result of cardiac or other proximal sources of emboli.

Cerebral venous thrombosis and venous infarct

Cerebral venous thrombosis is an important cause of stroke especially in children and young adults. It is more common than previously thought and frequently missed on initial imaging due to its nonspecific clinical presentation and subtle imaging findings:

- Noncontrast head CT may show a hyperdense sinus or a hyperdense cortical vein. Cerebral edema may also be seen.
- After contrast administration a filling defect in a sinus is present 1–4 weeks after sinus occlusion and seen as an "empty delta" especially in the superior sagittal sinus. Filling defects should not be confused with Pacchionian bodies (arachnoid granulations), which can be seen in essentially all dural sinuses and are especially common in the superior sagittal and transverse sinuses.
- Small venous occlusions are not reliably detected by CT.
- On MRI, venous sinus thrombosis is suspected when venous flow voids are lost and confirmed when the clot is observed.
- An acute clot is isointense on T1-WI and hypointense on T2-WI (this can mimic a flow void), becoming hyperintense on T1-WI in subacute stage.
- MR venography will demonstrate lack of flow in the affected sinus. Hypoplastic dural sinuses and slow flow within veins are potential MRI pitfalls in the diagnosis of venous occlusion.
- Cerebral edema can be identified even in the absence of neurological dysfunction or infarction.

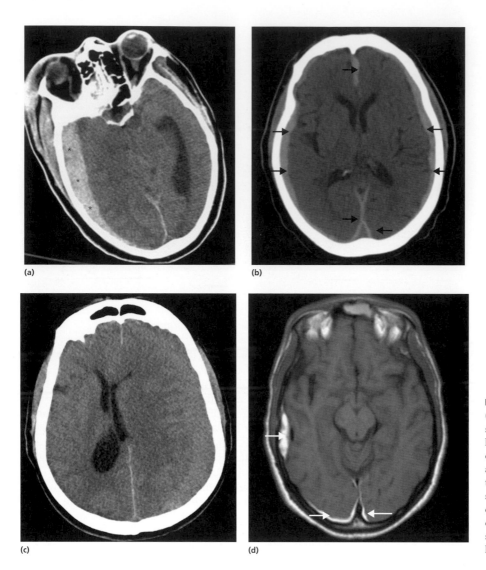

(a)

(b)

(c)

(d)

Figure 6.3 Subdural hematomas. Axial CT (a) shows acute right temporal hematoma, seen as a crescent-shaped extra-axial hyperdense collection (*) with mass effect. In other patient, axial CT (b) shows bilateral acute subdural hematomas extending along the fax (arrows). Axial CT (c) shows left subacute subdural hematoma (*), seen as an extra-axial collection isodense with the brain cortex. Axial T1-W MRI (d) shows high-signal-intensity bilateral subacute subdural hematomas (arrows) in a different patient.

Venous infarctions have a nonarterial distribution in the white matter and/or cortex and are often hemorrhagic. Bilateral cerebral involvement can occur, including the white matter of the convexities from superior sagittal sinus thrombosis, or in the basal ganglia and thalami from deep venous thrombosis in which the internal cerebral veins and vein of Galen may appear hyperdense on noncontrast CT (Figure 6.5).

Subarachnoid hemorrhage

Nontraumatic subarachnoid hemorrhage (**SAH**) is most commonly due to aneurysm rupture. Sudden, severe headache is the most common symptom.

Common locations of ruptured aneurysms include the region of the ACOM artery (33%), MCA (30%), PCOM artery (25%), and basilar artery (10%). Less commonly, they can occur in the ophthalmic artery or in the cavernous ICA or posterior inferior cerebellar artery (Figure 6.6):

- CT is over 90% sensitive for the detection of acute SAH due to the increased density of clotted blood.
- Prompt scanning is important, since the sensitivity CT for SAH decreases to 66% by day 3.
- Nontraumatic SAH requires further workup by CTA to identify an aneurysm.
- Hydrocephalus and vasospasm are common and potentially treatable complications of SAH.

Evaluation and management of aneurysmal SAH have changed considerably over the past 10 years due to wider application of CTA and endovascular coil embolization.

Hydrocephalus

Hydrocephalus is a potentially fatal yet treatable condition. Based on its underlying mechanisms, hydrocephalus can be classified into communicating and noncommunicating (obstructive). Both forms can be either congenital or acquired.

Obstructive hydrocephalus is caused by obstruction of the CSF flow, as in congenital stenosis of the cerebral aqueduct or obstruction secondary to tumor. Communicating hydrocephalus occurs when the CSF is overproduced (such as with a choroid plexus papilloma) or is not properly reabsorbed as it occurs in meningeal inflammation or hemorrhage.

Hydrocephalus can be distinguished from enlargement of the ventricular system related to atrophy by:

- A discrepancy in the degree of ventricular with respect to sulcal enlargement suggests hydrocephalus.
- Characteristic pattern of disproportionate temporal horn enlargement compared with the frontal horns suggests hydrocephalus.
- A founded appearance of the anterior portion of the third ventricle also suggests hydrocephalus.

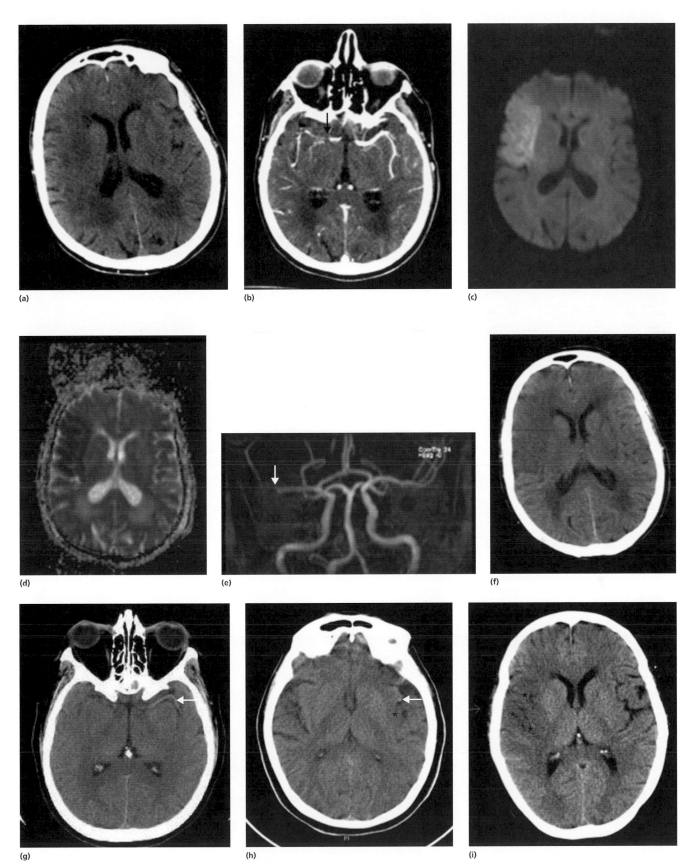

Figure 6.4 Acute infarct. Axial CT (a) shows small-vessel diseases and no signs of acute infarct, CT angiography (b) shows occlusion of the right MCA (arrow), DWI (c) MR and ADC map (d) show an area of restricted diffusion (*), MR angiography (3D TOF) (e) shows MCA occlusion (arrow), and the follow-up axial CT (f) demonstrates the typical findings of a subacute infarct(*). Axial CTs in two different patients (g and h, and i) show early signs of acute stroke: hyperdense MCA (arrow) (g), poor definition of the cortex in the insula (*) and also a hyperdense MCA ("dot sign") (arrow) (h), and loss of gray/ white matter distinction and effacement of the sulci (*)(i).

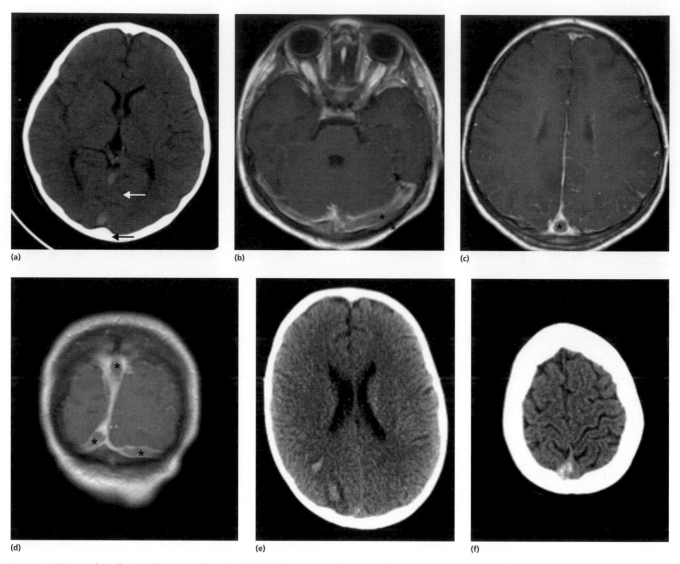

Figure 6.5 Venous thrombosis and venous infarct. Axial CT (a) shows hyperdense straight sinus (arrows), and axial (b and c) and coronal (d) postcontrast T1-W MR show a filling defect in transverse and superior sagittal sinuses (*). Axial CT in a different patient (e and f) show a hemorrhagic lesion (venous infarct) (arrow) and a hyperdense superior sagittal sinus (thrombosis) (*).

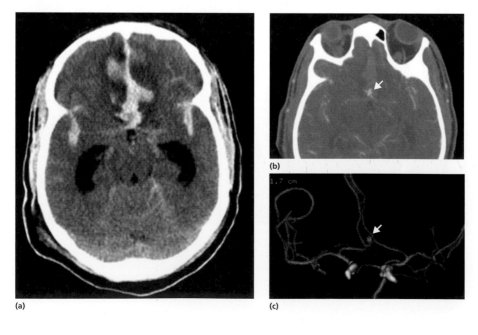

Figure 6.6 SAH due to aneurysm rupture SHA. Axial CT (a) shows diffuse SHA with hydrocephalus. Axial MIP (b) and 3D reconstruction (c) CT angiography show an ACOM aneurysm (arrows).

Coma

The **comatose or acutely confused** patient should undergo CT to identify any intracranial hemorrhages or other acute lesions. However, most these patients will not show an acute structural brain lesion, the encephalopathy is instead due to systemic metabolic abnormalities.

Trauma

Imaging of acute head trauma is best performed with CT to detect treatable lesions before secondary neurologic damage occurs. When performed in unconscious patients with severe head injury, the craniocervical junction should be included. MRI is the modality of choice for patients with subacute and chronic head injury or for patients with acute head trauma when neurologic findings are unexplained by CT.

Scalp soft tissue swelling is a reliable sign of the site of impact. **Subgaleal hematoma** is the most common manifestation of scalp injury and is seen as a soft tissue swelling of the scalp located beneath the subcutaneous fibrofatty tissue superficial to the temporalis muscle and skull.

Nondisplaced linear **fractures** of the skull are the most common type of fracture. Isolated linear skull fractures do not require treatment, while surgical management is usually indicated for depressed and compound skull fractures. Depressed fractures are frequently associated with an underlying brain contusion. Intracranial air (pneumocephalus) may be an indirect sign of fracture particularly one involving the skull base.

Traumatic head injury can be divided into primary and secondary. Primary lesions occur as a direct result of head trauma and include epidural, subdural, subarachnoid, and intraventricular hemorrhages as well as diffuse axonal injury (DAI), cortical contusions, intracerebral hematomas, subcortical gray matter injury, and direct injury of the cerebral vasculature. Secondary lesions result from mass effect or vascular compromise, such as cerebral swelling, brain herniation, hydrocephalus, ischemia or infarction, CSF leak, leptomeningeal cyst formation, and encephalomalacia. Secondary lesions are often preventable.

Primary brain injury

Epidural and **subdural hematomas** are described in the "Critical observations" section.

SAH results from a disruption of small subarachnoid vessels or direct extension into subarachnoid space of a contusion or hematoma. On CT, it appears as areas of high attenuation within the cisterns and sulci. SAH may lead to subsequent hydrocephalus by virtue of impaired CSF resorption.

Intraventricular hemorrhage (IVH) may result from rotationally induced tearing of subependymal veins on the surface of the ventricles or by direct extension of a parenchymal hematoma into the ventricular system. Additionally, it may result from retrograde flow of SAH into the ventricular system through the fourth ventricle foramina. On CT, IVH appears as hyperdense material layering dependently or completely filling the ventricular system. It may lead to hydrocephalus by obstruction at the level of the aqueduct or arachnoid villi.

DAI is characterized by widespread disruption of axons caused by acceleration, rotation, and/or deceleration injury. Direct impact does not necessarily cause DAI. DAI is one of the major causes of unconsciousness and persistent vegetative state after head trauma. DAI may or may not show up on a CT scan and is much better seen by MRI. Only hemorrhagic DAI lesions (about 30% of them) are visible on CT (Figure 6.7):

- On CT, small petechial hemorrhages at the gray/white matter cerebral junction or corpus callosum are the most common findings. Ill-defined areas of decreased attenuation may also be seen in nonhemorrhagic lesions.

In the brainstem, DAI is the most common type of primary injury. It affects the dorsolateral aspect of the midbrain and upper pons. The locations and the presence of subtle hemorrhage make these lesions difficult to diagnose on CT.

Cortical contusions are focal brain injuries primarily involving the cortical gray matter and have a better prognosis than DAI (Figure 6.8):

- They typically occur near bony protuberances, commonly involving the temporal bones above the petrous bone or posterior to the greater sphenoid wing and the frontal lobe above the cribriform plate, planum sphenoidale, and lesser sphenoid wing.
- They tend to be multiple and bilateral and may also occur at the margins of depressed skull fractures.
- CT appearance of contusions varies according to its age. Initially, they appear followed by development of surrounding edema, before gradually fading away leaving behind more or less obvious area of atrophy.

Occasionally, **intraparenchymal hemorrhages** not associated with contusions are present, and they represent shear-induced hemorrhage from rupture of small intraparenchymal blood vessels and are usually located in the frontotemporal white matter. These lesions can also present late secondary to delayed hemorrhage, which is a cause of clinical deterioration during the first week after head trauma.

Subcortical gray matter injury is an uncommon manifestation of head trauma. It is seen as multiple petechial hemorrhages affecting the basal ganglia and thalamus and is probably due to shearing of tiny perforating arteries.

Other **traumatic vascular injuries** include arterial dissections or occlusions, pseudoaneurysm formation, and acquired arteriovenous or dural fistulas (e.g., direct carotid cavernous fistula).

Secondary brain injury

Diffuse cerebral swelling is a common secondary brain injury, usually resulting from increase in tissue fluid content (edema) secondary to hypoxia that leads to generalize mass effect with effacement of sulci and basal cisterns, compression of the ventricles, and loss of gray/white matter differentiation. The cerebellum and brainstem are usually spared and may appear hyperdense relative to the cerebral hemispheres. Hypodensity in the brainstem is an ominous sign. Often, the falx and cerebral vessels appear dense, mimicking acute SAH (Figure 6.9).

Brain herniation is described in the "Critical observations" section.

As stated before, **hydrocephalus** may occur after SAH or IVH. Additionally, mass effect from cerebral swelling or hematoma can also cause hydrocephalus by compression.

Posttraumatic ischemia or infarction can result from raised intracranial pressure, embolization from arterial dissection, or direct mass effect on the cerebral vasculature from brain herniation. Infarctions caused by local mass effect include those affecting the ACA territory and caused by subfalcine herniation, PCA infarcts caused by uncal herniation, and PICA infarcts caused by cerebellar tonsillar herniation. Ischemia or infarction secondary to globally reduced cerebral perfusion tends to occur in "watershed zones,"

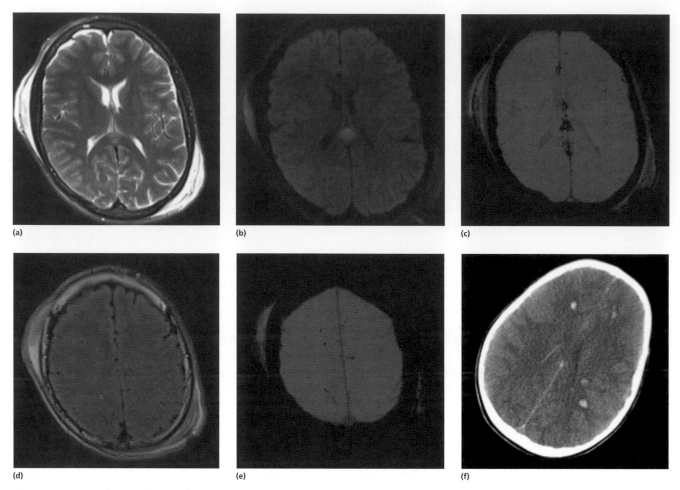

(a)

(b)

(c)

(d)

(e)

(f)

Figure 6.7 DAI. Axial T2-W (a), DWI (b), and SWI (c) MRI show hemorrhagic DAI at the corpus callosum with restricted diffusion (arrows). Axial FLAIR (d) shows petechial hemorrhages at the gray/white matter cerebral junction, better depicted on SWI (e) (arrows). Axial CT (f) in a different patient shows hemorrhagic DAI lesions (arrows).

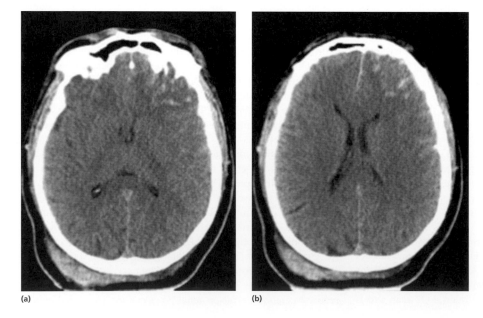

(a)

(b)

Figure 6.8 Cortical contusion involving the frontal lobe. Axial CT (a and b) (*).

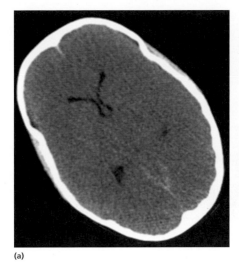 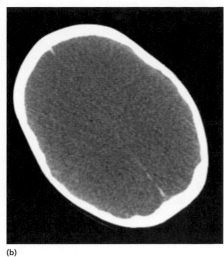

Figure 6.9 Posttraumatic diffuse cerebral edema. Axial CT (a and b) shows effacement of sulci and basal cisterns, compression of the ventricles, and loss of gray/white matter differentiation.

(a)   (b)

which are generally located parallel to the outer borders of the lateral ventricles.

Secondary brainstem injury includes infarction, compression usually due to uncal herniation, and hemorrhage, which is known as Duret hemorrhage and is a midline hematoma in the rostral pons and midbrain seen in descending transtentorial herniation.

Vascular lesions

Stroke is a clinical symptom that is caused by either brain infarction (75%) or hemorrhage (25%) and must be distinguished from other conditions causing abrupt neurologic deficits such as tumors.

Infarction is a permanent injury that occurs when tissue perfusion decreases long enough to cause necrosis, typically due to occlusion a feeding artery. Transient ischemic attack (TIA) is defined as transient neurologic signs or symptoms lasting less than 1 h and accompanied by normal DWI and MR perfusion imaging. It may serve as a "warning sign" as 10% of patients will go to develop infarctions in the first 90 days after it.

Ischemic strokes can be divided according to territory affected, and mechanism, namely embolism (from the heart, atherosclerotic from aortic arch or carotid arteries, and fat or air embolism) and thrombosis. Thrombi are formed at sites abnormal vascular endothelium typically over an area of atherosclerotic plaque or ulcers most commonly at the carotid artery bifurcation in the neck. Small-vessel thrombi frequently occur in diseased perforator vessels causing lacunar infarcts. There is overlap between the thrombotic and embolic groups since the majority of emboli begin as thrombi somewhere proximal in the cardiovascular tree (hence the practical term "thromboembolic disease"). Vasculitis, vasospasm, coagulopathies, global hypoperfusion, and venous thrombosis account for 5% of acute strokes but are important to recognize due differing treatments and prognosis.

The only imaging technique presently required before intravenous rtPA administration for treatment of ischemic stroke is an unenhanced head CT used to exclude:

- Intracranial hemorrhage (an absolute contraindication to thrombolytic treatment)
- Infarct size greater than one third of the MCA territory (a relative contraindication and predictor of increased hemorrhagic risk and poor outcome)

In most centers, CTA and CTP follow the nonenhanced head CT at admission to guide therapy. This protocol changes clinical outcome by increasing the number of patients adequately selected for thrombolysis.

Acute stroke is described in the "Critical observations" section.

In the subacute phase of ischemic stroke, edema leads to mass effect ranging from slight sulcal effacement to marked midline shift with brain herniation, depending on the size and location of infarct. Infarcts with volumes over 100 ml are considered "malignant" as they result in marked mass effect that generally leads to death. These changes peak at 3–7 days, and thereafter, there is progressive brain softening (encephalomalacia).

Reperfusion into infarcted tissues may secondarily lead to gross or microscopic hemorrhages seen in up to 50% of infarcts. The peak time for hemorrhagic transformation is at about 72 h postinfarction, and it is usually seen as a serpiginous area of petechial blood following the gyral contours of the infarcted cortex. More extensive hemorrhagic transformation may lead to the formation of a gross hematoma. These hematomas tend to occur earlier and are commonly associated with clinical deterioration and poor outcomes. Catastrophic hemorrhagic transformation may occur following thrombolysis.

The watershed or border zone regions are areas perfused by terminal branches of two adjacent arterial territories. When flow in one or both of parent vessels falls below a critical level, the brain in the watershed zone is first to infarct. Unilateral watershed infarcts may be seen in internal carotid occlusion or stenosis, while bilateral watershed infarcts occur in global hypoperfusion.

Cerebral venous infarction usually results from thrombosis of cortical veins, while occlusion of isolated dural venous sinuses results in symptoms of intracranial hypertension. Any dural sinus, deep cerebral vein, or cortical vein may be affected in isolation or combination. Venous thromboses usually occur in younger patients presenting with headache, sudden focal deficits, and seizures. Predisposing factors include hypercoagulable states, pregnancy, infection (spread from contiguous scalp, face, middle era, or sinus), dehydration, meningitis, trauma, and direct invasion by tumor. (Venous thrombosis and infarction imaging findings are described in the "Critical observations" section.)

Brain hemorrhages can be divided into subarachnoid and parenchymal. Imaging is critical in determining the site of

Table 6.1 Imaging characteristics of blood on magnetic resonance imaging according to the stage of the hemorrhage

Stage	Time	Hemoglobin	T1	T2
Hyperacute	<24h	Oxyhemoglobin	Iso	Hyper
Acute	1–3 days	Deoxyhemoglobin	Iso	Hypo
Early subacute	3–7 days	Methemoglobin in RBCs	Hyper	Hypo
Late subacute	>7 days	Methemoglobin free	Hyper	Hyper
Chronic	>14 days	Hemosiderin	Iso/hypo	Hypo

bleeding and showing any associated complications and pinpointing an underlying lesion:

- On CT, acute hemorrhage is hyperdense (typically 50–100 Hounsfield units). As blood becomes older and the globin molecule breaks down, the hematoma loses its hyperdense appearance, beginning at the periphery and working centrally. Clot contraction also contributes to this finding. A hematoma becomes isodense with the brain (4 days to 2 weeks, depending on clot size) and finally hypodense (>2–3 weeks) with respect to it.
- The MRI signal generated by blood depends mainly on the oxidation state of the hemoglobin, the chemical state of its iron-containing moieties, and the integrity of the red blood cell membrane (Table 6.1).

Patients with aneurysms may develop symptoms attributable to either local mass effect or bleeding (SAH), as described previously. Brain or spine arteriovenous malformations (AVMs) and vascular malformations involving the dura may also cause SAH but usually in combination with parenchymal or subdural bleeding.

Hematomas in the putamen, thalamus, medial cerebellum, and pons suggest hypertension, while a hemispheric hematoma, especially in patients older than 65 years, suggests amyloid angiopathy. In patients with no risk factors and under 55 years of age, a CTA should be performed to exclude any underlying vascular anomaly, such as AVM or tumor (Figure 6.10).

Neoplastic processes (benign/malignant)

In the presence of a potential brain tumor, there are questions that need to be answered as follows:

- Patient's age, since different tumors occur in different age groups (Table 6.2)
- Lesion location:
  - Is the lesion intra-axial, within the brain and expanding it, or extra-axial, outside the brain and compressing it?
  - Is the lesion supra or infratentorial? What is its specific location (e.g., sellar/suprasellar, pineal, or pontocerebellar region)?
- Is it a solitary mass or a multifocal disease?
- What are its tissue characteristics (calcifications, fat, cystic, density/intensity on CT/MRI and contrast enhancement)?

Roughly one third of CNS tumors are metastases, one third are gliomas, and one third are of nonglial origin, which tend to be extra-axial in location.

"Glioma" is a nonspecific term indicating that the tumor originates from glial cells like astrocytes, oligodendrocytes, and ependymal and choroid plexus cells. Astrocytoma is the most common glioma and can be subdivided into the low-grade (WHO 2), intermediate anaplastic type (WHO 3), and high-grade malignant glioblastoma (GB, WHO 4). GB is the most common type (50% of all astrocytomas). The nonglial cell tumors are a large heterogeneous group of tumors of which meningioma is most common.

Specific tumors occur under the age of 2 years and include mostly choroid plexus papillomas, anaplastic astrocytomas, medulloblastoma, and teratomas. In the first decade of life, medulloblastomas, astrocytomas, ependymomas, craniopharyngiomas, and gliomas are common, while metastases are rare. At this age, the most frequent metastases are from neuroblastoma and affect the skull. Conversely, in adults, about 50% of all CNS lesions are metastases.

In some cases, the distinction between intra- and extra-axial tumors is difficult to establish. Intra-axial masses are usually aggressive and less easily treated. The typical signs of an extra-axial tumor are (Figure 6.11):

- CSF cleft between the brain and mass.
- Inward displacement of the subarachnoid vessels that run on the surface of the brain.
- Gray matter between the lesion and the white matter.
- Widening of the subarachnoid space because the growth of an extra-axial lesion tends to push away the brain. In the posterior fossa, this is a reliable sign of an extra-axial mass.
- After contrast administration, extra-axial masses frequently show dural enhancement known as "dural tail."
- Adjacent bone changes such as remodeling.

In an adult, 80% of extra-axial lesions are either meningiomas or schwannomas. In the region of the cerebellopontine angle, 90% of extra-axial tumors are schwannomas. **Meningiomas** are located anywhere where meninges are found and in some places where only rest cells are presumed to be located (such as the carotid artery and jugular vein sheath). Common locations for meningioma are parasagittal, convexities, sphenoid ridge, olfactory groove, planum sphenoidale, and juxtasellar. Some features of meningioma follow (Figure 6.12):

- CT shows an extra-axial lesion usually slightly hyperdense to normal brain, with intense and homogeneous enhancement after contrast administration. Calcifications are seen in 20–30% of meningioma.
- Underlying skull hyperostosis is typical for meningiomas especially for those that abut the base of skull.
- On MRI, meningiomas are mostly of signal similar to gray matter in all sequences, which show significant contrast enhancement and high perfusion.
- Atypical and malignant subtypes may show frank brain invasion and restricted diffusion on DWI.

Cerebellopontine angle **schwannomas** are described in Chapter 8.

Multiple tumors in the brain are usually metastases. Primary brain tumors are typically single; nevertheless, some brain tumors like lymphoma, multicentric glioblastoma, and gliomatosis cerebri can be multifocal.

Additionally, multiple brain tumors can be seen in patients with phakomatoses such as:

- Neurofibromatosis I: optic gliomas and other astrocytomas, and neurofibromas
- Neurofibromatosis II: meningiomas, ependymomas, choroid plexus papillomas, and schwannomas
- Tuberous sclerosis: subependymal tubers, intraventricular giant cell astrocytomas, and ependymomas
- von Hippel–Lindau: hemangioblastomas and endolymphatic sac tumors

CT and MRI characteristics are important clues for the diagnosis of tumors as follows:

- Most brain tumors are hypodense on CT, hypointense on MRI T1-WI, and hyperintense on T2-WI.
- Some tumors can have a high density on CT and low T2-WI signal, indicating hypercellularity and malignant nature.

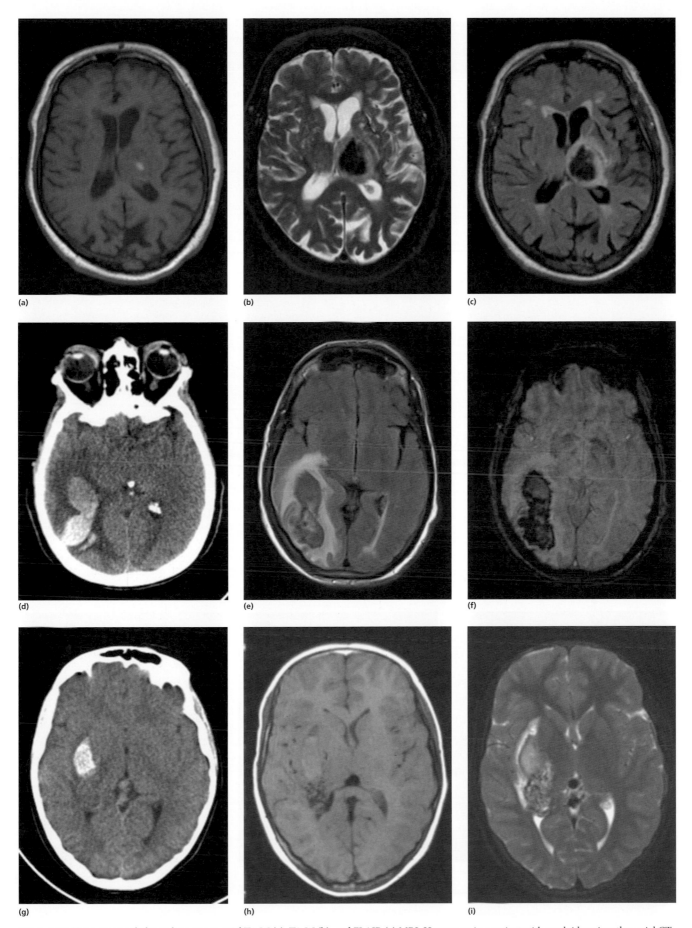

Figure 6.10 Hypertensive thalamic hematoma: axial T1-W (a), T2-W (b), and FLAIR (c) MRI. Hematoma in a patient with amyloid angiopathy: axial CT (d), axial FLAIR (e), and SWI (f) MR. Acute hematoma seen on axial CT (g) underlying an AVM depicted on T1-W (h) and T2-W (i) MRI.

- High signal on T1-WI may represent subacute hemorrhage, high protein content, melanin, or fat.
- Fat in a tumor is seen in lipomas, dermoid cysts, and teratomas.
- Calcification is seen in many CNS tumors (Table 6.3). It is better evaluated by CT.

An important consideration when assessing a tumor is its mass effect on the surrounding structures. Primary brain tumors are derived from brain cells and often have less mass effect for their size than would be expected, due to their infiltrative growth.

Table 6.2 Common ages for brain tumors.

	Astrocytomas				
Choroid plexus papilloma			Meningiomas		
Teratoma				Metastases	
Germinoma		Hemangioblastoma			
Craniopharyngioma			Schwannoma		
Medulloblastoma		Colloid cyst			
Ependymoma			Ependymoma		
		Oligodendroglioma			
10	20	30	40	50	60years

Table 6.3 Calcifications in brain tumors.

Commonly calcified tumors
- Oligodendroglioma
- Ependymoma
- Ganglioglioma
- Craniopharyngiomas
- Meningiomas
- Chordomas
- Chondrosarcomas

Less commonly calcified tumors
- Choroid plexus papilloma
- Astrocytoma
- Metastases

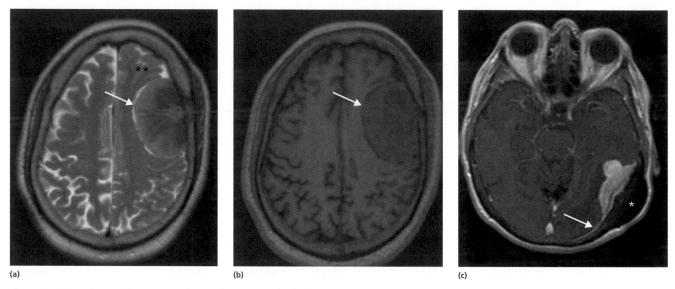

(a) (b) (c)

Figure 6.11 Typical signs of an extra-axial tumor (meningioma). Axial T1-W (a) and T2-W (b) show CSF cleft (arrows) with displacement of the subarachnoid vessels and gray matter between the lesion and the white matter (**). Coronal postcontrast T1-W (c) MRI of a different patient shows the "dural tail" (arrow) and exuberant hyperostosis (*) of the adjacent bone.

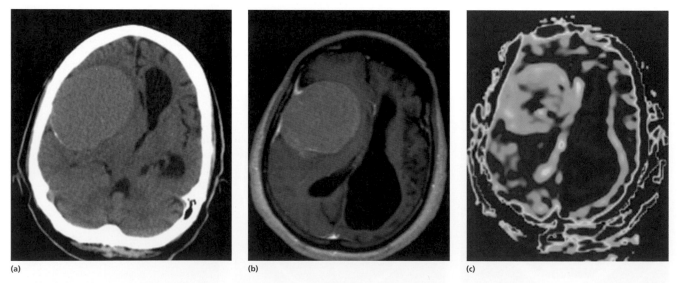

(a) (b) (c)

Figure 6.12 Meningioma. Axial CT (a) shows a meningioma with marginal calcifications, dural tail seen on postgadolinium T1-WI (b), and increased MR perfusions on CBV map (c).

Conversely, metastases and extra-axial tumors like meningiomas or schwannomas have significant mass effect.

The ability of tumors to cross the midline also limits the differential diagnosis. GB frequently crosses the midline by infiltrating the corpus callosum. Radiation necrosis (a complication of radiotherapy or radiosurgery) may have similar imaging features as recurrent tumor and also sometimes cross the midline. Primary brain lymphoma is usually located near the midline or along the walls of the ventricles. Meningioma can spread along the meninges to the contralateral side and even cross the falx and tentorium.

One of the most important roles of imaging is to assess the extent of a tumor. Astrocytomas spread along the white matter tracts and do not respect the boundaries of the lobes. Because of this infiltrative growth, in many cases the tumor is actually larger than can be depicted and commonly extends microscopically beyond the MRI abnormalities.

Some tumors show subarachnoid seeding and form nodules on the brain and spinal cord. This is seen for example in medulloblastoma or ependymomas. In these cases, spine imaging is necessary for disease staging.

DWI has been used to study gliomas and brain abscesses and to differentiate between arachnoid cysts and epidermoid cysts. In most tumors, there is no restricted diffusion. However, highly malignant tumors such as GB, lymphoma, and medulloblastoma may show restricted DWI, which is an important clue for their diagnosis. This restricted diffusion indicates hypercellularity (Figure 6.13).

MRI perfusion is useful in the management of primary brain tumors by predicting most malignant portion of the tumor, which guides biopsy, determines the biologic nature of the lesion, and correlates with prognosis. Increased CBV correlates with tumor angiogenesis and hence high tumor grade. Caveats include angiogenesis-modifying chemotherapeutic agents that can alter the CBV of treated high-grade tumors as well as benign vascular tumors that can mimic high-grade tumors (Figure 6.14).

Many nontumoral lesions can mimic a brain tumor, such as abscesses that may be difficult to distinguish by imaging from metastases or GB. Tumefactive demyelinating lesions may present as a mass-like areas with contrast enhancement but show low perfusion contrary to the high perfusion seen in malignant tumors.

Infectious conditions

Patients with **bacterial meningitis** usually present with a relatively acute onset of fever, neck stiffness, irritability, and headache, followed by a decline in mental status. CSF studies are usually diagnostic, and the CT is performed for complications or to rule out increased intracranial pressure before performing a lumbar puncture. In meningitis, imaging may show:

- CT may show a hyperdense exudate within the subarachnoid space and ventricles. On MRI, this exudate is hyperdense on FLAIR images and accompanied by pial contrast enhancement.
- Diffuse cerebral edema is sometimes seen.
- Hydrocephalus is the most common complication and can be easily identified with CT.
- Abscess and subdural/epidural empyemas are better evaluated with MRI, which shows peripheral contrast enhancement and restricted diffusion on ADC maps.

Brain abscesses are potentially life-threatening conditions requiring rapid treatment and prompt imaging identification. MRI is the preferred imaging modality. Clinical presentation is nonspecific with many patients having no convincing inflammatory/septic symptoms. Four stages of abscess formation are recognized, which have distinct pathological and imaging features: early cerebritis, late cerebritis, early capsule, and late capsule:

- Early cerebritis may be invisible on CT or as a poorly marginated cortical or subcortical hypodensity with mass effect with little or absent contrast enhancement.
- Late cerebritis is seen as an irregular incompletely ring-enhancing lesion with a hypodense center, better defined than early cerebritis.
- Early capsule is seen as ill-defined and often incomplete ring-enhancing mass.
- Late capsule stage (mature abscess) is seen as a ring-enhancing lesion thin nonnodular capsule with a necrotic central cavity (Figure 6.15).
- DWI shows restricted diffusion (low signal on ADC), which permits the differential diagnosis with other rim-enhancing lesions such as GB and metastases that show no restricted diffusion.
- MRS may show elevation of a succinate peak that is relatively specific but not present in all abscesses; high lactate, acetate, alanine, valine, leucine, and isoleucine levels peak may be present as by-products of bacterial metabolism; Cho/Cr and NAA peaks are reduced.
- Ventriculitis may be present, seen as enhancement of the ependyma.

Herpes simplex encephalitis is the most common viral encephalitis. It spreads from the oral and nasal mucosa to the trigeminal and olfactory ganglion cells and then transdurally to the brain. The most common locations of brain involvement are the medial temporal lobes adjacent to the trigeminal ganglia and the orbital frontal regions adjacent to the olfactory bulbs. Imaging features of herpes infection are as follows:

- Early diagnosis is difficult and a "normal" CT should not dissuade from instituting treatment.
- Early CT findings include subtle low density in affected areas, usually bilateral and symmetric. Later, changes may become more obvious, and hemorrhage may occur.
- MRI may show edema in affected regions. If complicated by hemorrhage, areas of hyperintense signal on T1-WI and hypointense on T2-WI and SWI may be seen. Restricted diffusion is common due to cytotoxic edema.
- Enhancement is usually absent early on. Later, enhancement is variable in pattern and may be gyral, leptomeningeal, ring, or diffuse.

Inflammatory conditions

Multiple sclerosis (MS) is a relatively common acquired chronic relapsing primary demyelinating disease involving the CNS. It is by definition disseminated in space (i.e., multiple lesions) and in time (i.e., lesions of different age). Diagnosis is supported by clinical studies, which include visual, somatosensory, or motor-evoked potentials and analysis of CSF for oligoclonal bands, immunoglobulin G index, and presence of myelin basic protein.

Several variants are recognized, each with specific imaging findings and clinical presentation, including classic, tumefactive, acute malignant Marburg type, Schilder type (diffuse cerebral sclerosis), and Balo concentric sclerosis. Neuromyelitis optica (Devic disease),

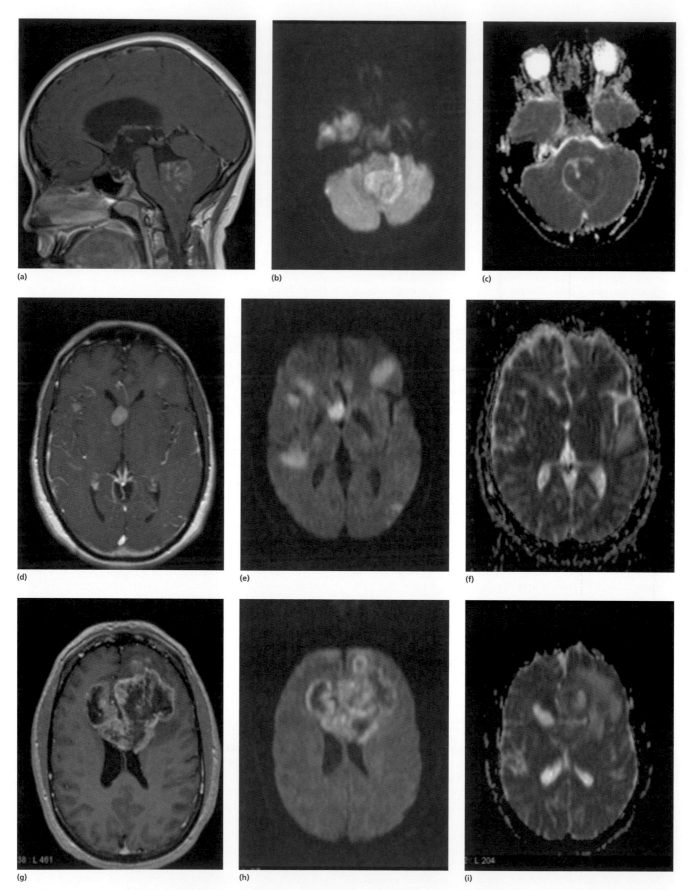

Figure 6.13 DWI on brain tumors. Sagittal postcontrast T1-WI (a), axial DWI (b), and ADC map (c) of a medulloblastoma with restricted diffusion. Axial postcontrast T1-WI (d), DWI (e), and ADC map (f) of a lymphoma with restricted diffusion. Axial postcontrast T1-WI (g), DWI (h), and ADC map (i) of a glioblastoma with restricted diffusion.

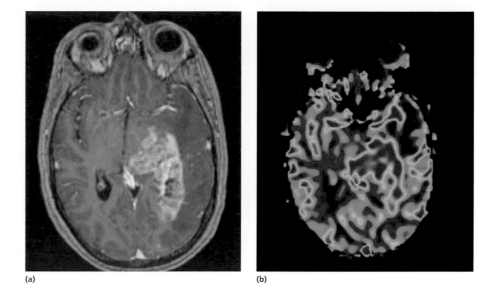

Figure 6.14 High-grade glioma (GB) seen on postcontrast T1-W MRI (a) as a heterogeneous enhanced mass with increased perfusion on CBV map (b).

(a)

(b)

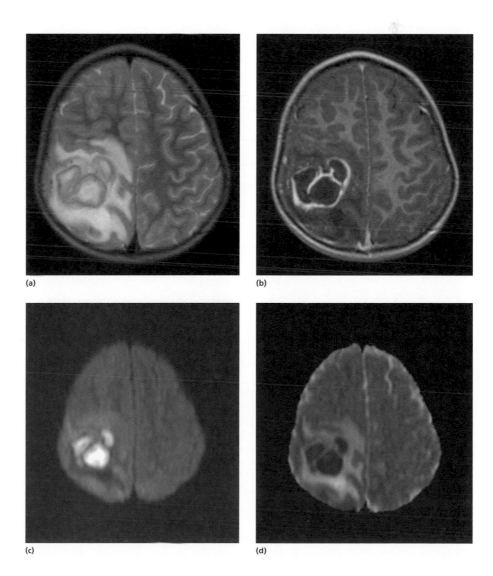

Figure 6.15 Abscess. Axial T2-W (a) and postcontrast T1-WI (b) show a ring-enhancing lesion with a necrotic central cavity and restricted diffusion on DWI (c) and ADC map (d).

(a)

(b)

(c)

(d)

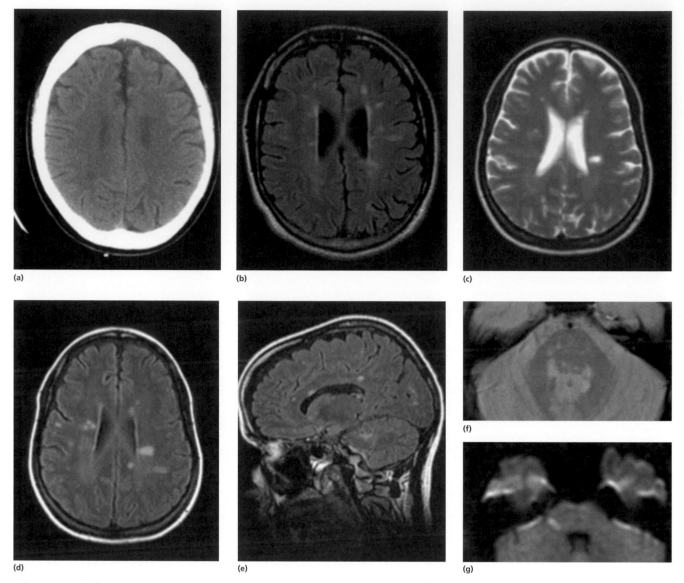

Figure 6.16 Multiple sclerosis (MS). Axial CT (a) and FLAIR (b) in a patient with MS show the differences in diagnostic acuity of the two techniques. Axial T2-WI (c) and FLAIR (d) and sagittal FLAIR (e) in a different patient (arrows). Another patient with MS has a lesion in the right middle cerebellar peduncle that demonstrates high signal on axial T2-WI (f) with restricted diffusion (g).

which affects only the optic nerve and spinal cord, was considered a MS variant but is now recognized necrotizing and not demyelinating process.

Regarding classic MS, CT features are usually subtle and nonspecific as follows:

- CT may show homogeneously hypoattenuating white matter lesions, with contrast enhancement in the active phase and eventually brain atrophy in chronic patients. Most of the lesions are periventricular in location.

MRI is the imaging technique of choice used for diagnosis and surveillance of MS patients and may show the following abnormalities (Figure 6.16):

- Plaques are typically round or ovoid with a periventricular or juxtacortical location. Posterior fossa structures are also involved especially the middle cerebellar peduncles.
- Periventricular lesions are usually aligned perpendicular to the long axis of the ventricles, known as "Dawson fingers."

- Lesions along the callosal–septal interface and in the cerebellar peduncles, the corpus callosum, medulla, and spinal cord are typical.
- All plaques, regardless of age, are hyperintense on T2-WI and FLAIR.
- Active lesions show contrast enhancement, often as an incomplete rim, called the "open ring sign" and show peripheral restricted diffusion.
- MRS may show reduced NAA peaks within lesions and elevated choline implying active inflammation.
- Hypointense lesions on T1-WI, often referred as "dark lesions or holes," are significant because they reflect loss of underlying neuronal tissue rather than simple demyelination.
- Additionally, in chronic patients, brain atrophy and thinning of the corpus callosum are seen.
- Optic neuritis is often the first manifestation of MS. On MRI, acute optic neuritis shows hyperintense T2-WI signal in an enlarged and enhancing optic nerve.

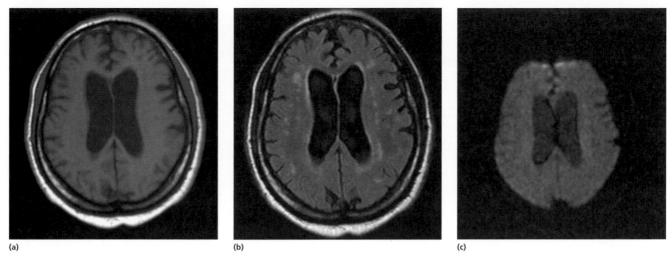

(a)   (b)   (c)

Figure 6.17 Small-vessel diseases. Axial T1-WI (a), T2-WI (b), and DWI (c) show multiple lacunar infarcts without restricted diffusion (arrows).

Generalized conditions

Age-related demyelination and atrophy
Small-vessel ischemic changes within the deep cerebral white matter are seen with increasing frequency especially over 50 years of age and are associated to hypertension and diabetes. The deep white matter is more susceptible to ischemic injury than gray matter because it is supplied by long, small caliber, penetrating end arteries, without significant collateral blood supply. A small amount of these changes has no clinical correlations, but large burdens are seen in individuals who can cognitively impaired. Mild diffuse general atrophy may be present and may be age appropriate (patients older than 65 years with normal cognitive function), named **age-appropriate volume loss**.

Dementia
Patterns of MRI atrophy may be helpful to distinguish different types of dementia.

Alzheimer's disease (AD) is the most common cause of dementia. Neuroimaging studies demonstrate:
- Diffuse atrophy, particularly affecting the medial temporal and parietal lobes.
- Enlargement of the temporal horns, suprasellar cisterns, Sylvian fissures, and central sulcus may be useful in discriminating AD from normal age-related atrophy.
- Nuclear medicine techniques, such as PET and single photon emission CT, have shown reduction in temporoparietal metabolism or blood flow in patients with AD.
- Perfusion MRI has also shown reduced perfusion (CBV) in the temporoparietal and sensorimotor cortices of AD patients.
- Tractography is being used for the early diagnosis and follow-up of AD patients, based on evidence from animal, pathological, and imaging studies that disruption of white matter occurs in the course of AD and may be an early event.

Vascular dementia (VaD) is thought to be the second most common cause of dementia after AD. It can sometimes be distinguished from AD by a more sudden onset and association with vascular risk factors. Imaging is characterized by infarctions, especially cortical ones, of different ages. Cognitive dysfunction in VaD can be the result of large-vessel infarctions, watershed infarctions in the dominant hemisphere, and small-vessel disease: multiple lacunar infarctions involving the white matter, basal ganglia, and thalami (Figure 6.17).

Parkinson disease is the most common movement neurodegenerative basal ganglia disorder. It is characterized clinically by tremor, muscular rigidity, and loss of postural reflexes. About 25% of Parkinson patients also develop dementia especially at the end of their lives. On conventional anatomic imaging, no findings are seen, and imaging serves to exclude other causes for movement disorders.

Headache
Patients with "thunderclap" headaches should undergo emergent head CT, while those with chronic headaches should be imaged with MRI. Acute severe headaches may be related to SAH, acute hydrocephalus, or an enlarging intracranial mass. Typical uncomplicated migraine does not require imaging.

Seizures
For the evaluation of first seizure, an intracranial tumor, infection, or other acute processes must be excluded, and CT scan should be performed first.

If the seizure disorder is chronic and particularly if it is refractory to therapy, a detailed MRI is needed. In this case, the imaging study should wait until clinical seizure semiology and electrical studies results are available. Detailed examinations of the brain help identify abnormal hippocampi and/or cortical dysplasias, which may be amenable to surgical resection.

Suggested reading
Al-Okaili, R.N., Krejza, J., Wang, S. *et al.* (2006) Advanced MR imaging techniques in the diagnosis of intraaxial brain tumors in adults. *Radiographics*, **26**, 525–551.

Brant, W.E. & Helms, C.A. (2012) *Fundamentals of Diagnostic Radiology*, fourth edn. Lippincott Williams & Wilkins, Philadelphia, PA.

Laughlin, S. & Montanera, W. (1998) Central nervous system imaging: when is CT more appropriate than MRI? *Postgraduate Medicine*, **104** (5).

Smirniotopoulos, J.G., Murphy, F.M., Rushing, E.J. *et al.* (2007) From the archives of the AFIP. Patterns of contrast enhancement in the brain and meninges. *Radiographics*, **27** (2), S173–189.

Tomandl, B.F., Klotz, E., Handschu, R. *et al.* (2003) Comprehensive imaging of ischemic stroke with multisection CT. *Radiographics*, **23** (3), 565–592.

Yousem, D.M., Zimmerman, R.D. & Grossman, R.I. (2010) *Neuroradiology: The Requisites*. St Mosby, Elsevier, Philadelphia, PA.

CHAPTER 7

Spine imaging

Joana N. Ramalho[1,2] and Mauricio Castillo[2]
[1]Department of Neuroradiology, Centro Hospitalar de Lisboa Central, Lisboa, Portugal
[2]Department of Radiology, University of North Carolina, Chapel Hill, USA

Introduction

Spine pathology can be grossly divided into degenerative and non-degenerative diseases that may be clinically indistinguishable as symptoms commonly overlap. Patients with spine disorders may present with focal or diffuse back pain, radiculopathy, or myelopathy. Myelopathy describes any neurologic deficits related to disease in the spinal cord while radiculopathy generally results from impingement of the spinal nerves along their course. Focal back pain without neurologic compromise or fever is not usually an emergency and does not require emergent imaging. However, vertebral metastases or infectious discitis may cause isolated focal back pain, and if neurological deficits accompany them, immediate imaging is indicated. When the history and physical findings are nonspecific, as frequently they are in clinical practice, imaging findings become central to the diagnosis and treatment.

Imaging modalities

Conventional radiography was the initial imaging procedure in spine evaluation, but with computed tomography (CT) and magnetic resonance imaging (MRI) now widely available, radiographs are no longer considered adequate. Radiographs are still useful for acute trauma screening, for localization purposes during surgery procedures (plain films and fluoroscopy), and for dynamic imaging (flexion and extension). CT myelography and MRI with myelographic and neurographic sequences have also replaced conventional myelography.

Spinal CT is the modality of choice for evaluation of the bone structures and calcifications, while MRI is better to evaluate the details of spinal anatomy, including the intraspinal contents (spinal cord, *conus medullaris* and *cauda equina*, dural sac epidural, subdural and subarachnoid spaces), neural foramina, joints, ligaments, intervertebral discs, and bone marrow. Sagittal and axial images should be acquired through the cervical, thoracic, and lumbar segments of the spine, as they are generally considered complementary. The addition of coronal images may also be useful, especially in patients with scoliosis.

A standard spine MRI protocol comprises sagittal and axial T1- and T2-weighted sequences and fluid-sensitive MR images (which include short tau inversion recovery (STIR) or fat-saturated T2-weighted sequences), complemented by postcontrast T1-WI if tumor, inflammation, infection, or vascular diseases are suspected.

Diffusion-weighted imaging (DWI) is challenging in the spine, largely due to physiological cerebrospinal fluid (CSF) flow-induced artifact and distortion from magnetic susceptibilities. It has been used in the diagnosis of spinal cord infarct. Similar to the brain, spinal cord infarcts show restricted diffusion, seen as bright lesions on DWI with low signal on apparent diffusion coefficient (ADC) maps. It has also been used to distinguish benign from pathologic vertebral body compression fractures, but its usefulness and efficacy in this setting remains controversial.

Diffusion tensor imaging (DTI) evaluates the direction and magnitude of extracellular water molecules movement within the white matter fibers and enables the visualization of the major white matter tracts in the brain and spine. Spine DTI has been used to evaluate the integrity of the extent of neural damage in patients with acute or chronic spinal cord injury and also to distinguish between infiltrative and localized tumors because the latter are easier to resect.

Nuclear medicine bone scans and PET/CT are used to screen the entire skeleton for metastasis. They are highly sensitive but nonspecific, since degenerative and nondegenerative processes may show increased uptake.

Ultrasound (US) has limited applications in adults, except during surgery after removal of the posterior elements. In this setting, it may be used to image the spinal cord. However, in neonates, the nonossified posterior elements provide the acoustic window through which the spinal anomalies can be readily evaluated.

Conventional digital subtraction angiography (DSA) can be performed for spinal vasculature evaluation, since spinal CT and MR angiography are difficult to interpret and have limited application. The major indications for spinal DSA are evaluation of suspected arteriovenous fistulas (AVF), arteriovenous malformations, and localization of the arterial cord supply before surgery.

Critical Observations in Radiology for Medical Students, First Edition. Katherine R. Birchard, Kiran Reddy Busireddy, and Richard C. Semelka.
© 2015 John Wiley & Sons, Ltd. Published 2015 by John Wiley & Sons, Ltd.
Companion website: www.wiley.com/go/birchard

Appearance of the normal spine study

Vertebral anatomy varies somewhat by region, but the basic components are the same as follows:

- Vertebral body with vertebral end plates that define the intervertebral space, which contains the intervertebral disc
- Posterior vertebral arch that includes a pair of pedicles, a pair of laminae, and 7 processes: 2 superior articular processes, 2 inferior articular processes, 2 transverse processes, and 1 posterior midline spinous process

The cervical spine comprises the first seven superior vertebrae of the spinal column. C1, also known as the atlas, and C2, also known as the axis, are unique. The other cervical vertebrae are similar in size and configuration. C1 is a ring-shaped vertebra, composed of anterior and posterior arches and two lateral articular masses, without a central vertebral body. The vertebral arteries commonly traverse the lateral masses of C1. C2 is also a ring-shaped vertebra but has a central body and a superiorly oriented odontoid process, also known as the dens, which lies posterior to the anterior arch of C1. The normal distance between the dens and anterior arch of C1 is approximately 3 mm in adults and 4 mm in children as they are held together mainly by the transverse ligament. Exclusive to the cervical spine are bilateral uncovertebral joints, also named Luschka joints formed by the articulation of the uncinate process between two adjacent vertebral bodies. The transverse foramen (also known as the *foramen transversarium*) located in the transverse processes of the cervical vertebrae gives passage to the vertebral artery, the vertebral vein, and a plexus of sympathetic nerves generally from C6 up to C1.

The discs of the cervical and thoracic spine are much thinner compared with the lumbar discs. In the lumbar spine, the posterior margins of the discs tend to be slightly concave at upper levels, straight at L4/5 level, and slightly convex at the lumbosacral spinal junction. This appearance should not be confused with pathologic bulging.

The main ligaments of the spine are the anterior longitudinal ligament (ALL), posterior longitudinal ligament (PLL), and posterior ligamentous complex (PLC) that include the supraspinous and interspinous ligaments, articular facet capsules, and *ligamentum flavum*.

The spinal canal contains the thecal sac formed by the dura mater and surrounded by the epidural space, which contains epidural fat and a large venous plexus. The thecal sac houses the spinal cord, *conus medullaris*, and *cauda equina* (lower lumbar and sacral nerve roots), surrounded by freely flowing CSF within the subarachnoid space.

The spinal cord is composed of a core of gray matter surrounded by the white matter tracts. In the axial plane, the gray matter has a "butterfly shape" given by its anterior and posterior horns joined in the midline by a commissure. The *conus medullaris* normally ends around L1–L2 vertebral level. The *filum terminale* is a strand of pial–ependymal tissues, proceeding downward from the apex of the *conus medullaris to the coccyx*.

Throughout the spine, the intervertebral foramina, or neural foramina, contain the nerve roots and its sleeve, the dorsal root ganglion, fat, and blood vessels.

On MRI, the appearance of different structures varies according to the sequence used. The vertebral body contains bone marrow, which signal varies with age, reflecting the gradual conversion of red marrow to fatty marrow. The normal mature bone marrow shows high T1-WI and fairly high T2-WI signal intensity, related with the presence of fat. Tumor infiltration, radiation therapy, increased hematopoiesis, or any disease that affects the bone marrow may alter the normal bone marrow signal. Peripherally, the bone marrow is surrounded by low T1- and T2-WI signal of the cortical bone. Intervertebral discs demonstrate slightly less signal than the adjacent vertebral bodies on T1-WI, but the differentiation of the centrally located nucleus pulposus and peripheral annulus fibrosis of the discs is difficult on this sequence. On T2-WI, the normally hydrated nucleus pulposus composed of water and proteoglycans shows high signal centrally with lower signal from the less hydrated annulus fibrosis. CSF demonstrates low signal on T1-WI and high signal on T2-WI that provides contrast with the adjacent spinal cord and nerve roots within the spinal canal, which show intermediate signal on both sequences. The periphery of the spinal canal is lined by high T1 signal intensity epidural fat. The spinal ligaments and dura show low signal intensity on T1- and T2-WI.

As elsewhere in the body, bones and calcifications appear hyperdense on CT. Paraspinal muscles have intermediate density, while CSF spaces are hypodense. As stated before, the differentiation between intraspinal contents cannot be made on CT.

CT and MRI scans of the normal spine are shown in Figure 7.1.

Critical observations

Myelopathy

Myelopathy results from compromise of the spinal cord itself, generally due to compression, intrinsic lesions, or inflammatory process known as "myelitis." It is most commonly caused by compression of the spinal cord by intradural or extradural tumors (most frequently bone metastases), trauma (spinal cord injury), and degenerative cervical or dorsal spondylosis. Many primary neoplastic, infectious, inflammatory, neurodegenerative, vascular (arteriovenous malformation, dural fistulae, infarct, or hematoma), nutritional (vitamin B12 deficiency), congenital (neural tube defects), and idiopathic disorders result in myelopathy, though these are very much less common. Despite the clinical situation, MRI is the procedure of choice for spinal cord evaluation.

In an acute setting, imaging evaluation is primarily focused on extrinsic cord compression or presence of intramedullary spinal cord hematoma, since the resultant myelopathy may be reversible, particularly if treated earlier and aggressively. With regard to imaging of myelopathy, the following should be kept in mind:

- MRI shows mass effect upon the cord and sometimes areas of high T2-WI signal inside the cord (Figure 7.2).
- Keep in mind that this T2-WI sign is inconstant, may appear late, and, when present, is associated with poor prognosis even after therapy. DTI has been used recently to overcome this limitation, by showing abnormalities of the white matter tracts before the T2-WI abnormalities being evident but is generally not used routinely in clinical practice.

Epidural abscess

Epidural abscess represents a rare but important neurosurgical emergency requiring immediate action. Most result from hematogenous spread from infections elsewhere in the body and are primarily located in the posterior aspect of the spinal canal. Abscesses from direct spread from neighboring structures, such as spondylodiscitis, are often located in the anterior aspect of the spinal canal. The following are imaging features of abscesses (Figure 7.3):

- On MRI, abscesses typically display intense peripheral rim enhancing surrounding a heterogeneous nonenhancing central zone of necrosis, and/or pus, with restricted diffusion.
- The dura represents a relative mechanical barrier, so infections tend to spread in a craniocaudal fashion within the epidural space.
- Epidural abscesses have little room to expand axially and compression of the thecal sac and spinal cord may be seen. Spinal cord high T2-WI signal may develop representing edema, myelitis, or ischemia secondary to cord compression.

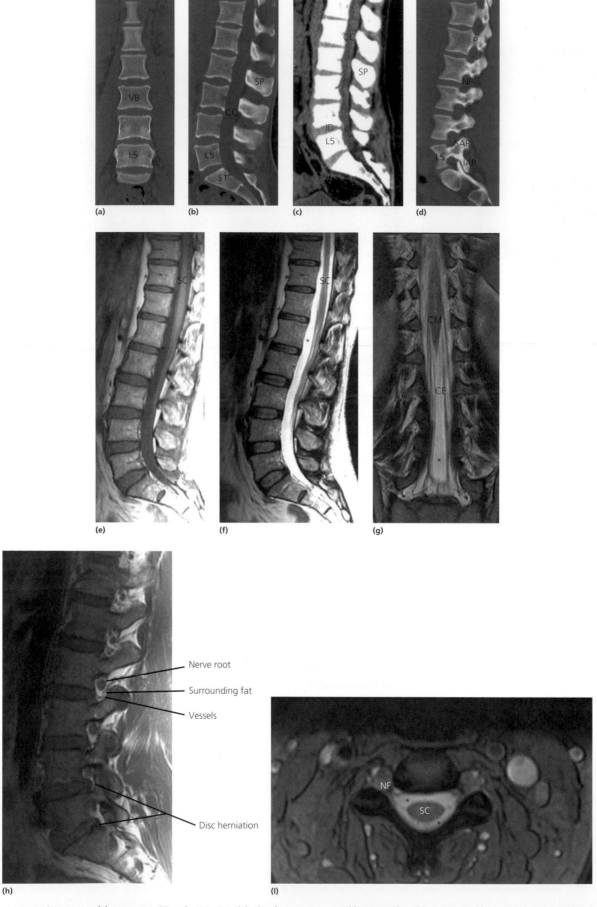

Figure 7.1 Normal anatomy of the spine on CT and MRI. CT of the lumbar spine: coronal bone window (a), midsagittal bone window (b), and soft tissue window(c) at the level of the central canal (CC) and sagittal bone window (d) at level of the neural foramina (NF). MR of the lumbar spine: midsagittal T1-WI (e) and T2-WI (f), coronal T2-WI (g), and sagittal T1-WI (h) at the level of the neural foramen. Axial T2-WI at the level of the cervical spine (i), conus medullaris (j), and cauda equina (k). CE, cauda equina; CM, conus medullaris; * CSF; IAP, inferior articular process; ID, intervertebral disc; P, pedicle; SAP, superior articular process; SC, spinal cord; SP, spinous process; VB, vertebral body.

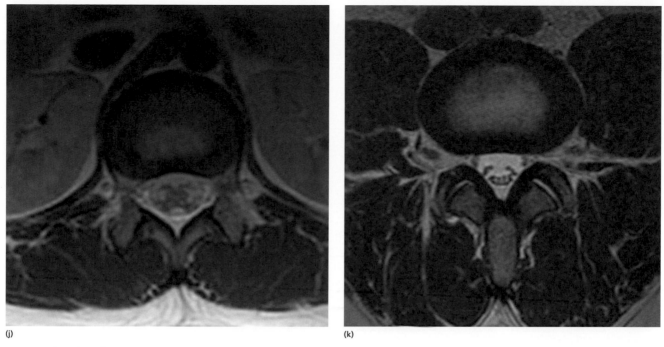

(j)   (k)

Figure 7.1 (*continued*)

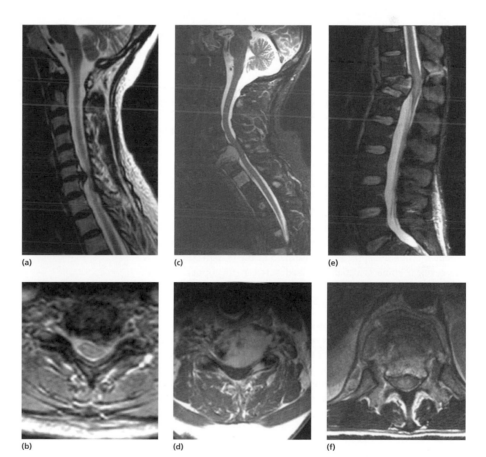

(a)   (c)   (e)

(b)   (d)   (f)

Figure 7.2 Cord compression. Sagittal and axial cervical T2* (a and b) show a disc herniation with cord compression. Sagittal STIR (c) and axial postcontrast T1-WI (d) show a cervical spine metastatic tumor. Sagittal STIR (e) and axial T2-WI (f) show a thoracic burst fracture.

Trauma

The screening examination for low-risk traumatic spine injuries consists of radiographs, supplemented by CT to further characterize or detect fractures. After severe trauma however, CT should be immediately performed, since unstable fractures can compromise the diameter of the central canal leading to cord compression. MRI is used to assess the nerve roots, soft tissues, and the spinal cord itself, particularly in patients who have neurologic symptoms unexplained by CT. MRI can detect posterior ligamentous injuries, traumatic disc herniation, and spinal epidural hemorrhage difficult to visualize on CT.

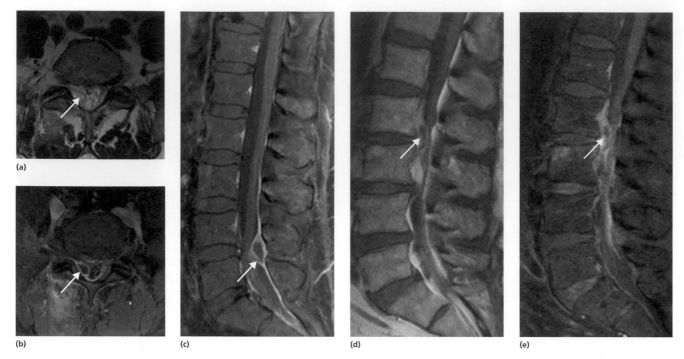

Figure 7.3 Epidural abscess. Axial T2-WI (a) and axial (b) and sagittal (c) postcontrast T1-WI show a posterior epidural abscess. Sagittal postcontrast T1-WI (d) and postcontrast FS T1-WI (e) show an anterior epidural abscess (arrows).

Mechanical stability is a critical factor for treatment planning in patients with traumatic spine injury. Spine stability is defined as the ability to prevent the development of neurologic injury and progressive deformity in response to physiologic loading and a normal range of movement. Spine stability relies on the integrity of both bone and ligamentous components, and injury to either or both can result in instability and require surgical stabilization.

Cervical spine

The cervical spine is highly susceptible to traumatic injury, because it is extremely mobile with relatively small vertebral bodies and supports the head, which is heavy and acts as a lever. Different classification systems have been developed in an attempt to predict instability, to standardize injury nomenclature and to define a consistent therapeutic approach. Regardless of the classification used, the cervical spine is usually divided between the upper cervical spine, with its unique anatomy and the subaxial cervical spine.

Upper cervical spine

Atlanto-occipital dissociation injuries are severe and include both atlanto-occipital dislocations and atlanto-occipital subluxations. On imaging studies, a gross disruption of the normal alignment of the atlanto-occipital joints may be seen. A number of lines and distances on the cervical spine plain films and CT may help the diagnosis: (i) basion-dens interval (BDI) greater than 12 mm in adults, (ii) basion-axial interval (BAI) greater than 12 mm in adults, and atlantodental interval (ADI) greater than 3 mm (adults males) and greater than 2.5 mm (adults females; Figure 7.4).

Occipital condyle fractures may be divided into (i) type I, an impaction fracture, which is a result of axial loading and lateral bending; (ii) type II, a basilar skull fracture that extends into the occipital condyle; and (iii) type III, a tension injury, resulting in an avulsion of the occipital condyle.

Atlas fractures are common (representing 10% of all cervical fractures) and usually associated with other cervical spine fractures.

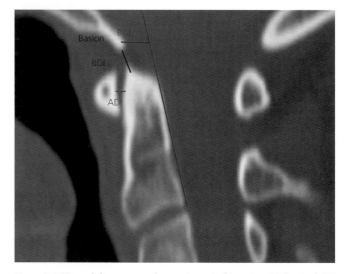

Figure 7.4 Normal distances on the craniocervical junction. Midsagittal CT demonstrates the posterior axial line drawn along the posterior cortex of the body of the axis and extended cranially. The BAI is the distance between the basion and this line. BDI is the distance from the most inferior portion of the basion to the closest point of the superior aspect of the dens. ADI is the distance between the posterior aspect of the anterior arch of C1 and the most anterior aspect of the dens.

These fractures are classified based upon their location. Posterior arch fractures are typically bilateral, are the most common, and are stable. Lateral mass fractures are usually unilateral and may have instability if there is associated ligamentous injury. The burst fracture is commonly called a Jefferson fracture and has a characteristic pattern of fractures in both the anterior and posterior arches, which widen rather than narrow the spinal canal (Figure 7.5).

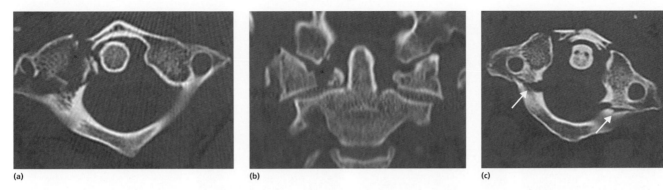

(a)   (b)   (c)

Figure 7.5 Atlas (C1) fractures. Axial (a) and coronal (b) CT show a right lateral mass fracture (*). Axial (c) CT show a Jefferson fracture (fractures in the anterior and posterior arches) (arrows).

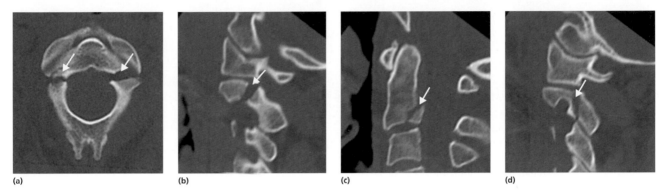

(a)   (b)   (c)   (d)

Figure 7.6 Hangman's fracture. Axial (a), sagittal at the level of the right pars interarticularis (b), midsagittal (c), and sagittal at the level of the left pars interarticularis (d) CT scans (arrows).

Odontoid fractures also known as the dens fractures are common fractures (representing 20% of all cervical fractures), usually classified as (i) type I, a fracture of the upper part of the odontoid process; (ii) type II, a fracture at the base of the odontoid, usually unstable and with a high risk of nonunion; and (iii) type III, a fracture of the odontoid, which extends into the body of C2.

Hangman's fracture is a term frequently used to describe traumatic spondylolisthesis of the axis. The fracture involves both pars interarticularis of C2 and is as a result of hyperextension and distraction. Despite the name, which hearkens to the era of judicial hangings, this fracture is virtually never seen in suicidal hanging, and major trauma such as high-speed motor vehicle accident is in fact the most common association. It is the most severe cervical fracture that can be sustained with preservation of life (Figure 7.6).

Subaxial cervical spine

Subaxial cervical spine injuries represent a broad of injury patterns and degrees of instability. The most accepted classification systems are based on the mechanism of injury.

Flexion–compression injuries represent a continuum of injury patterns, with minor degrees of trauma producing simple vertebral body compression fractures and more severe injuries resulting in a triangular "teardrop" fracture (fracture of the anteroinferior vertebral body—teardrop sign) or a quadrangular fracture with posterior ligamentous disruption. The most severe pattern results in posterior subluxation of the posterior vertebral body into the canal, acute kyphosis, and disruption of the ALL, PLL, and posterior ligaments, associated with a high incidence of cord damage.

Flexion–distraction injuries also represent a spectrum of pathology from mild posterior ligamentous strains to bilateral facet dislocations.

Facet dislocation refers to anterior displacement of one vertebral body onto another and may occur in variable degrees as follows (Figure 7.7):
- Facets subluxation—the superior facet slides over the inferior facet.
- Perched facets—the inferior facet appears to sit "perched" on the superior facet of the vertebra below.
- Locked facets—when one facet "jumps" over the other and becomes locked in this position.
- The naked facet sign refers to the CT appearance of an uncovered facet when the facet joint is completely dislocated.

Complications include cord injury (especially with bilateral involvement or in the setting of canal stenosis) or vertebral artery injury, such as dissection or thrombosis.

Vertical compression-type injuries are most commonly manifested as a cervical vertebral burst fracture. Axial loading of the cervical spine results in compression of the vertebral body with resultant retropulsion of the posterior wall into the canal.

Hyperextension injuries also represent a continuum of injury patterns with mild trauma resulting in widening of the disc space with disruption of the ALL and disc injury. In more severe cases, a teardrop fracture, characterized by the avulsion of the anteroinferior corner of the vertebral body, may be seen. Extension teardrop is not as severe as its counterpart, the flexion teardrop fracture. However, posterior ligaments disruption with displacement of the cephalad vertebrae into the spinal canal may also occur.

Thoracolumbar spine

Three different biomechanical regions can be defined: (i) the upper thoracic region (T1–T8) that is rigid and stable due to the ribcage; (ii) the transition zone (T9–L2) between the rigid and kyphotic

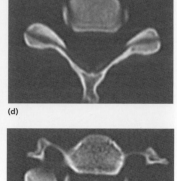
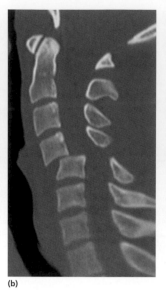
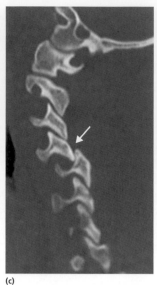
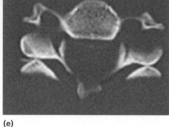

(a)   (b)   (c)   (d)

(e)

Figure 7.7 Facets dislocation. Sagittal at the level of the right articular processes (a), midsagittal (b), and sagittal at the level of the left articular processes (c) show locked facets (arrows). Axial (d and e) CT shows normal facet joints and naked facet, respectively.

upper thoracic part and the flexible lordotic lumbar spine, where most injuries occur; and (iii) the L3–sacrum zone, a flexible segment where axial loading injuries usually occur.

Numerous thoracolumbar spine injury classification systems have been developed, most of them based on the three-column concept devised by Denis.

According to Denis' classification, the anterior column comprises the ALL and the anterior half of the vertebral body, the middle column comprises the posterior half of the vertebral body and the PLL, and the posterior column comprises the pedicles, the facet joints, and the supraspinous ligaments. In his model, stability is dependent on at least two intact columns. The Denis system also classifies spinal trauma as minor (fractures of transverse processes, articular processes, pars interarticularis, and spinous processes that do not lead to acute instability) and major injuries (compression fracture, burst fracture, seat belt injury, and fracture–dislocation), according with injury morphology and mechanism. As of lately, this classification has fallen out of favor with neurosurgeons and spine surgeons.

Recently, the Spine Trauma Study Group proposed the thoracolumbar injury classification and severity score (TLICS). The TLICS is both a scoring and a classification system, based on three injury categories that are independently critical and complementary for appropriate treatment recommendations: (i) injury morphology, (ii) integrity of the PLC, and (iii) neurologic status of the patient. Within each category, subgroups are arranged from least to most significant, with a numeric value assigned to each injury pattern. Point values from the three main injury categories are totaled to provide a comprehensive severity score (Table 7.1). One distinguishing feature of the TLICS is its emphasis on injury morphology rather than the mechanism of injury, since various mechanisms can lead to similar injury patterns.

Independently of the different classifications systems, morphologic description of the fractures seen on imaging studies must be reported as follows:

- *Compression fracture*—vertebral collapse, defined as a visible loss of vertebral body height or disruption of the vertebral end plates. Less severe compression injuries may involve only the anterior portion of the vertebral body.

Table 7.1 The thoracolumbar injury classification and severity score with its subcategories and respective scoring.

Injury category	
Injury morphology	
Compression	1
Burst	2
Translation and rotation	3
Distraction	4
PLC status	
Intact	0
Injury suspected or indeterminate	2
Injured	3
Neurologic status	
Intact	0
Nerve root involvement	2
Spinal cord injury	
Incomplete	3
Complete	2
Cauda equine syndrome	3

Source: From Khurana et al. (2013).

- *Burst fractures*—a type of compression fracture with disruption of the posterior vertebral body, varying degrees of retropulsed fragments in the spinal canal and bone shards of the vertebra penetrating surrounding tissues (Figure 7.8).
- *Translation injuries*—defined as a horizontal displacement or rotation of one vertebral body with respect to another. These injuries are characterized by rotation of the spinous processes, unilateral or bilateral facet fracture–dislocation, and vertebral subluxation. Anteroposterior or sagittal translational instability is best seen on lateral images, while instability in the mediolateral or coronal plane is best seen on anteroposterior views.
- *Distraction injuries*—identified as anatomic dissociation along the vertical axis that can occur through the anterior and posterior supporting ligaments, the anterior and posterior osseous elements, or a combination of both.

A basic description of injury features includes the degree of comminution, percentage of vertebral height loss, retropulsion

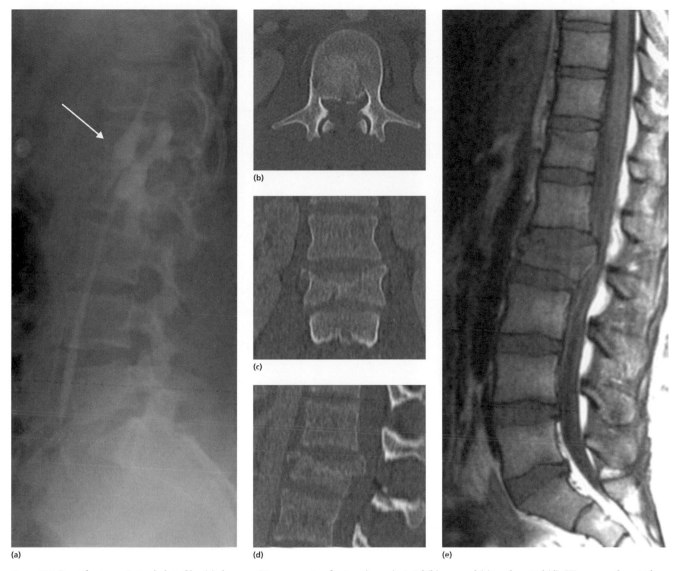

Figure 7.8 Burst fractures. Lateral plain film (a) shows an L2 compression fracture (arrow). Axial (b), coronal (c), and sagittal (d) CT scans and sagittal T1-W MRI (e) of the same patient.

distance, percentage of canal compromise, and other contiguous or noncontiguous vertebral injuries. Osseous retropulsion alone does not imply neurologic injury. In the thoracic spine, retropulsion may cause significant neurologic injury because the spinal canal is narrow and blood supply to the cord is sparse. In contrast, in the lumbar spine, a burst fracture may cause marked displacement of the *cauda equina* without neurologic deficits since the central canal is wide and the spinal cord generally ends at the level of L1.

The PLC serves as the posterior "tension band" of the spinal column and protects it from excessive flexion, rotation, translation, and distraction. Disruption of the PLC is seen on radiographs and CT or MR images as follows:

- Splaying of the spinous processes (widening of the interspinous space), avulsion fracture of the superior or inferior aspects of contiguous spinous processes, widening of the facet joints, empty ("naked") facet joints, perched or dislocated facet joints, or vertebral body translation or rotation.

The PLC must be directly assessed at MRI regardless of the severity of vertebral body injury seen at CT, because there is an inverse relationship between osseous destruction and ligamentous injury (Figure 7.9). With respect to spinal soft tissue injuries, keep in mind the following:

- On MRI, the ligamentum flavum and supraspinous ligament are seen as a low-signal-intensity continuous black stripe on sagittal T1-WI or T2-WI. Disruption of these stripes indicates a supraspinous ligament or ligamentum flavum tears.
- Fluid in the facet capsules or edema in the interspinous region on fluid-sensitive MR images (which include STIR or fat-saturated T2-weighted sequences) reflects a capsular or interspinous ligament injury, respectively.

Spinal cord injury

Spinal cord injury usually occurs at sites of fractures, secondary to bony impingement and cord compression. However, cord injury may also occur in the absence of bone fractures, caused by hyperflexion and hyperextension mechanism and associated vascular insults.

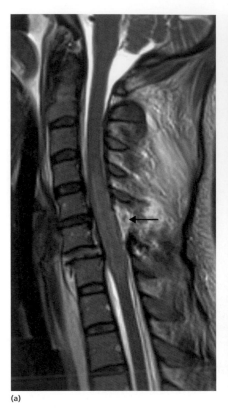
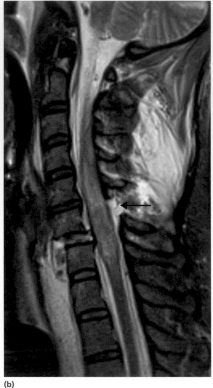
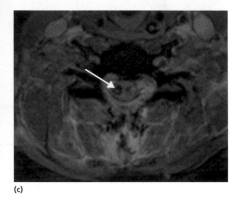

(a)   (b)   (c)

Figure 7.9 Hyperflexion cervical injury. Sagittal T2-WI (a and b) shows disruption of the posterior ligamentous complex (arrows), cord edema and hemorrhage, better depicted on axial T2* (c) (arrow).

There are two types of spinal cord injury:
- Nonhemorrhagic—seen on MRI as areas of high T2-WI signal that represents edema
- Hemorrhagic—seen on MRI as areas of low signal intensity on T2-/T2*-WI within the area of edema that represents hemorrhage (see Figure 7.9)

There is a strong correlation between the length of the spinal cord edema and the clinical outcome with patients who have over two vertebral segments doing poorly. However, the most important prognostic factor is the presence of hemorrhage, which has an extremely poor outcome.

Specific types of trauma, such as sudden distracted forces along the long axis, may lead to cord avulsion, more common at the junction of the cervical and thoracic cord. These injuries are more common in children.

Extramedullary hematomas

Extramedullary hematomas can follow trauma or be spontaneous. Subdural hematomas are rare and are usually related to coagulopathies. Epidural hematomas are more common, since the ventral epidural space contains a rich venous plexus susceptible to tearing injuries, even without vertebral fractures. MRI is the modality of choice to depict epidural and subdural hematomas.

Nerve root avulsion

The traumatic lesions described earlier may also affect nerve roots and result in radiculopathies. An additional form of direct trauma to the nerve roots is avulsion from their connection to the cord.

Brachial plexus nerve roots are most commonly affected resulting in upper extremity neurologic deficits. Birth trauma is a classic example of nerve root avulsion at the cervicothoracic junction. CT myelography or MRI may confirm the diagnosis as follows:
- MRI allows the direct visualization of nerve roots, CSF leaks through avulsed nerve roots sleeves, and associated cord injuries (edema and cord hematoma in acute stage, myelomalacia in the chronic stage).
- Postcontrast enhancement of nerve roots suggests functional impairment even if the nerve appears continuous and is due to disruption of the nerve–blood barrier. Abnormal enhancement of paraspinal muscles is also an indirect sign of root avulsion.
- The steady-state coherent gradient echo sequences (MR myelography) can easily identify nerve roots and the meningocele sac as do T2-weighted images.
- Diffusion-weighted neurography is a new MRI technique that may also show postganglionic injuries, as a discontinuation of the injured nerves. It is not currently used in routine clinical practice.

Vascular lesions

Spinal cord infarct

Spinal cord infarct is uncommon, but it is usually associated with devastating clinical symptoms and poor prognosis. It can be a complication of aortic aneurysm surgery or stenting; however, in the majority of patients, no obvious cause is identified. Patients usually present with acute paraparesis or quadriparesis, depending on the level of the spinal cord involvement.

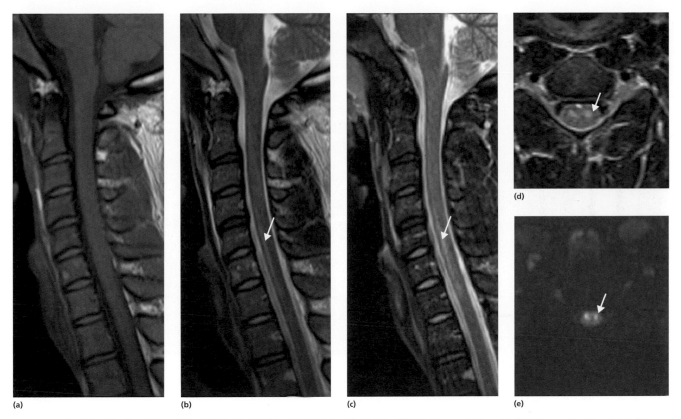

Figure 7.10 Spinal cord infarct. Sagittal T1-WI (a), T2-WI (b) and STIR (c), and axial T2-WI (d) show a spinal cord infarct (arrows) with restricted diffusion (e) (arrows).

MRI should be obtained in all patients with suspected spinal cord infarction, not only to confirm the diagnosis but also to exclude other more readily treated causes of cord impairment, such as compression. The following are the imaging features of cord infarctions (Figure 7.10):

- The hallmark of spinal cord infarction is a high T2-WI signal lesion within the cord, most commonly located centrally (anterior spinal artery territory). On axial images, a characteristic snake-eye appearance may be seen due to the prominent high signal involving the anterior gray matter horns. Central involvement can be more extensive and the white matter can also be affected.
- Restricted diffusion, when present, establishes the diagnosis.
- Spinal cord enlargement may be seen during the acute phase, while cord atrophy may be seen during the chronic phase.

Cord ischemia due to venous hypertension or arterial steal can be seen in spinal vascular malformations.

Spinal vascular malformations

Spinal arteriovenous malformation is a generic term used to cover any abnormal vascular complex that has a direct connection between the arterial system and the venous system without intervening capillaries.

Intramedullary AVMs have a congenital nidus of abnormal vessels within the spinal cord. Hemorrhage or ischemia (related with steal phenomenon) may be seen. Flow voids may be depicted on MRI within the substance of the spinal cord. They are exceedingly rare.

Extramedullary AVMs are located in the pia (**intradural AVMs**, located outside the substance of the spinal cord) or in the dura (**spinal dural** AVF). An AVF represents an abnormal connection between an artery and a vein in the dura of the nerve root sleeve. They are the most common type of AVMs in adults and the symptoms are related with venous hypertension and cord congestion with edema. The dilated venous plexus can be visualized on MRI as multiple flow voids and the cord shows high T2 signal and contrast enhancement.

Degenerative conditions

Degenerative disease of the spine

CT continues to be used widely in the examination of degenerative spinal disorders, and only a few differences between CT and MRI have been noted concerning diagnostic accuracy in the lumbar spine. CT remains superior in the evaluation of osseous features, such as osteophytes, spinal stenosis, facet hypertrophy, or sclerosis associated with degenerative disorders. MRI is the preferred procedure for evaluating the cervical spine as well as intervertebral disc disease.

As disc degeneration progresses, the water content of the disc decreases and fissures develop in the annulus. This results in decreased disc space height, posterior bulging of the disc annulus, and low signal of the disc on T2-WI. Further degeneration results in disc space collapse, misalignment, and nitrogen accumulation within the disc. Alterations in adjacent vertebral body marrow often occur with disc degeneration and appear as bands of altered signal intensity on MRI paralleling the narrowed disc (Figure 7.11).

The nomenclature of disc disease is controversial. Different definitions have been given to disc bulges, herniations, protrusions, extrusions, sequestrations, and migrations. The recommendations

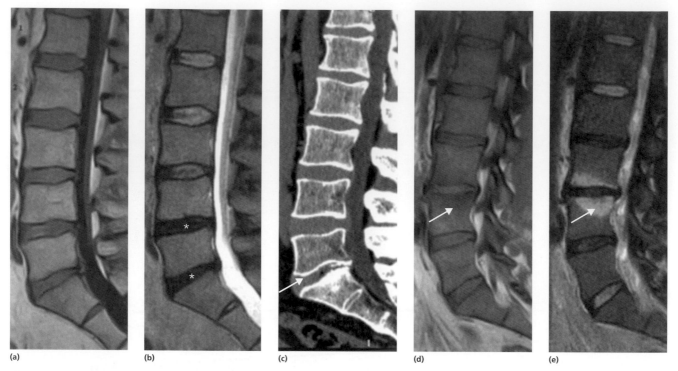

Figure 7.11 Degenerative disease of the spine. Sagittal T1-WI (a) and T2-WI (b) show decreased disc space height and low signal of the disc on T2-WI (*). Sagittal CT (c) shows disc space collapse and nitrogen accumulation within the disc (arrow). Sagittal T1-WI (d) shows a parallel band of low T1 signal adjacent to the end plates, with high signal intensity on T2-WI (e) (arrows).

from the American Society of Spine Radiology, the American Society of Neuroradiology, and the American Spine Society are:

- Disc bulge—bulging of the annulus fibrosus that involves more than half of the circumference of an intervertebral disc (>180°).
- Disc herniation—displacement of intervertebral disc material beyond the normal confines of the disc but involving less than half the circumference (to distinguish it from a disc bulge). Herniations are further divided into protrusions and extrusions. The distinction between a protrusion and an extrusion is made on the basis of the size of the "neck" versus the size of the "dome" of the herniation as well as its relationship to the disc level:
  - Protrusion has a broader neck than its "dome" and does not extend above or below the disc level. Disc protrusions are further divided into broad based, in which the base involves between 90 and 180° of the circumference, and focal, in which the base involves less than 90° of the disc circumference.
  - Extrusion has a narrower neck than dome and/or extends above or beyond the vertebral end plates. Extrusion can be in any axial direction and may migrate either superiorly or inferiorly. If the extrusion migrates but becomes separated from the rest of the herniation, it is known as an intervertebral disc sequestration.

Herniations may also be described in terms of its axial position, into central, subarticular, foraminal, extraforaminal, or anterior (Figure 7.12).

More important than the terminology used is the description of the disc disease, the relationship between the disc and the neuronal structures, and other associated findings, such as facet diseases, spondylolysis and spondylolisthesis, and central canal or neuroforaminal stenosis.

Degenerative joint diseases of the facets include bony hypertrophy, some facet slippage, and ligamentum flavum hypertrophy, a common cause of central canal and neuroforaminal stenosis.

Spondylolysis is a defect in the bony pars interarticularis and can be the source of low back pain and instability and generally involves the L5 segment. Prior to disc surgery or other back surgery, identification of spondylolysis is imperative. Spondylolisthesis represents a forward displacement of a vertebra and occurs from either bilateral spondylolysis or degenerative joint diseases of the facets with slippage of the facets (Figure 7.13).

It is not unusual to have patients with disc herniations or stenosis that appears severe on imaging, but who have no symptoms; thus, any imaging findings must be matched with clinical findings. Central canal measurements are no longer considered a valid indicator of disease by themselves.

Failed back surgery is common especially after lumbar spine operations. Identifiable causes of recurrent symptoms after surgery include inadequate surgery (including missed free disc fragments), development of fibrosis (scar tissue), recurrent or residual disc herniations, arachnoiditis, and spinal stenosis. Scar tissue located in the epidural space has been shown to enhance homogeneously on MRI after contrast administration, regardless of the time since surgery, while recurrent or residual herniated disc or disc fragments show only minimal peripheral enhancement presumably related with inflammation. Furthermore, a recurrent or residual disc herniation should cause mass effect upon the thecal sac and/or nerve roots, while scar generally surrounds the neural tissue.

Inflammatory conditions

Multiple sclerosis (MS) is the most common primary demyelinating disease. The majority of patients have brain and spinal cord involvement. Isolated spinal cord disease occurs in less than 20% of cases. Imaging plays an important role in MS diagnosis as included in McDonald criteria, introduced in 2001, then revised and simplified

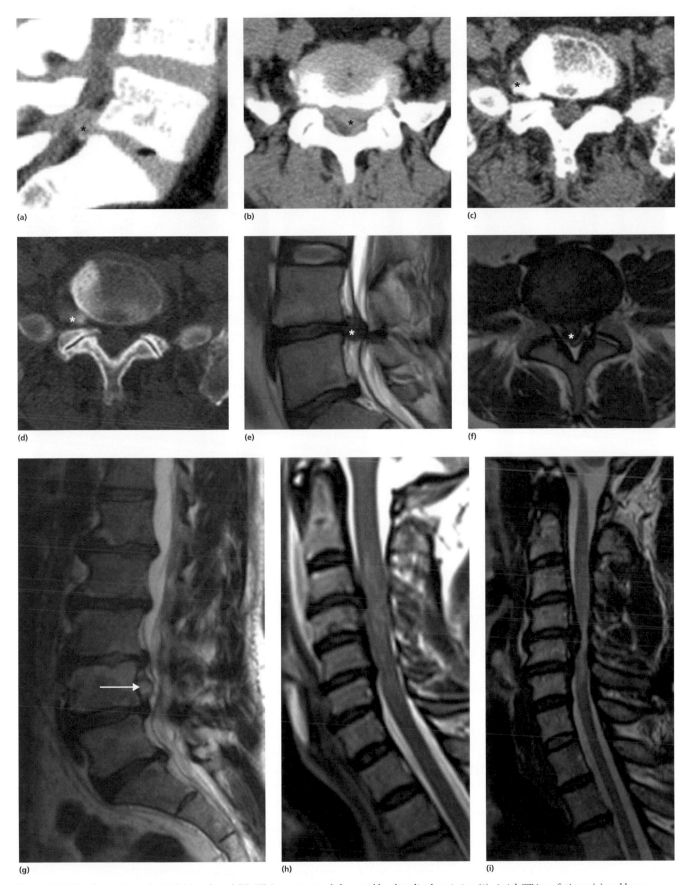

Figure 7.12 Disc herniations. Sagittal (a) and axial (b) CT demonstrate a left central lumbar disc herniation (*). Axial CT in soft tissue (c) and bone window (d) show a right extraforaminal calcified lumbar disc herniation (*). Sagittal (e) and axial T2-WI (f) show a subligamentous extrusion (*). Sagittal T2-WI (g) shows a sequestered disc (arrow). Sagittal T2-WI (h and i) in two different patients with cervical disc herniation, central canal stenosis, and cord compression with edema (*) (spondylotic myelopathy).

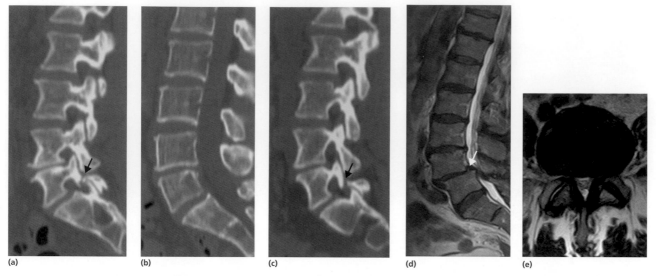

(a)   (b)   (c)   (d)   (e)

Figure 7.13 Spondylolysis and spondylolisthesis. Sagittal at the level of the right articular processes (a), midsagittal (b), and sagittal at the level of the left articular processes (c) bone window CT show bilateral defect in the L5 (arrow) pars interarticularis (spondylolisthesis). Sagittal T2-WI (d) shows forward displacement of L4 over L5 (arrow) caused by degenerative joint diseases of the facets (spondylolysis) well seen on axial T2-WI (e) with lumbar central canal stenosis.

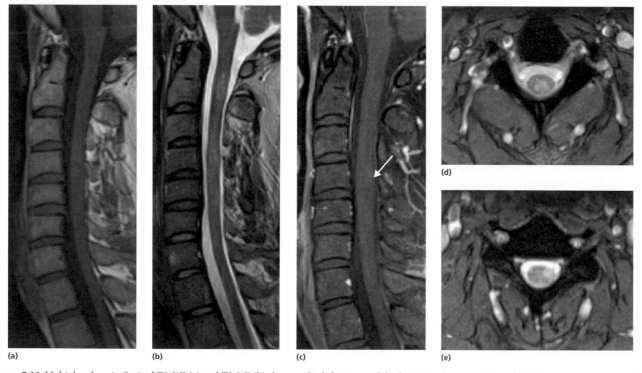

(a)   (b)   (c)   (e)

Figure 7.14 Multiple sclerosis. Sagittal T1-WI (a) and T2-WI (b) show multiple lesions with high T2 signal (arrows). One of the lesions shows minimal enhancement after gadolinium administration (arrow) (c). Axial T2-WI (d and e) demonstrates typical location of the lesions (arrows).

in 2005 and 2010. In McDonald criteria, MRI is used to demonstrate lesion dissemination in time and space (Figure 7.14):

- CT has poor sensitivity for detection, evaluation, and characterization of MS lesions. MRI offers by far the most sensitive technique for MS diagnosis and follow-up.
- On MRI, demyelinating lesions appear as high-signal T2-WI areas, typically triangular in shape and mostly located dorsally or laterally, involving the white matter tracts, generally with less than 2 vertebral bodies in length. However, as in the brain, both white matter and gray matter can be affected.

- Active lesions usually demonstrate enhancement after gadolinium administration and may show extensive edema with associated focal enlargement of the spinal cord.
- Classic chronic lesions do not show contrast enhancement and may demonstrate focal cord atrophy.

Primary and secondary neoplasms of the spinal cord (e.g., astrocytomas, ependymomas), other demyelinating diseases (acute disseminated encephalomyelitis (ADEM), transverse myelitis (TM)), neuromyelitis optica (NMO), infection, acute infarction, sarcoidosis, and systemic lupus erythematosus may mimic MS.

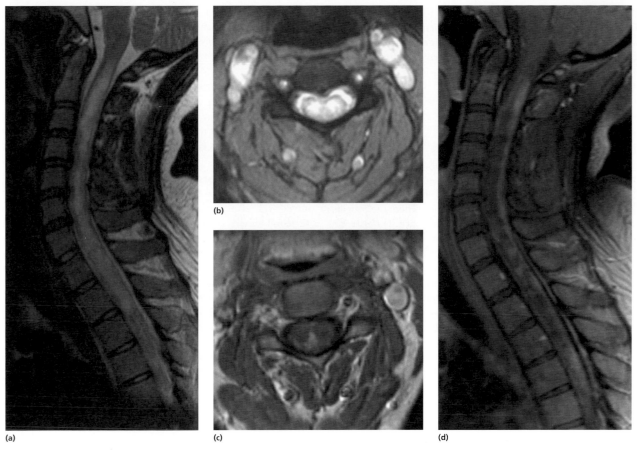

Figure 7.15 Neuromyelitis optica. Sagittal (a) and axial (b) T2-WI show a long lesion with patchy enhancement on axial (c) and sagittal (d) postcontrast T1-WI.

Neuromyelitis optica (NMO), also known as **Devic disease**, is no longer considered an MS variant. It is recognized as a distinct entity characterized by bilateral optic neuritis and myelitis, with blindness and paraplegia. NMO is an autoimmune demyelinating and necrotizing disease induced by a specific autoantibody, the NMO-IgG, which targets a transmembrane water channel (aquaporin 4). Imaging features of NMO follow (Figure 7.15):

- MRI shows typical features of optic neuritis: enlarged optic nerves hyperintense on T2-WI with enhancement after contrast administration. Bilateral involvement and extension of the signal back into the chiasm is particularly suggestive of NMO.
- Spinal lesions extend over long distances (>3 vertebral segments, often much more), usually involve the central part of the cord (MS lesions tend to involve individual peripheral white matter tracts), and after contrast administration may show patchy enhancement. Thin ependymal enhancement similar to ependymitis may be seen.
- Brain lesions follow the distribution of aquaporin 4 in the brain, which is particularly found in the periependymal brain adjacent to the ventricles.

ADEM is an immunologically mediated allergic inflammatory disease of the central nervous system (CNS), resulting in multifocal demyelinating lesions affecting the gray and white matter of the brain and spinal cord. It is typically seen in young children usually 4 weeks after a viral infection or vaccination. ADEM is characteristically monophasic, but multiphasic forms may be seen in 10% of cases. In 50% of ADEM patients, the antimyelin oligodendrocyte glycoprotein (MOG) IgG test is positive and supports the diagnosis. The imaging features of ADEM are:

- MRI usually shows diffuse high T2-WI signal of the spinal cord with cord swelling and variable enhancement after contrast administration.
- Brain imaging appearances vary from small "punctate" lesions to tumefactive lesions. Lesions are usually bilateral but asymmetrical. Brain lesions generally show no contrast enhancement.
- Compared to MS, involvement of the callososeptal interface is unusual. Involvement of the cerebral cortex; subcortical gray matter, especially the thalami; and the brainstem is also not very common, but if present are helpful in distinguishing from MS.

Transverse myelitis (TM) is a focal inflammatory disorder of the spinal cord resulting in motor, sensory, and autonomic dysfunction. TM may occur without apparent underlying cause (idiopathic) or in the setting of another illness. Idiopathic TM is assumed to be the result of abnormal activation of the immune system against the spinal cord. Underlying causes of TM include systemic inflammatory disease, such as Sjögren's syndrome; lupus (SLE) and neurosarcoidosis; infectious diseases like herpes simplex virus, herpes zoster virus, cytomegalovirus (CMV), Epstein–Barr virus (EBV), human immunodeficiency virus (HIV), enteroviruses, influenza, syphilis, tuberculosis, or Lyme diseases; and vascular diseases, such as thrombosis, vasculitis, or arteriovenous malformations. It can also be a paraneoplastic syndrome or the initial manifestation of MS, NMO, or ADEM. Remember that:

- MRI shows T2-WI hyperintense lesions involving more than 2/3 of the spinal cord cross-sectional area with focal enlargement and variable enhancement after contrast administration.

Infectious conditions

Infections may be classified according to their causative organism or according to their anatomic location. Spine pyogenic infections are usually secondary to bacteremia (arterial dissemination). However, some organisms may reach the lower spine through Batson venous plexus, and direct inoculation may occur in postsurgery patients or children with spinal dysraphism.

Osteomyelitis/discitis

Spondylodiscitis is a combination of discitis, inflammation of the intervertebral disc space, and spondylitis, inflammation of the vertebrae. In adults, the primary site of hematogenous infection is the vertebral end plates, due to its richest blood supply. First, vertebral osteomyelitis develops affecting the end plates. Then, the pyogenic infection progresses and extends into the disc space. This osteomyelitis/discitis complex is usually known as "pyogenic spondylodiscitis." If the infection is left untreated, the disc space is rapidly destroyed, with collapse and destruction of adjacent bone. The imaging features of osteomyelitis and discitis are:

- CT may show disc space narrowing and irregularity/ill definition of the end plates with surrounding soft tissue swelling.
- Characteristic MRI findings are low T1-WI and high T2-WI signal in disc space (fluid), low T1-WI and high T2-WI signal in adjacent end plates (bone marrow edema), loss of the normal cortical end plate definition, and high signal in paravertebral soft tissues.
- The T2-WI changes described earlier are particularly well seen on STIR or fat-saturated T2-WI.
- Peripheral enhancement around fluid collection(s), enhancement of vertebral end plates, and enhancement of perivertebral soft tissues are usually depicted on postcontrast T1-WI.

  Epidural phlegmon or abscess may accompany spondylodiscitis as follows (Figure 7.16):

- Epidural phlegmons are characteristically hypointense or isointense on T1-WI and slightly hyperintense on T2-WI with homogenous enhancement after contrast administration, while abscesses show rim enhancing and restricted DWI as described previously (see section "Critical observations").
- The adjacent dura and epidural venous plexus usually enhance intensely and appear thick.
- Epidural phlegmon and/or abscess typically compress the thecal sac and spinal cord, displacing the cord posteriorly. T2-WI signal abnormalities hyperintensity may develop in the cord. Direct invasion or hematogenous spread of the infectious processes into the spinal cord may occur but is rare.
- Paraspinal or psoas abscesses may also be seen.

Nonpyogenic infections, such as tuberculosis and some fungal infections, can show a more indolent clinical course and may mimic neoplastic diseases.

  Tuberculosis of the spine, or "Pott" disease, usually spreads by a subligamentous route involving multiple vertebral bodies, often with relative sparing of the intervening discs. Vertebral collapse, paraspinal calcification, and proliferative new bone formation with a kyphotic or "gibbus" deformity are usually seen and may lead to cord compression. Large paraspinal abscesses without severe pain or pus are common and are called "cold abscesses." Tuberculosis may also affect the intradural spinal compartment, resulting in an inflammatory arachnoiditis that can spread to the cord and nerve roots.

  Subdural empyemas are rare and tend to be associated with surgery or other violation of the dura. Subdural infections can rapidly spread through the arachnoid layer, resulting in meningitis.

Direct **spinal cord infections** are uncommon and are usually caused by viruses, such as varicella-zoster virus, HIV, CMV, or EBV and in immunocompromised patients by bacteria and fungi.

Neoplastic processes (benign/malignant)

Mass lesions of the spine are classified according to their locations as intramedullary, intradural–extramedullary, and extradural. The location is critical for the differential diagnosis. MRI is unquestionably the imaging procedure of choice in these patients.

Extradural tumors

Neoplasm is the second most frequent cause of an extradural mass, after disc herniation and other degenerative diseases. Primary vertebral tumors, such as chordomas, giant cells tumors, hemangiomas, and sarcomas, are discussed elsewhere in this book. The most common extradural neoplasms are **vertebral body metastases** generally from breast, lung, and prostate carcinoma. Imaging features of vertebral metastases are (Figure 7.17):

- Bone metastases appear as low-signal areas on T1-WI with high signal on T2-WI, because of their higher water content compared with the normal bone marrow fat. Nearly all metastases enhance.
- Densely sclerotic metastases, often seen in prostate cancer, can be dark on all sequences.

Distinguishing between benign osteoporotic and pathologic vertebral body compression fractures may be difficult, particularly when only one vertebra is involved. The following imaging findings are helpful:

- Most vertebral compression fractures, regardless of whether they are benign or malignant, show low T1- and high T2-WI signal intensities and may enhance after contrast material administration.
- In the chronic stage, the bone marrow of benign vertebral compression fractures returns to its normally high T1-WI signal intensity, whereas the bone marrow infiltrated by tumor remains hypointense on T1-WI.
- The most reliable MRI sign suggesting benign etiology is visualizing the fracture line as a T2- or postcontrast T1-WI linear hypointensity in the compressed vertebral body.
- Other signs that favor benign compression fractures include the presence of intervertebral fluid, an intervertebral vacuum cleft, absence of accompanying soft tissue masses, lack of pedicle abnormalities, solitary vertebral involvement, preservation of the posterior cortical margin, and a wedge-shaped deformity. Unfortunately, these signs cannot be found in all patients.
- In theory, malignant compressive fractures may show restricted diffusion caused by the infiltrating tumor cells, and benign osteoporotic fractures may show increased diffusion caused by the increased extracellular water. However, infiltrated vertebrae may show areas of both patterns, confusing the diagnosis (Figure 7.18).

Direct extension of paraspinous tumors

Any retroperitoneal and mediastinal tumor can invade the vertebral column and spinal canal by direct extension.

  Neuroblastoma, ganglioneuroma, and ganglioneuroblastoma arise from primitive paraspinous neural remnants, similar to fetal neuroblasts, and frequently involve the spinal canal extending through the neural foramina. In adults, lung cancer commonly does this.

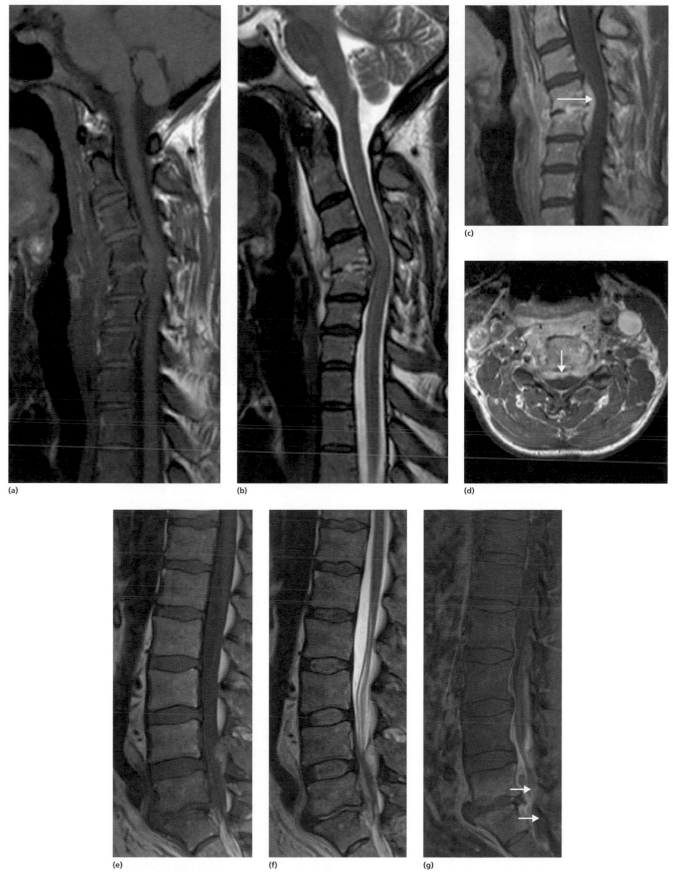

Figure 7.16 Spondylodiscitis. SagittalT1-WI(a), sagittalT2WI(b), and sagittal(c) and axial(d)postcontrastT1-WI show cervical spondylodiscitis with epidural phlegmon (arrows). Sagittal T1-WI (e), T2-WI (f), and postcontrast T1-WI (g) show lumbar spondylodiscitis with epidural abscesses in a different patient (arrows).

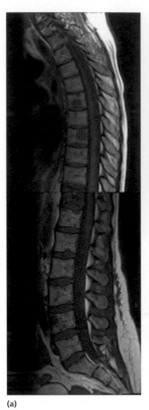
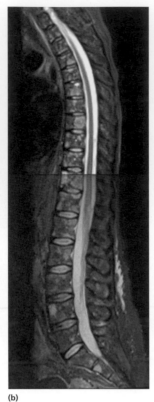
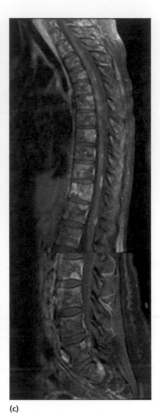

(a)   (b)   (c)

Figure 7.17 Bone metastases. Sagittal T1-WI (a), T2-WI (b), and postcontrast FS T1-WI (c) of a thoracic and lumbar spine.

Hematologic tumors

Leukemias show diffuse involvement or replacement of the normal bone marrow with tumor. Solid leukemia (chloromas) can be seen in the epidural space and may cause cord compression and also occur in the paraspinal regions.

Multiple myeloma is the most common primary malignant bone neoplasm in adults. Four main patterns are recognized: (i) disseminated form with multiple focal lesions predominantly affecting the axial skeleton; (ii) diffuse skeletal osteopenia; (iii) solitary plasmacytoma, which is a single expansile lesion most commonly in a vertebral body or in the pelvis; and (iv) osteosclerosing myeloma.

Solitary plasmacytoma usually appears as a lytic lesion with thinning and destruction of cortex and often has a nonspecific appearance. It is also one of the differential diagnoses for vertebra plana (totally collapsed vertebral body), along with eosinophilic granuloma (which tends to occur in children), leukemia, and severe osteoporosis.

Hodgkin and B-cell-type **lymphomas** are the most common lymphomas in the CNS. Spinal involvement is usually secondary. Lymphoma more commonly involves the vertebral body and paraspinal tissues or epidural compartment or both. Epidural lesions present usually as large masses that can mimic epidural infections.

Intradural–extramedullary tumors

Tumors within the thecal sac but outside the spinal cord (intradural and extramedullary) most often are nerve sheath tumors (schwannomas and neurofibromas) or meningiomas.

Most **nerve sheath tumors** arise from the dorsal sensory roots. Seventy percent are intradural–extramedullary in location, 15% are purely extradural, and 15% have both intradural and extradural components ("dumbbell" lesions).

Schwannomas are composed almost entirely of Schwann cells and typically grow within a capsule and remain extrinsic to the parent nerve, causing symptoms by compression. Thus, they may be resected with minimal damage to the underlying nerve.

By contrast, **neurofibromas** contain all the cellular elements of a peripheral nerve, including Schwann cells, fibroblasts, perineurial cells, and axons. The tumor cells grow diffusely within and along nerves and usually cannot be dissected from the parent nerve. These tumors may undergo malignant changes.

Neurofibromas are associated with neurofibromatosis type I, while schwannomas are associated with neurofibromatosis type II. Imaging alone cannot consistently differentiate these two types of nerve tumors. Imaging features of these tumors follow:

- MRI shows well-defined T1-WI hypointense/T2-WI hyperintense mass with enhancement after contrast administration.
- Adjacent bone remodeling is usually seen resulting in widening of the neural foramen and posterior vertebral body scalloping.
- When large, they may either align themselves with the long axis of the cord, forming "sausage"-shaped masses, which can extend over several levels, or may protrude out of the neural foramen, forming a "dumbbell"-shaped mass.
- A hyperintense rim surrounding a central area of low T2-WI signal ("target sign") was initially believed to be pathognomonic of neurofibroma, but it has been observed in both neurofibromas and schwannomas and has even been reported in malignant peripheral nerve sheath tumors.
- Schwannomas are usually round, whereas neurofibromas are more commonly fusiform.
- Schwannomas are frequently associated with hemorrhage, intrinsic vascular changes, cyst formation, and fatty degeneration, seen as mixed signal intensity on T2-WI.

Meningiomas are most commonly located in the thoracic spine followed by the cervical region especially the craniocervical junction, and despite being usually small, significant neurologic dysfunction may occur due to cord compression. CT and MRI

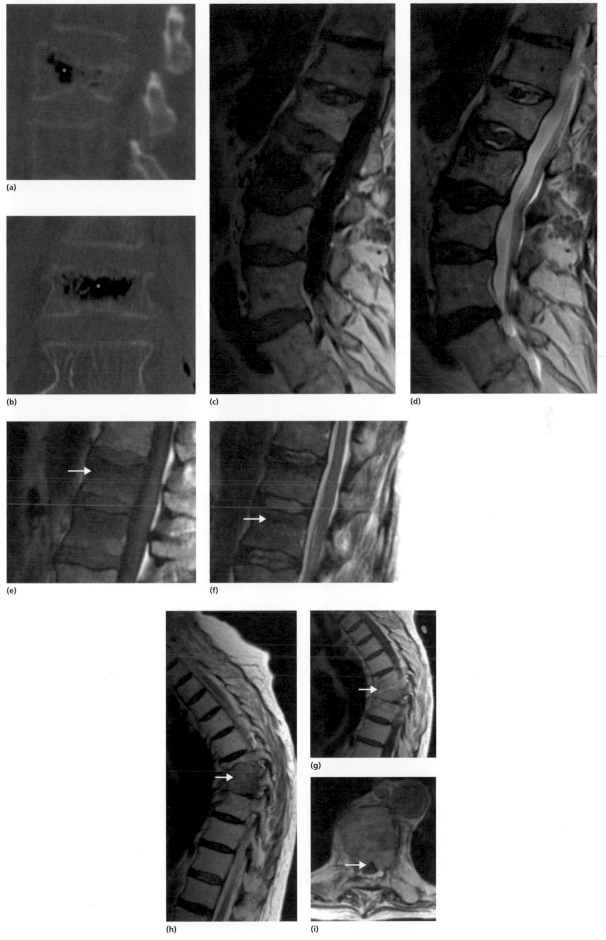

Figure 7.18 Benign and malignant compressive fractures. Sagittal (a) and coronal (b) CT, sagittal T1-WI (c), and T2-WI (d) of thoracic vertebrae show a benign compressive fracture with intravertebral vacuum cleft (*). Sagittal T1-WI (e) and T2-WI (f) of a different patient show the characteristic fracture line (arrows). Sagittal T1-WI (g), sagittal (h), and axial (i) postcontrast FS T1-WI show a malignant fracture from thyroid cancer (arrows).

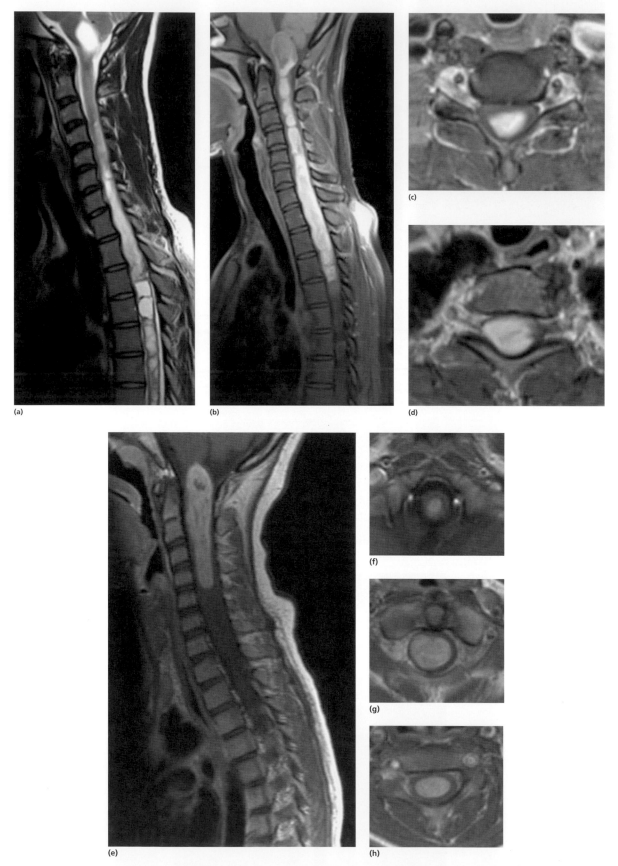

Figure 7.19 Astrocytoma and ependymoma. Sagittal T2-WI (a) and sagittal (b) and axial (c and d) postcontrast T1-WI show an astrocytoma. Sagittal (e) and axial (f, g, and h) postcontrast T1-WI show an ependymoma.

findings are similar to that of intracranial meningiomas, showing strong enhancement and dural tails.

Intramedullary tumors

Intramedullary tumors are usually astrocytomas, ependymomas, or, less frequently, hemangioblastomas.

The distinction between **astrocytomas and ependymomas** may be difficult as follows (Figure 7.19):

- Both are expansible low T1-WI and high T2-WI signal intensity lesions with variable enhancement after contrast administration.
- Involvement of the entire cord diameter and longer cord segments favors astrocytoma.
- Most astrocytomas occur in the cervical and upper to midthoracic cord.
- The presence of cysts and hemorrhage favors ependymoma.

Histologically, ependymomas are usually benign, but a complete curative excision is commonly not possible, except for the filum terminale ependymomas, which are known as myxopapillary ependymomas due to their unique histology.

Hemangioblastomas occur in the spine as well as the posterior fossa; both are associated with von Hippel–Lindau syndrome.

- They are usually located in the thoracic cord, followed by the cervical cord.
- MRI usually shows hypointense T1-WI and hyperintense T2-WI intramedullary lesions, eccentrically located with a variable exophytic component and surrounding edema. Discrete nodules are the most common presentation, but diffuse cord expansion is not uncommon.
- An associated tumor cyst or syrinx is seen in 50–100% of cases.
- Hemosiderin around the edges of the tumors may be present.
- Intrinsic focal flow voids may be seen, especially in larger lesions.
- The tumor nodule enhances vividly on postcontrast T1-WI.
- Conventional angiography shows the characteristic enhancing nidus with associated dilated arteries and prominent draining veins. Endovascular embolization may be performed to reduce intraoperative blood loss.

Care should be taken to image the entire neuraxis to ensure that no other lesions are present.

Suggested reading

Brant, W.B. & Helms, C.A. (2012) *Fundamentals of Diagnostic Radiology*, fourth edn. Lippincott Williams & Wilkins, Philadelphia, PA.

Fardon, D.F. & Milette, P.C. (2001) Nomenclature and Classification of Lumbar Disc Pathology. Recommendations of the Combined Task Forces of the North American Spine Society, American Society of Spine Radiology, and American Society of Neuroradiology. *Spine*, **26** (5), E93–E113.

Jindal, G. & Pukenas, B. (2011) Normal spinal anatomy on magnetic resonance imaging. *Magnetic Resonance Imaging Clinics of North America*, **19**, 475–488.

Khurana, B., Sheehan, S.E., Sodickson, A. *et al.* (2013) Traumatic Thoraco-lumbar spine injuries: what the spine surgeon wants to know. *Radiographics*, **33** (7), 2031–2046.

Rojas, A.C., Bertozzi, J.C., Martinez, C.R. *et al.* (2007) Reassessment of the Craniocervical Junction: Normal Values on CT. *American Journal of Neuroradiology*, **28**, 1819–1823.

Yousem, D.M., Zimmerman, R.D. & Grossman, R.I. (2010) *Neuroradiology: The Requisites*. St Mosby, Elsevier, Philadelphia, PA.

CHAPTER 8

Head and neck imaging

Joana N. Ramalho[1,2], Kiran Reddy Busireddy[1], and Benjamin Huang[1]
[1] Department of Radiology, University of North Carolina, Chapel Hill, USA
[2] Department of Neuroradiology, Centro Hospitalar de Lisboa Central, Lisboa, Portugal

Paranasal sinus and nasal cavity

Computed tomography (CT) is the first-line imaging modality for evaluation of the paranasal sinuses. The primary goals of imaging are identification of critical anatomic landmarks or variants and identification of abnormal soft tissue disease and any extension beyond the sinonasal cavities. Magnetic resonance imaging (MRI) is used to evaluate tumors and to assess disease extension into adjacent soft tissues, the cavernous sinus, or the intracranial compartment. Plain films are no longer considered adequate in assessment of sinus pathology.

Anatomic considerations

Nasal anatomy can be extremely variable (Figure 8.1). Anatomic changes, which alter normal airflow or mucociliary clearance, may predispose to inflammatory disease or may modify surgical approaches. Furthermore, under the age of two, not all the sinuses are pneumatized.

The major components of the nasal cavity are the midline septum and the lateral walls. The septum is composed of the perpendicular plate of the ethmoid bone, the vomer, and the quadrangular cartilage. The lateral walls are the most functionally significant components, as they contain the ostia, which drain the paranasal sinuses into the nasal cavity, as well as the superior, middle, and inferior turbinates, which divide the nasal cavities into their respective meatuses.

Although they are usually not clinically significant, anatomic variants such as an aerated turbinate (concha bullosa), variant ethmoid cells (e.g., Haller and agger nasi cells), or deviation of the nasal septum can predispose to sinusitis by obstructing normal drainage (Figure 8.2).

The paranasal sinuses are air-filled spaces surrounding on the nasal cavity, which may function to lighten the weight of the head, humidify and heat inhaled air, increase the resonance of speech, or serve as a protective crumple zone in the event of facial trauma.

The *frontal sinuses* are housed in the frontal bone superior to the orbits in the forehead. They are absent at birth and are formed by the upward movement of anterior ethmoid cells after the age of 2. They drain into the middle meatuses through the frontal recesses.

The *maxillary sinuses* are the largest paranasal sinus and lie inferior to the orbits in the maxillary bone. They are the first sinuses to develop. They drain into the middle meatus through the ethmoid infundibulum. The infraorbital nerves run through the infraorbital canals along the roof of each sinus.

Behind the posteromedial wall of each maxillary sinus lies the pterygopalatine fossa, a small space that houses several important neurovascular structures and communicates with several skull base foramina, becoming an important route for intracranial spread of sinus diseases.

The *sphenoid sinuses* originate in the sphenoid bone and are the most posteriorly located sinuses. They reach their full size by the late teenage years. Each drains into the superior meatus. Important surgical relations of the sphenoid sinus include the carotid artery along its lateral walls, the sella turcica posterosuperiorly, and the optic nerve superolaterally.

The *ethmoid sinuses* arise in the ethmoid bone, forming several distinct air cells. They continue to grow and pneumatize until the age of 12. Ethmoid cells are divided into anterior and posterior cells by the bony basal lamellae of the middle turbinates. Anterior ethmoid cells drain into the middle meatus, while posterior ethmoid cells drain into the superior meatus.

The ostiomeatal complex is the major area of mucociliary drainage for the frontal and maxillary sinuses and anterior ethmoid cells. It comprises the maxillary sinus ostium, the ethmoid infundibulum, the uncinate process, the ethmoid bulla and anterior ethmoid cells, the semilunar hiatus, the frontal recess, and the middle meatus.

The neurosensory cells for smell reside in the olfactory epithelium along the roof of the nasal cavity. The axons of these cells extend through the cribriform plate of the ethmoid bone into the paired olfactory bulbs at the anterior end of the *olfactory nerves*. Each nerve courses posteriorly through the anterior cranial fossa in the recesses known as the olfactory grooves.

Critical Observations in Radiology for Medical Students, First Edition. Katherine R. Birchard, Kiran Reddy Busireddy, and Richard C. Semelka.
© 2015 John Wiley & Sons, Ltd. Published 2015 by John Wiley & Sons, Ltd.
Companion website: www.wiley.com/go/birchard

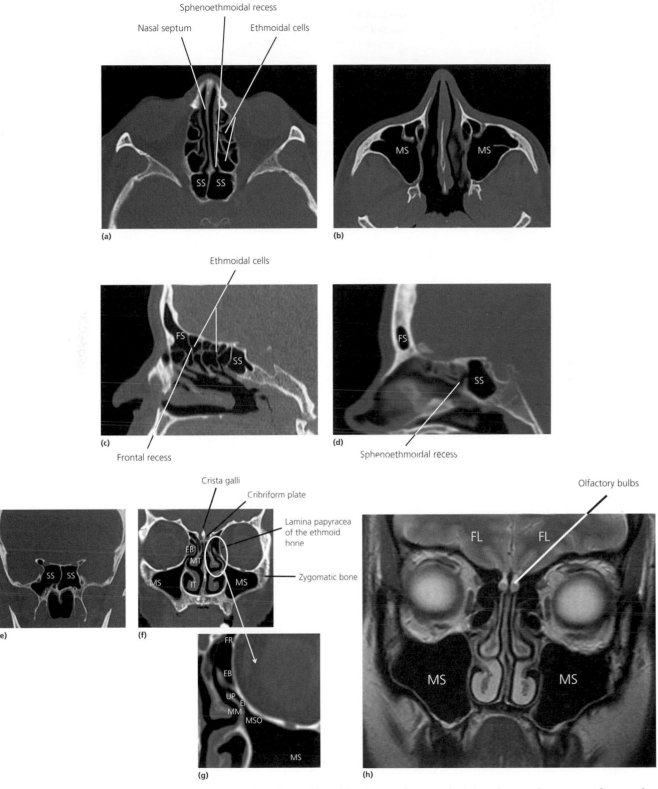

Figure 8.1 Normal anatomy. Axial (a and b), sagittal (c and d), and coronal (e and f) CT images (bone window) show the normal appearance of paranasal sinus and nasal cavity (EB, ethmoid bulla; FS, frontal sinus; IT, inferior turbinate; MS, maxillary sinus; MT, middle turbinate; SS, sphenoid sinus). The detailed ostiomeatal complex (circle on f) is shown on (g). It includes the maxillary sinus ostium (MSO), the ethmoid infundibulum (EI), the uncinate process (UP), the ethmoid bulla (EB), the semilunar hiatus (not shown), the frontal recess (FR), and the middle meatus (MM). Coronal T2-W MRI (h) at the level of the olfactory bulbs (FL, frontal lobe).

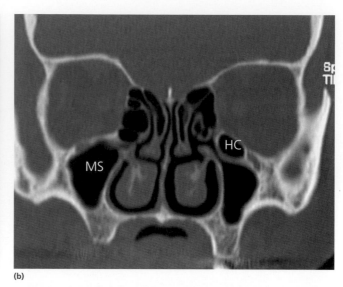

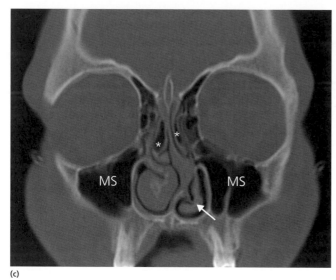

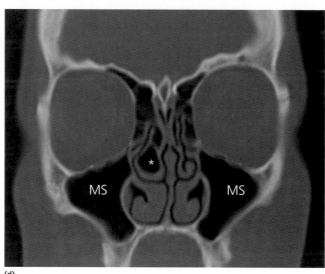

Figure 8.2 Anatomic variants. Axial CT (a) shows deviation of the nasal septum (arrow) and Onodi cell (OC). Also known as sphenoethmoid cell, OC is a posterior ethmoid cell lateral and superior to the sphenoid sinus that has a close relationship with the optic nerve. Coronal CT (b) shows a left Haller cell. Coronal CT (c) shows a paradoxal left inferior turbinate (arrow). Note also the deviation of the nasal septum and the left Haller cell. Coronal CT (d) shows a right aerated middle turbinate (concha bullosa) (*), also seen bilaterally in the previous patient (c).

Critical observations

Acute invasive fungal sinusitis

Acute invasive fungal sinusitis is a rapidly progressive fungal infection defined by the presence of fungal hyphae within the mucosa, submucosa, bone, or blood vessels of the paranasal sinuses. It typically develops in immunocompromised patients and is a source of significant morbidity and mortality. The infection spreads from the sinus by vascular invasion, and orbital and intracranial extension develops rapidly if it is not appropriately treated (Figure 8.3):

- CT shows soft tissue attenuation with hypoattenuating mucosal thickening of the involved paranasal sinus and nasal cavity. There is a predilection for unilateral involvement of the ethmoid and sphenoid sinuses.
- Bone erosion and mucosal thickening may be extensive or very subtle. Attention should be paid to the presence of obliteration of the perisinus fat planes and invasion of adjacent structures such

as the maxillofacial soft tissues, orbit, pterygopalatine fossa, and anterior cranial fossa.

- MRI is the modality of choice to assess soft tissue extension. The findings within the sinus itself are variable and range from mucosal thickening to complete opacification of the sinus with T1-WI and T2-WI intermediate to low signal.

Complications of acute invasive fungal sinusitis include vascular invasion and thrombosis, intracranial hemorrhage, meningitis, epidural or cerebral abscesses, cavernous sinus thrombosis, orbital infection, and osteomyelitis.

Trauma

CT is the modality of choice in the assessment of facial trauma. Patients with facial fractures frequently have concurrent intracranial injuries. Contrast administration is only performed in cases of suspected vascular injury.

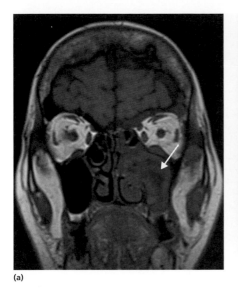
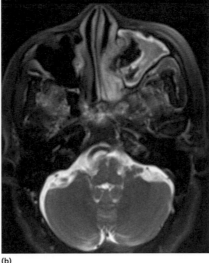
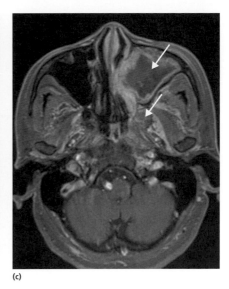

(a) (b) (c)

Figure 8.3 Acute invasive fungal sinusitis. Coronal T1 (a), axial T2 (b) and axial postcontrast T1-W MRI (c) show left acute invasive sinusitis (arrows) extending behind the paranasal sinus.

The facial bones and the adjacent aerated sinuses are difficult to visualize on MRI because they produce relatively little signal. However, MRI is useful for assessing potential vascular complications such as arterial dissections, pseudoaneurysms, and arteriovenous fistulas. Angiography may also be indicated in this setting.

Indirect signs of facial injury such as soft tissue swelling and paranasal sinus opacification can help provide evidence of trauma and may help to localize the site of impact or suggest the presence of an occult fracture.

Nasal bone fractures are the most common type of facial fractures. Radiologic confirmation is not needed, but they are often missed when significant facial swelling is present.

Le Fort fractures are fractures of the midface, which collectively involve separation of all or a portion of the maxilla from the skull base. Three different patterns are described according to the plane of injury, with all including a fracture through the pterygoid plates (Figure 8.4). Since multiple and different combinations of Le Fort fracture patterns may occur at the same time, in clinical practice, it is probably better to describe the specific bones fractured rather than classify the fractures into a specific category.

Nasoethmoid complex injury covers a wide variety of different fractures that may include the lamina papyracea, orbital roof, orbital rim, frontal or ethmoid sinus, nasal bone, frontal process of the maxilla, and sphenoid bone. These fractures have also been called nasoethmoid-orbital fractures because of the importance of the often associated orbital injuries.

The zygoma articulates with the frontal, maxillary, sphenoid and temporal bone. Zygomatic arch fractures may occur as an isolated finding or as part of a *zygomaticomaxillary complex fracture*, also known as "tripod," "quadripod," or "trimalar" fracture. Quadripod fracture is probably the most accurate term as it involves all four zygomatic articulations.

Mandibular fractures are extremely common in patients with maxillofacial injury. They can be classified in either simple or compound. Simple fractures are most common in the ramus and condyle and do not communicate externally or with the mouth. Compound fractures are those that communicate internally through a tooth socket or externally through a laceration with a resultant vulnerability to infection.

Degenerative/inflammatory/infectious conditions

Sinusitis

Inflammatory disease is the most common pathology involving the paranasal sinus and nasal cavity. Mild mucosal thickening, mainly in the maxillary and ethmoid sinus, is common even in asymptomatic individuals.

Acute sinusitis is an acute inflammation of the nasal and paranasal sinus mucosa that lasts less than 4 weeks. It is typically caused by a viral upper respiratory tract infection.

Diagnostic criteria (Figure 8.5) are:
- On CT peripheral mucosal thickening, airfluid levels, and air bubbles within the sinus secretions are typically seen.
- At MRI, T1-WI can differentiate mucosal thickening, which is isointense, from soft tissue and fluid, which are hypointense. Both are hyperintense in T2-WI. The inflamed mucosa shows contrast enhancement, while sinus secretions do not.

Sinusitis complications can occur, namely, bone erosion with subperiosteal abscess formation, cavernous sinus thrombosis, and intracranial extension with meningitis, subdural empyema, or cerebral abscess formation. Sphenoid sinusitis is of particular clinical concern, as it may easily extend intracranially owing to the presence of valveless veins.

Chronic sinusitis is an inflammation of the nasal and paranasal sinus mucosa that lasts for at least 8 weeks, despite treatment attempts. Chronic sinusitis can result from recurring episodes of acute sinusitis or can be caused by other health conditions like asthma and allergic rhinitis, immune disorders, or structural abnormalities such as a deviated septum or nasal polyps.

Diagnostic criteria are:
- CT shows sinus secretions and mucoperiosteal thickening of the sinus walls.
- On MRI, chronic sinus secretions that have become desiccated are hypointense on both T1- and T2-WI and may mimic an aerated sinus.

Fungal sinusitis is a relatively common, often misdiagnosed type of sinusitis with particular clinical and imaging findings. It is broadly categorized as either invasive or noninvasive, based on the presence

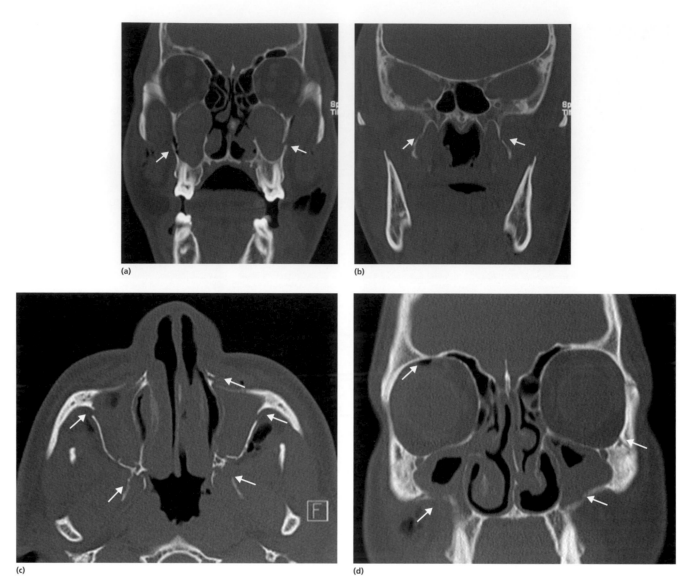

(a)

(b)

(c)

(d)

Figure 8.4 Facial fractures. Coronal CT (a and b) shows Le Fort fracture type 1, in which the fracture line passes through the alveolar ridge, lateral nose, and inferior wall of maxillary sinus. Axial and coronal CT (c and d) shows type 2 Le Fort fracture, in which the fracture arch passes through posterior alveolar ridge, lateral walls of maxillary sinuses, inferior orbital rim, and nasal bones.

or absence of fungal hyphae within the mucosa, submucosa, bone, or blood vessels of the paranasal sinuses. Fungal infections tend to occur in immunocompromised patients but can also occur in patients with healthy immune systems.

Acute invasive fungal sinusitis is the most aggressive form of fungal sinusitis (previousely described in Critical observations section).

Allergic fungal sinusitis is the most common form of fungal sinusitis particularly common in warm and humid climates such as the southern United States. The underlying cause is thought to be a hypersensitivity reaction (type 1, IgE-mediated hypersensitivity reaction) to certain inhaled fungal organisms resulting in a chronic noninfectious, inflammatory process. Typically, this form affects immunocompetent individuals with history of atopy including allergic rhinitis and asthma.

- The disease tends to be bilateral, usually involving multiple sinuses and the nasal cavity. The majority of the sinuses show near-complete opacification.
- On CT, the sinuses are typically opacified by centrally (often serpiginous) hyperdense material (hyperattenuating allergic mucin) with a peripheral rim of hypodense mucosa.

- Some patients may have expansion of an involved sinus with remodeling and thinning of the bony sinus walls or even erosion.
- On MRI, variable T1-WI signal intensity of sinus contents can be seen. There is characteristic low T2 signal. The inflamed mucosal lining is hypointense on T1-WI and hyperintense on T2-WI with contrast enhancement. There is no enhancement in the center or in the majority of the sinus contents.

Although the condition is not considered invasive, intracranial or intraorbital extension may occur if it is left untreated. Surgical treatment is usually required to restore the normal sinus drainage.

Inflammatory polyps

Inflammatory nasal polyps are benign sinonasal mucosal lesions.

Nasal polyps represent hyperplasia of the mucosa in response to chronic inflammation, usually secondary to chronic sinusitis.

Antrochoanal polyps are solitary polyps arising within the maxillary sinus and extending to the nasopharynx. Although they

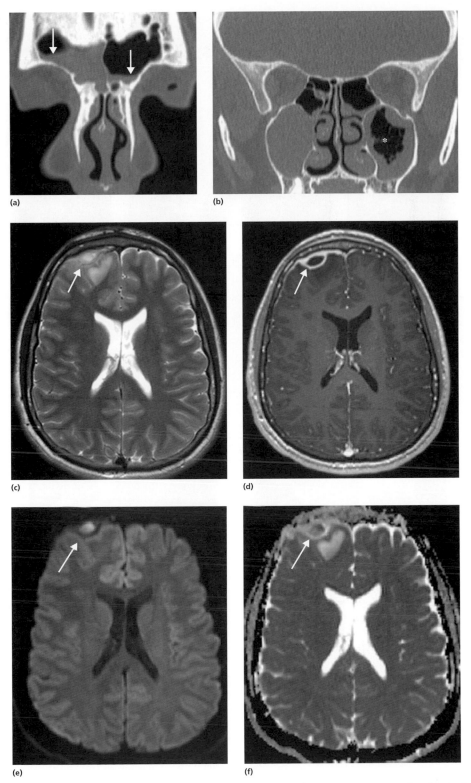

Figure 8.5 Acute sinusitis. Coronal CT of two different patients (a and b) with acute sinusitis, showing sinus secretions. Note the air–fluid level in the frontal sinus (arrow) (a) and air bubbles within the left maxillary sinus (*) (b). Axial T2 (c), axial (d) T1 postcontrast MRI, diffusion (e), and ADC map (f) show a right frontal epidural abscess with underlying parenchymal edema and restricted diffusion (arrows) of a different patient with complicated acute sinusitis.

represent reactive mucosal thickening as nasal polyps, they are usually found in nonatopic patients and for that reason have been recently considered a distinct entity (Figure 8.6):

- On CT, *solitary inflammatory polyps* are well-defined masses with mucoid density.

- *Sinonasal polyposis* is seen as polypoid masses involving nasal cavity and paranasal sinus mixed with chronic inflammatory secretions. Remodeling of sinonasal bones is common in severe cases. Polyps may have a higher density if they are long standing and/or have an associated fungal infection.

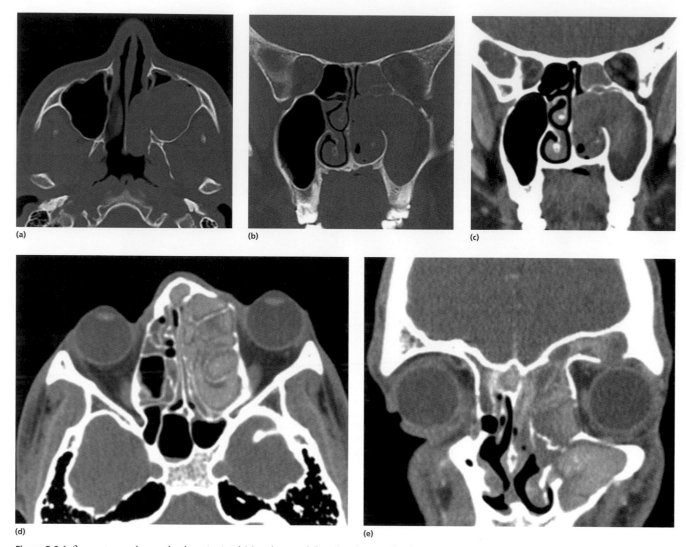

Figure 8.6 Inflammatory polyps and polyposis. Axial (a) and coronal (b and c—bone and soft tissue windows, respectively) CT show a left antrochoanal polyp. Axial (d) and coronal (e) CT in a patient with sinonasal polyposis.

- An *antrochoanal polyp* arises within the maxillary sinus and extends into the nasal cavity and nasopharynx by passing through and widening the major or accessory maxillary ostium. Similar polyps arising in the sphenoid sinus and extending into the naso-pharynx, are called sphenochoanal polyps. These cause smooth sinus enlargement.
- On MR, inflammatory polyps are intermediate to low signal inten-sity on T1-WI with high homogeneous T2-WI signal intensity, which aids in distinction from tumors. The signal may vary if they are chronic and/or if fungal infection is present. Postcontrast T1-WI show peripheral enhancement without central enhancement.

Mucous retention cysts and mucoceles

Mucous retention cysts result from the accumulation of mucus within the soft tissue that lines the sinuses as a result of obstruction of a duct or gland within the epithelial layer. They are usually dis-covered incidentally as a rounded, dome-shaped, soft tissue mass, most commonly situated on the floor of the maxillary sinus. Though usually asymptomatic, they may be associated with headaches or facial pain. If located in the ostium, they may obstruct drainage and lead to infection.

A mucocele is similar to retention cysts but occupies the entire sinus instead of being confined to a single mucous gland. The characteristic feature of a mucocele is expansion of the involved sinus with associated sinus wall bony thinning and remodeling. The frontal sinus is the most commonly affected sinus followed by the ethmoids. Large mucoceles may breach bone and extend into nasal cavity, orbit, or intracranial cavity.

When a mucocele becomes infected, it is referred to as mucopyo-cele. These lesions frequently require surgical decompression. Delay in diagnosis and treatment can lead to complications including orbital abscess, meningitis, subdural empyema, or cavernous sinus thrombosis. At imaging they are similar with mucoceles but demon-strate peripheral enhancement.

Neoplastic processes

Benign neoplasms

Inverted papilloma is an uncommon sinonasal tumor, almost inva-riably unilateral, that originates in the lateral nasal wall. It is named based on its histologic appearance, since the neoplastic nasal epithelium inverts and grows into the underlying mucosa. It is a benign tumor; however, it has an unlimited growth potential and may degenerate into squamous cell carcinoma (Figure 8.7):

- CT features are nonspecific, showing a soft tissue density mass with slightly enhancement. The location of the mass is one of the few clues toward the correct diagnosis. Calcification and focal hyperostosis, which tend to occur at the site of tumor origin, are sometimes observed. Bone erosion may be present, similar to that seen in squamous cell carcinoma.
- MRI often demonstrates a distinctive appearance, referred to as convoluted cerebriform pattern seen on both T2- and contrast-enhanced T1-WI that represents alternating lines of high and low signal intensity. This signal is seen in the majority of cases, and it is uncommon in other sinonasal tumors.

Unfortunately, imaging is unable to confidently distinguish between inverted papillomas from inverted papilloma with malignancy or pure malignancy.

Juvenile nasopharyngeal angiofibroma is a rare benign but locally aggressive vascular tumor, typically seen in male adolescents presenting with epistaxis. It is important to have a high clinical suspicion for this lesion, because life-threatening hemorrhage may result if a biopsy or limited resection is attempted (Figure 8.7):

- On CT, it is typically seen as a lobulated nonencapsulated soft tissue mass. Although these masses are thought to arise from the region of the sphenopalatine foramen, which is often widened, they are usually sizeable at diagnosis, frequently with extension into the nasopharynx and pterygopalatine fossa and over time into the orbit, paranasal sinuses, intracranial cavity, and infratemporal fossa. There is marked enhancement following contrast administration.
- Bone is remodeled or resorbed rather than destroyed. This feature may be helpful in differentiating from other more aggressive lesions.
- MRI is excellent at evaluating tumor extension into the orbit and intracranial compartments. The presence of prominent flow voids leads to a salt-and-pepper appearance on most sequences and is characteristic of these lesions.
- Angiography may be useful for defining the vascular supply of the tumor and for preoperative embolization.

Malignant neoplasms

Simplistically, MRI can differentiate malignant neoplasms from inflammatory masses and sinusitis, since most malignant sinonasal tumors have intermediate T2-WI signal intensity whereas inflammatory lesions and sinus secretions have markedly increased signal intensity on T2-WI.

Primary nasal neoplasms can originate from any of the intrinsic nasal tissues, including squamous epithelium, minor salivary glands, neuroectoderm, soft tissue, bone, cartilage, and lymphoid tissue.

Because the entire upper aerodigestive tract is lined with squamous epithelium, *squamous cell carcinoma* is the most common malignancy (80–90%) of the paranasal sinuses and nasal cavity and also of the entire head and neck. It is often clinically silent until quite advanced. Imaging findings are nonspecific and do not allow differentiation from other malignancies. They usually present as soft tissue masses with bone destruction.

Minor salivary glands are dispersed throughout the upper aerodigestive tract but are most highly concentrated in the palate. The most common minor *salivary malignancies* include adenoid cystic carcinoma, pleomorphic adenoma, and mucoepidermoid carcinoma.

Olfactory neuroblastoma (historically referred to as *esthesioneuroblastoma*) is a neural crest-derived neoplasm arising from the olfactory mucosa in the superior nasal fossa:

- On CT, these tumors are usually seen as a homogeneous, enhancing mass that primarily remodels bone. Calcifications can be seen.
- On MRI, these tumors have intermediate signal intensity on all imaging sequences, with enhancement after contrast administration. Intracranial extension through the cribriform plate into the anterior cranial fossa is not uncommon and suggests the diagnosis.
- When intracranial extension is present, peritumoral cysts between it and the overlying brain are often present. This may be helpful in distinguishing it from other entities.

Orbits

CT is the first-line imaging modality for orbital evaluation and is suitable for the evaluation of fractures, calcifications, and radiopaque foreign bodies. MRI is preferred for the evaluation of orbital soft tissues, including the visual pathways and the other cranial nerves. The presence of an orbital metallic foreign body is a contraindication to MRI because of the risk of migration and heating, and resultant damage to ocular structures.

Anatomic considerations

The orbit is a conical craniofacial cavity oriented with its apex directed posteriorly. It is formed by the frontal, sphenoid, ethmoid, palatine, maxillary, zygomatic, and lacrimal bones. It contains the globe; the optic nerve (CN II); the ophthalmic artery; the inferior and superior ophthalmic veins; the extraocular muscles (medial rectus, superior rectus, inferior rectus, lateral rectus, superior oblique, and inferior oblique); the levator palpebrae superioris muscle; cranial nerves III, IV, and VI; branches of CN V; sympathetic nerves; fat; and part of the lacrimal apparatus.

The orbit can be subdivided into the ocular compartment (or globe), the muscle cone, and the intraconal and extraconal spaces. The extraocular muscles (except the inferior oblique muscle) form the muscle cone, which converge posteriorly on a tendinous ring (the annulus of Zinn) at the orbital apex.

The major orbital foramina are the optic canal (traversed by CN II and the ophthalmic artery), the superior orbital fissure (traversed by cranial nerves III, IV, V1, and VI and the superior ophthalmic vein), and the inferior orbital fissure (traversed by CN V2 and the infraorbital artery and vein).

The optic canal communicates with the middle cranial fossa, while the superior orbital fissure connects the orbit with the cavernous sinus and Meckel's cave. The inferior orbital fissure forms a pathway between the orbit and the deep soft tissues of the face and the pterygopalatine fossa.

The orbital septum (palpebral ligament) is a membranous sheet that acts as the anterior boundary of the orbit. It extends from the orbital rims to the eyelids and represents an important anatomic landmark to define and classify orbital disease and to plan surgery.

Like the olfactory nerve, the *optic nerve (CN II)* is histologically a white matter tract. The optic sheath has all three meningeal layers (pia, cerebrospinal fluid (CSF)-filled arachnoid, and dura), and the space within the sheath is continuous with the suprasellar cistern. CN II includes four anatomic segments: retinal, orbital, canalicular, and

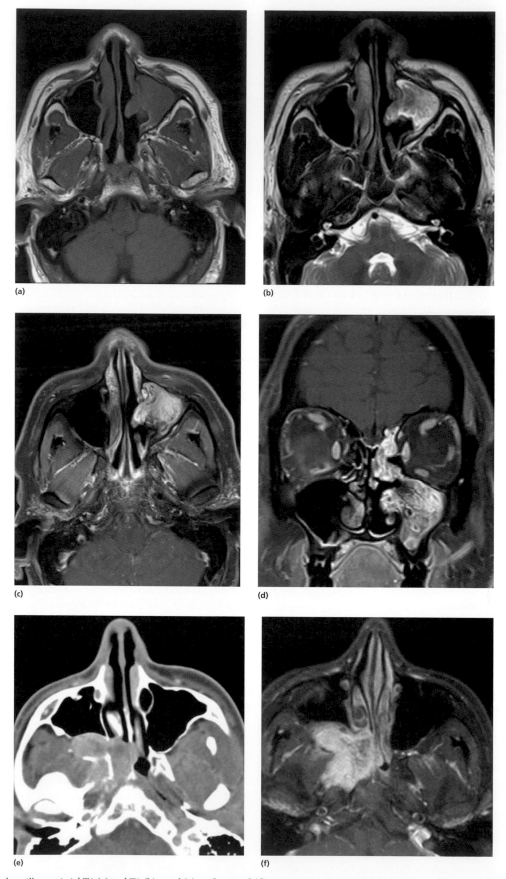

Figure 8.7 Inverted papilloma: Axial T1 (a) and T2 (b), axial (c), and coronal (d) postcontrast T1-W MRI. Juvenile angiofibroma: axial CT soft tissue window (e) and axial postcontrast T1-W MRI (f).

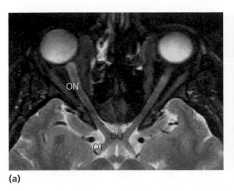
(a)

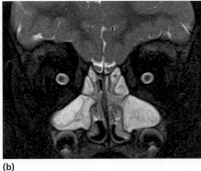
(b)

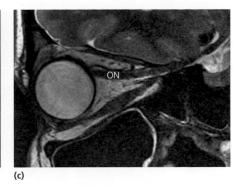
(c)

Figure 8.8 Axial (a), coronal (b), and sagittal (c) T2-W MRI show the optic nerve (ON), optic chiasm (OQ), and optic tract (OT).

cisternal (Figure 8.8). The orbital segment travels through the center of the fat-filled orbit. The canalicular segment is the portion that lies in the optic canal. The cisternal segment of the nerve can be visualized in the suprasellar cistern, where the nerve leads to the optic chiasm. The optic nerve terminates at the optic chiasm, where the two nerves meet, decussate, and form the optic tracts. The optic tracts travel around the cerebral peduncles, after which most axons enter the lateral geniculate body of the thalamus, loop around the inferior horns of the lateral ventricles (Meyer loop), and enter the visual cortex in the occipital lobe.

Critical observations

Periorbital and orbital cellulitis

Periorbital cellulitis, also known as preseptal cellulitis, is limited to the soft tissues anterior to the orbital septum and often results from contiguous spread of an infection of the face, teeth, or ocular adnexa. On CT, diffuse soft tissue thickening and areas of enhancement anterior to the orbital septum are seen. Periorbital cellulitis is treated with oral antibiotic therapy.

The term *orbital cellulitis* refers to a postseptal infection that typically results from extension of a paranasal infection (Figure 8.9). Complications of orbital cellulitis include superior ophthalmic vein thrombosis, cavernous sinus thrombosis, vision loss, meningitis, and intracranial abscess. Orbital cellulitis is treated with intravenous antibiotic therapy. If a subperiosteal abscess is present, surgical drainage may be necessary.

Optic neuritis

Optic neuritis is an inflammatory demyelinating process that causes acute, usually monocular, visual loss. It can also be idiopathic or as associated with other processes, including multiple sclerosis, systemic lupus erythematosus, viral infection, radiation therapy, and infection or inflammation of adjacent structures such as paranasal sinuses. Usually, diagnosis is made clinically and direct imaging of the optic nerves is reserved for atypical cases. On MRI, acute optic neuritis typically shows hyperintense T2-WI signal in an enlarged and enhancing optic nerve.

Perineuritis is defined as inflammation of the optic nerve sheath. It may mimic optic neuritis clinically, but at imaging, perineuritis is characterized by thickening and enhancement of the optic nerve sheath with a normal appearance of the nerve itself.

Carotid cavernous fistula

A carotid cavernous fistula is an abnormal connection between the internal carotid artery (ICA) and the venous cavernous sinus. This aberrant connection may result from trauma, surgery, or dural sinus thrombosis, and some cases are idiopathic:

- Proptosis, engorgement of the superior ophthalmic vein, cavernous sinus distention, and abnormal flow voids within the cavernous sinuses on MR images.
- Conventional angiography is necessary to identify the exact location of the carotid cavernous fistula so as to plan definitive treatment. Complications include vision loss and, in rare cases, ischemic ocular necrosis.

Superior ophthalmic vein thrombosis

Superior ophthalmic vein thrombosis is most commonly associated with an infectious process such as sinusitis and frequently occurs with cavernous sinus thrombosis. Contrast-enhanced CT and MR images demonstrate filling defects (thrombus) within the superior ophthalmic vein that is usually enlarged, exophthalmos, engorgement of the extraocular muscles, and periorbital edema. Potentially complications include vision loss.

Trauma

CT is the imaging modality of choice for evaluation of orbital trauma. Penetrating foreign bodies such as bullets, metal fragments, glasses, or other sharp objects account for a significant amount of injury to the orbit.

An *orbital blowout fracture* is a fracture of one of the walls of orbit with an intact orbital rim. A direct blow to the central orbit from a fist or ball is typically the cause. Blowout fractures can occur through one or more of the walls of the orbit.

Inferior blowout fractures are the most common. Orbital fat and the inferior rectus muscle may prolapse into the maxillary sinus (Figure 8.10). In approximately 50% of cases, inferior blowout fractures are associated with fractures of the medial wall.

Medial blowout fractures are the second most common type, occurring through the lamina papyracea. Orbital fat and the medial rectus muscle may prolapse into the ethmoid air cells.

Pure *superior blowout fractures* are uncommon and are usually seen in patients with pneumatization of the orbital roof. CSF leaks and meningitis may occur.

Lateral blowout fractures are rare as the bone is thick and bounded by muscle.

Rarely, fragments from an orbital floor fracture buckle upward into the orbit are referred to as a *"blow-in" fracture*.

In addition to evaluating the location and extent of the orbital fracture, other features need to be assessed, including the presence of emphysema, which is an indirect sign of fracture; intraorbital

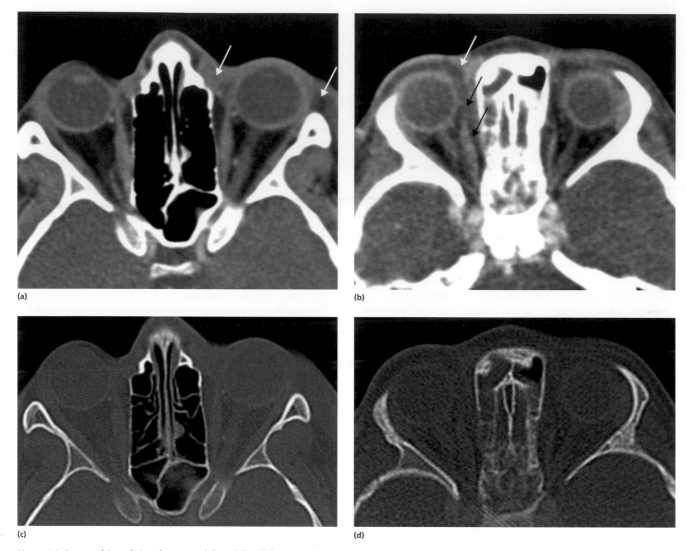

(a)   (b)   (c)   (d)

Figure 8.9 Preseptal (a and c) and postseptal (b and d) cellulitis. Axial CT soft tissue windows show diffuse soft tissue thickening anterior to the orbital septum (a) and beyond it (b) (arrows). Axial CT bone window (d) shows paranasal infection, not seen on the preseptal cellulitis case (c).

hemorrhage, which may result in stretching or compression of the optic nerve; globe injury or rupture; and extraocular muscle entrapment, which should be suspected if there is an acute change in the angle of the muscle.

Vascular lesions

Cavernous malformations (also known as cavernous hemangiomas) are thought to be congenital vascular anomalies that are present at birth, do not spontaneously involute, and grow slowly over time (Figure 8.11):
• They typically appear as a well-circumscribed, ovoid intraconal mass on cross-sectional images. On MRI, they are isointense on T1-WI and hyperintense on T2-WI with no flow voids with poor on enhancement on early arterial-phase images, owing to the scant arterial supply. Delayed venous-phase images demonstrate progressive filling of the mass from periphery to center, with complete filling within 30 min.

This pattern allows differentiation of cavernous malformations from other vascular lesions with rich arterial supply, such as capillary hemangiomas and arteriovenous malformations.

Capillary hemangiomas, also known as "strawberry hemangioma," develop in infants (<1 year) and are usually diagnosed within the first weeks of life. Although these lesions may grow rapidly in size, they typically plateau during the first year or two and then regress spontaneously. Radiology is required when the diagnosis is unclear:
• CT shows a homogeneous enhancing lobulated and infiltrative mass, usually located anterior to the globe, in the eyelid. It may involve the extraocular muscles and lacrimal glands and may extend intracranially through the optic canal or superior orbital fissure.
• On MRI, it is usually slightly hypointense on T1-WI and iso- to hyperintense on T2-WI with multiple flow voids and homogeneous enhancement after gadolinium administration. Ultrasound is mostly useful for smaller and limited lesions.

Lymphangiomas occur in an older group of children (3–15 years).
• Unencapsulated, multilobulated masses consist of vascular and lymphatic channels that may have intraconal and extraconal components and may cause bone remodeling.
• Its propensity to bleed produces the classic MRI appearance of multiple cysts containing fluid levels on T2-WI.

Orbital varices are the most common cause of spontaneous orbital hemorrhage and represent slow-flow congenital venous malformations.

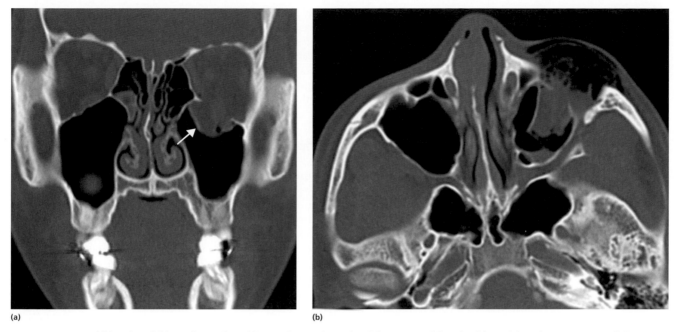

(a)

(b)

Figure 8.10 Coronal (a) and axial (b) CT show inferior blowout fracture (arrow) with herniation of the orbital fat and the inferior rectus muscle into the maxillary sinus.

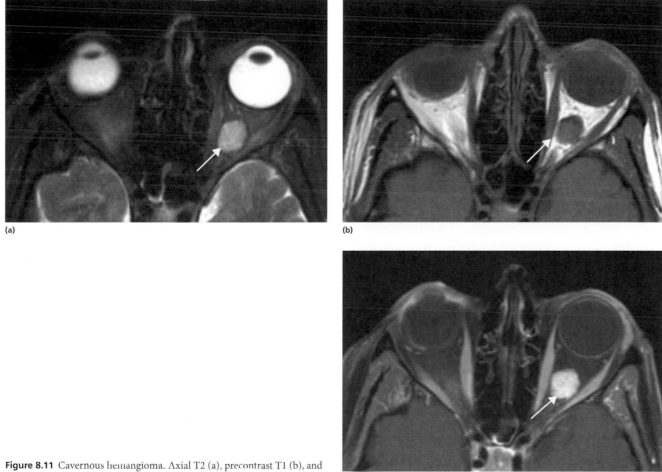

(a)

(b)

(c)

Figure 8.11 Cavernous hemangioma. Axial T2 (a), precontrast T1 (b), and postcontrast fat-saturated (FS) T1-W MRI (c) (arrows).

Most orbital varices have a large communication with the venous system, resulting in orbital varix distention and increased proptosis during the Valsalva maneuver or postural change. Imaging findings may be subtle, and imaging during the Valsalva maneuver may be necessary to elicit the characteristic appearance of an enhancing dilated vein.

Degenerative/inflammatory/infectious conditions

Graves ophthalmopathy is the most common cause of exophthalmos in adults. It usually occurs 5 years after the onset of Graves thyroid disease and is postulated to be an autoimmune condition unrelated to thyroid function.

Imaging findings include spindle-shaped enlargement of the extraocular muscles, with sparing of the tendinous insertion. The muscles involved, in decreasing order of frequency, are the inferior, medial, superior, and lateral rectus muscles (mnemonic "I'M SLow" reminds one of the order of muscle involvement and the typical orbital symptoms of Grave disease, namely lid lag and limitation of orbital movement). Most patients have bilateral and symmetric muscle involvement. In some cases, muscles may be normal and exophthalmos is the result of increased retrobulbar fat (Figure 8.12).

Idiopathic orbital inflammatory syndrome, also known as orbital pseudotumor, is the second most common cause of exophthalmos. It is an idiopathic inflammatory process that manifests with acute onset of orbital pain associated with proptosis, diplopia, restricted mobility, and decreased visual acuity:

- The imaging findings vary widely and can include orbital fat stranding; myositis; a focal poorly marginated, infiltrative, enhancing intraorbital mass; lacrimal gland inflammation and enlargement; diffuse orbital involvement; or involvement of the optic nerve sheath complex, uvea, and sclera.
- Unlike Graves ophthalmopathy, there is tendinous involvement of the extraocular muscles, and the superior and medial muscles are most commonly affected (Figure 8.13).

Neoplastic processes

Neoplasms

MRI is particularly valuable for evaluation of orbital neoplasms, as it provides critical anatomic information about ocular structures involved, perineural spread, and intracranial extension.

Lymphoma is the third most common adult orbital mass lesion, following pseudotumor and cavernous hemangioma. Lymphoma and pseudotumor may present with similar imaging findings: diffusely infiltrating lesions capable of involving and extending into any retrobulbar structures. However, lymphoma tends to present with painless proptosis, while pseudotumor presents with painful proptosis, chemosis, and ophthalmoplegia. Nevertheless, the distinction between these two entities frequently remains very difficult.

Neoplasms that arise from the optic nerve or its sheath include *glioma* and *meningioma*.

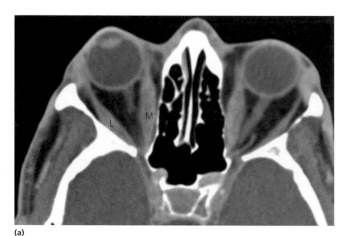

(a)

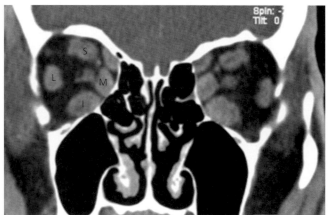

(b)

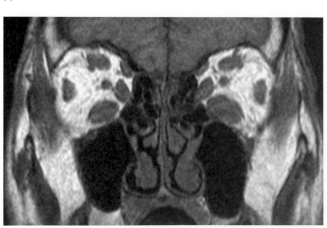

(c)

Figure 8.12 Graves ophthalmopathy. Axial (a) CT shows enlargement of the medial rectus muscles, with sparing of the tendinous insertion. Coronal CT (b) and T1-W MRI (c) show the typical order of involvement of the extraocular muscles: inferior (I), medial (M), superior (S), and lateral (L) rectus muscles.

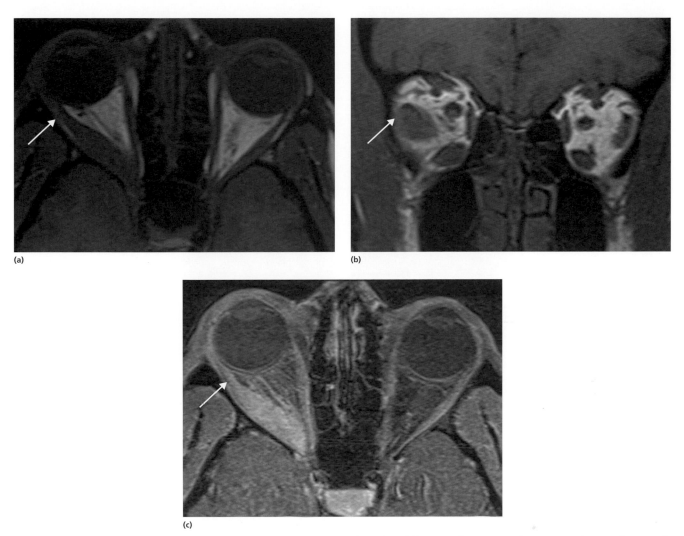

(a)

(b)

(c)

Figure 8.13 Orbital pseudotumor. Axial (a) and coronal (b) T1 FS precontrast MRI and axial (c) T1 FS after contrast administration show involvement of the lateral rectus muscle without sparing of the tendinous insertion (arrows).

Optic nerve gliomas are the most common tumors of the optic nerve. They are highly associated with neurofibromatosis type 1, particularly when bilateral. On imaging, gliomas may cause tubular, fusiform, or eccentric expansion of the optic nerve with kinking (Figure 8.14).

Meningiomas arise from hemangioendothelial cells of the arachnoid layer of the optic nerve sheath and grow in a circular and linear fashion along the optic nerve. In contrast with optic nerve gliomas, meningiomas classically have a "tram-track" configuration, whereby the contrast-enhancing tumor is seen alongside the nonenhancing optic nerve. Additionally, meningiomas may invade and grow through the dura and may calcify (Figure 8.15).

Neoplasms that derive from peripheral nerves include *schwannoma* and *neurofibroma*.

Schwannomas are encapsulated, slowly progressive, benign proliferations of Schwann cells that are typically extraconal and located at the superior orbit, owing to their frequent origin from the frontal branch CN V1. The lesions often abut orbital apertures, assuming a cone shape if the orbital apex is involved or a dumbbell shape when the superior orbital fissure is involved. On MRI, they typically appear as a well-circumscribed mixed solid and cystic mass with heterogeneous enhancement after contrast administration.

Neurofibromas are benign, slow-growing, peripheral nerve tumors composed of an admixture of fibroblasts, Schwann cells, and axons.

Localized, diffuse, and plexiform types may occur in the orbit. Plexiform neurofibromas are the most common type of peripheral nerve sheath tumor and are essentially pathognomonic for NF-1. Similar to schwannomas, neurofibromas are more commonly extraconal, owing to their frequent origin from sensory branches of the trigeminal nerve. On MRI, they are typically hyperintense on T2-WI with variable signal on T1-WI. Plexiform types may involve large portions of the face with a bag-of-worms appearance, while solitary types are difficult to distinguish from schwannomas.

A variety of lesions may involve the globe. In children, *retinoblastoma* is the most common primary ocular malignancy, habitually presenting with leukocoria and a calcified ocular mass. Other rare conditions are developmental abnormalities (persistent hyperplastic primary vitreous tumor and Coats' disease), acquired retinal lesions (retinopathy of prematurity), and infection. In adults, common ocular pathology includes retinal and choroidal detachment, uveal melanoma, and metastases.

Recognition of *retinal and choroidal detachments* in the acute setting is crucial to patient care, not for the evaluation of the detachment itself but rather for the detection of an underlying cause such as an intraocular tumor.

Orbital melanoma arises from the uveal tract, which consists of the choroid, ciliary body, and iris. The majority of lesions (90%)

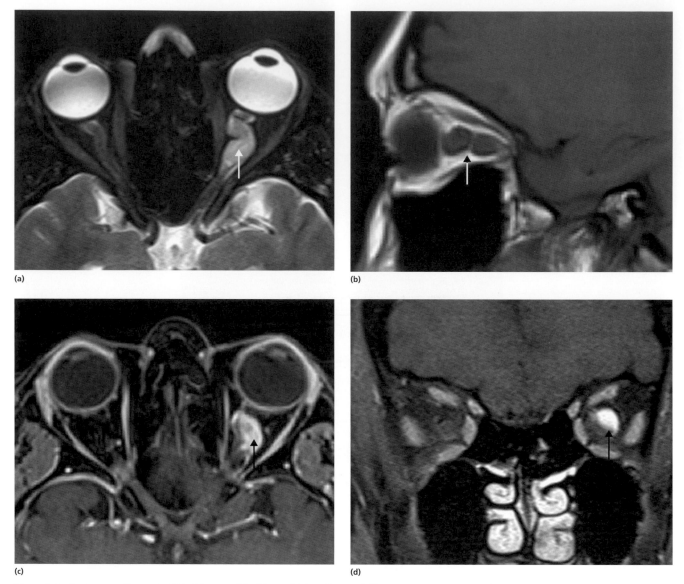

(a)   (b)

(c)   (d)

Figure 8.14 Optic nerve glioma. Axial T2 (a), sagittal T1 (b), axial (c), and coronal (d) postcontrast T1-W MRI (arrows).

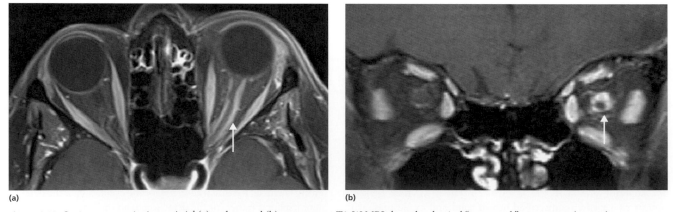

(a)   (b)

Figure 8.15 Optic nerve meningioma. Axial (a) and coronal (b) postcontrast T1-W MRI show the classical "tram-track" appearance (arrows).

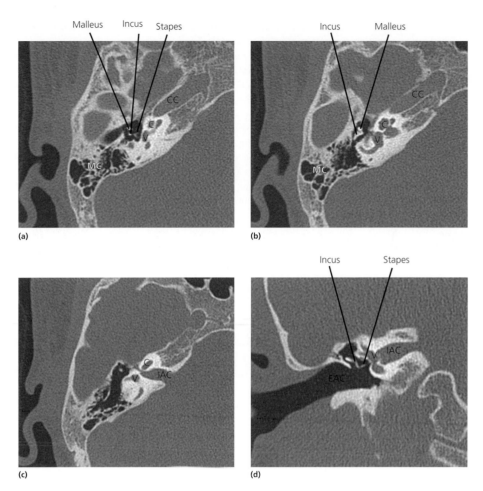

Figure 8.16 Temporal bone anatomy. Axial (a, b, and c) and coronal (d) CT bone windows (C, cochlea; CC, carotid canal; EAC, external auditory canal; IAC, internal auditory canal; V, vestibule).

derive from the choroid. Melanin has intrinsic T1- and T2-shortening effects, classically manifesting with increased T1 and decreased T2 signal intensity, but approximately 20% of melanomas are amelanotic, thereby lacking these features. MRI is also important for characterization of lesion size, extraocular extension, and ciliary body infiltration, all of which are associated with poor prognosis.

Metastases also occur in the orbit. The most common tumor that metastasizes to the orbit is breast cancer, followed by metastatic prostate carcinoma, melanoma, and lung cancer. Metastases to the globe most frequently involve the choroid, and metastatic lung cancer is the most common type of tumor involving the globe.

Temporal bone

CT is the imaging modality of choice for most of the pathologic conditions of the temporal bone, especially for those of the middle ear. MRI is more useful for diseases of the inner ear, internal auditory canal (IAC), and cerebellopontine angle, as well as for evaluation of tumors and other invasive diseases.

Anatomic considerations

The *external ear* consists of the auricle, or pinna, and the external auditory canal (EAC). The pinna collects sound waves, and the EAC conducts these vibrations to the tympanic membrane.

The *middle ear* or tympanic cavity can be structurally divided into three parts: the mesotympanum that lies at the level of the tympanic membrane, the epitympanic recess (attic) that lies above the level of the tympanic membrane, and the hypotympanum that lies inferior to the tympanic membrane. The tympanic cavity houses three ossicles: the malleus, the incus, and the stapes. The ossicular chain transmits and amplifies vibrations incident on the tympanic membrane across the middle ear cavity, causing deflection of the oval window, which is attached to the footplate of the stapes (Figure 8.16).

The *inner ear* consists of a bony and a membranous labyrinth. The bony labyrinth is made of cavities forming the cochlea, vestibule, and semicircular canals. The membranous labyrinth is a membranous sac within the osseous labyrinth that includes the vestibular utricle and saccule, the semicircular ducts, the scala media of cochlea, and the endolymphatic duct and sac. Fluid within the bony labyrinth called perilymph surrounds the membranous labyrinth, which contains its own unique fluid, the endolymph. There are three semicircular canals emanating from the vestibule: lateral, posterior, and superior. The cochlea has a conical, snaillike shape with approximately two and one-half turns.

The IAC runs medially from the base of the cochlea and vestibule to the cerebellopontine angle cistern on the posterior aspect of the petrous bone.

The *facial nerve (CN VII)* is a motor and sensory nerve (muscles of facial expression, parasympathetic to all glands of the head except the parotid, sensory for the ear and tympanic membrane, and taste of the anterior two-thirds of the tongue) that emerges from the lateral aspect of the pons, traverses the cerebellopontine angle cistern, runs through the IAC, and then enters the facial canal via the fallopian aqueduct. After a complex course within the petrous bone, the facial nerve exits the skull base through the stylomastoid foramen and enters the substance of the parotid gland.

The *vestibulocochlear nerve (CN VIII)* is a sensory nerve that conducts two special senses: hearing (cochlear) and balance (vestibular). The cochlear nerve originates in the organ of Corti, while the superior and inferior vestibular nerves originate in Scarpa's ganglia. The three nerves travel along the IAC with the facial nerve and merge into the vestibulocochlear nerve. The vestibulocochlear nerve crosses the cerebellopontine angle cistern and enters the brainstem at the junction of the pons and medulla lateral to the facial nerve.

Critical observations

Complicated acute otitis media

Acute otitis media (AOM) is the most common infection of the temporal bone and is most prevalent among children. It usually occurs as a sequela of a viral upper respiratory infection with disruption of the mucosal barrier that prevents bacteria in the nose and nasopharynx from spreading to the middle ear:

- On CT, AOM shows nonspecific findings with partial or total fluid opacification of the middle ear.

Although imaging is unnecessary in uncomplicated otitis media, it is important for evaluation of complications. Important complications include coalescent mastoiditis, subperiosteal abscess, dural sinus thrombosis, intracranial abscess and empyema, meningitis, facial nerve involvement, labyrinthitis, and petrous apicitis (Figure 8.17). The same complications can occasionally occur in patients with chronic otomastoiditis.

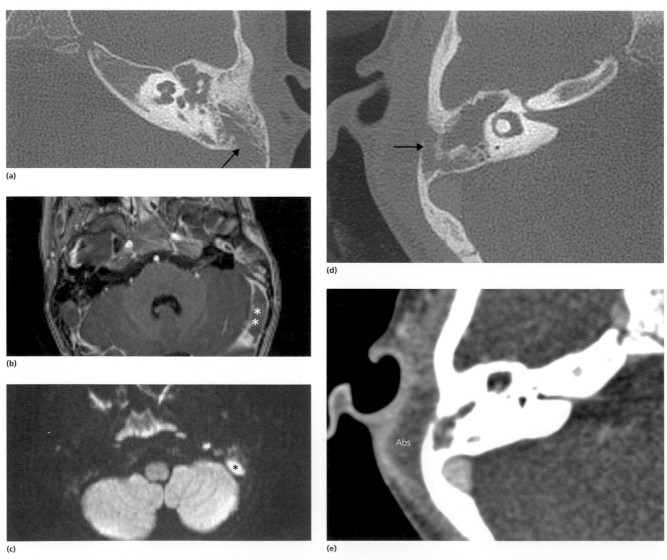

(a)

(b)

(c)

(d)

(e)

Figure 8.17 Acute ottis media. Axial CT (a) shows pacification of the middle ear with bone erosion (arrow). Axial T2 (b) and postcontrast T1-W (c) MRI show a filing defect (**) within the lateral sinus suggestive of sinus thrombosis. DWI (c) shows an abscess (*) with restricted diffusion. Axial CT bone window (d) and postcontrast soft tissue window (e) of another patient show coalescent mastoiditis with subperiosteal abscess (Abs).

Trauma

Historically, temporal bone fractures were classified into two main categories, longitudinal and transverse, so named based on the orientation of the fracture line relative to the long axis of the petrous bone. Longitudinal fractures run parallel to this axis and typically traverse the middle ear cavity, frequently disrupting the ossicular chain and causing conductive hearing loss. Transverse fractures run perpendicular to the long axis of the petrous bone and may traverse the fundus of the IAC or the bony labyrinth, resulting in sensorineural hearing loss.

In reality most fractures have an oblique course or have both longitudinal and transverse components. Other complications related to temporal bone fractures include facial nerve injury, perilymphatic fistula, vertigo, CSF, meningitis, and acquired cholesteatoma.

Recent classification schemes have been proposed describing temporal bone fractures with respect to involvement of the otic capsule.

Degenerative/inflammatory/infectious conditions

In addition of AOM, several inflammatory conditions may affect the temporal bone. At imaging, infectious or inflammatory processes can be described according to the degree of involvement of the four anatomic regions: external ear, middle ear and mastoid, inner ear, and petrous apex.

Chronic otomastoiditis typically occurs as a result of long-standing eustachian tube dysfunction. Both AOM and chronic otitis media can result in the development of acquired cholesteatomas in the middle ear.

Cholesteatoma is an epidermoid cyst composed of desquamating stratified squamous epithelium that enlarges due progressive accumulation of epithelial debris within its lumen. It can be either congenital (2%) or acquired (98%). Acquired cholesteatomas typically arise from the pars flaccida (superior portion) of the tympanic membrane and are centered in the Prussak space in the epitympanum:

- On CT, cholesteatoma classically manifests as soft tissue mass causing underlying bone erosion. The soft tissue density of the cholesteatoma may be difficult to differentiate from fluid attenuation in the middle ear related with chronic otitis media or other inflammatory/infectious conditions.
- Diffusion-weighted MRI cholesteatoma shows restricted diffusion allowing the diagnosis.

When pneumatized, the petrous apex can become involved by middle ear infections. A *cholesterol granuloma* results from a foreign body giant cell reaction to the deposition of cholesterol crystals in the air cells with fibrosis and vascular proliferation:

- CT shows a mass lesion with smooth margins.
- MR shows high signal intensity on T1-WI and T2-WI owing to the cholesterol crystals and methemoglobin from repeated hemorrhage.

Neoplastic processes

The most common tumor of the temporal bone at the cerebellopontine angle is the *vestibular schwannoma*.

- MRI shows a mass lesion centered in the porus acusticus, isointense to hypointense on T1-WI and slightly hyperintense on T2-WI with homogeneous enhancement after gadolinium administration.

Less commonly *meningioma* may occur in the cerebellopontine angle and involve the IAC. The imaging findings are similar to meningiomas elsewhere in the cranium, including the more common olfactory groove, sphenoid wing, planum sphenoidale, and supratentorial meningiomas.

Paragangliomas, also known as glomus tumors, are the second most common tumor to involve the temporal bone and the most common tumor of the middle ear. A paraglioma arising within the middle ear is referred to as a glomus tympanicum. These usually appear as enhancing soft tissue masses situated along the cochlear promontory.

Skull base

Imaging plays a central role in the management of skull base disease because this region is generally not amenable to clinical evaluation.

Anatomic considerations

The skull base is composed of five bones: ethmoid, sphenoid, occipital, temporal, and frontal bones. Viewed from above, the skull base demonstrates three well-defined regions: the anterior, middle, and posterior cranial fossae. Viewed from below, it is more complex, without clear internal boundaries facing the facial and neck structures.

The cranial base contains many foramina through which both vessels and nerves pass. These foramina are potential routes of spread of diseases between intra- and extracranial compartments.

Major foramina of the skull base include the following: the foramen cecum, anterior and posterior ethmoidal foramina, and foramina of the cribriform plate in the anterior cranial fossa; the optic canals, superior orbital fissure, carotid canals, foramen rotundum, foramen ovale, foramen spinosum, foramen lacerum, and vidian canal in the central skull base; and the internal acoustic meatus, jugular foramen, hypoglossal canal, foramen magnum, and stylomastoid foramen in posterior skull base. Cranial nerves IX, X, and XI exit the skull through the jugular foramen and the XII CN through the hypoglossal canal.

Trauma

Facial fractures may extend through the anterior or middle cranial fossa, which may lead to CSF leakage, intracranial hemorrhage, or intracranial infection.

Pneumocephalus may be seen associated with skull base fractures and may help the diagnosis.

Neoplastic processes

Skull base tumors arise from the cranial base or spread there from an intracranial or extracranial site. They may originate from the neurovascular structures of the base of the brain and the basal meninges (e.g., meningioma, pituitary adenoma, schwannoma, paraganglioma), the cranial base itself (e.g., chordoma, chondrosarcoma), the subcranial structures of the head and neck (e.g., nasopharyngeal carcinomas), or the remote sites (metastases).

Primary benign neoplasms

Glomus jugulare tumors are slow-growing tumors arising from nonchromaffin paraganglion cells (part of the sympathetic system) along the course of Arnold's nerve in the jugular foramen (Figure 8.18):

- CT often demonstrates an irregular "moth-eaten" erosion of the bony margins of the jugular fossa. Eventually, as the tumor

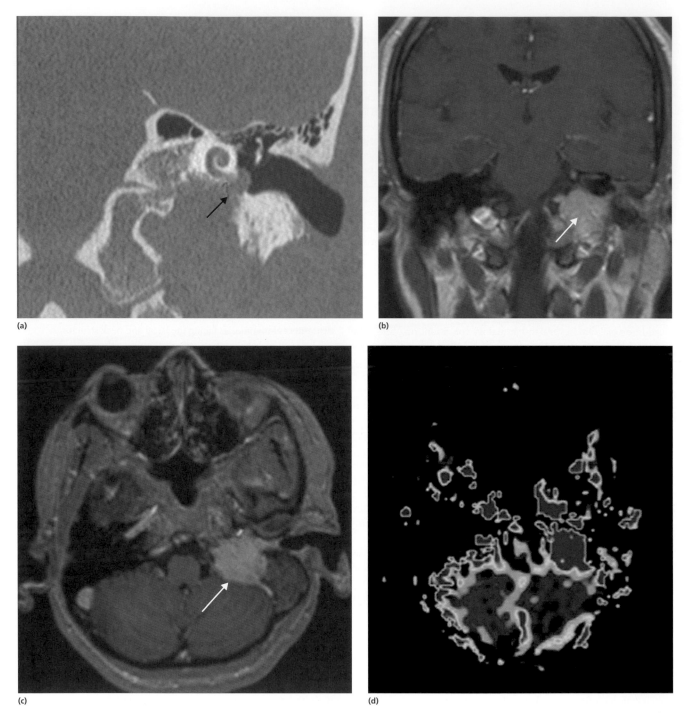

(a)

(b)

(c)

(d)

Figure 8.18 Glomus jugulotympanicum. Coronal CT (a) shows irregular "moth-eaten" erosion (arrow). Coronal (b) and axial (c) postcontrast T1-W MRI (d) of a different patient show avid enhancement (arrows). MRI perfusion (cerebral blood volume) shows hyperperfusion (*).

enlarges, the mass extends into the middle ear, as well as inferiorly into the infratemporal fossa.

- MRI shows the characteristic "salt-and-pepper" pattern on T1- and T2-WI representing blood products from hemorrhage and flow voids due to high vascularity with avid enhancement on post contrast T1-WI. This pattern may not be seen in smaller glomus tumors.
- Angiography demonstrates an intense tumor blush. It is useful to characterize the arterial supply as well as for preoperative embolization.

Schwannomas are well-demarcated soft tissue masses, with the characteristic dumbbell configuration that causes smooth expansion of the jugular foramen. Cystic components may be seen. Smaller lesions demonstrate intense homogeneous enhancement, while larger lesions tend to have heterogeneous enhancement.

Primary malignant neoplasms

Primary malignant neoplasms are relatively uncommon. In addition to the entities discussed in the following, malignancies of the skull base can include rhabdomyosarcoma, metastasis, myeloma, and plasmacytoma. Differentiating these lesions based on imaging findings may be challenging.

Chordomas are uncommon malignant tumors that originate from embryonic remnants of the primitive notochord. They can be found along the axial skeleton distributed among three locations: sacrococcygeal (30–50%), spheno-occipital (30–35%), and vertebral body (15–30%). They are locally aggressive but rarely metastasize:

- On CT, chordomas are midline expansile soft tissue masses, with marked enhancement after contrast administration and associated bony destruction. They may appear heterogeneous due to cystic necrosis or hemorrhage. Marginal sclerosis and irregular intratumoral calcifications may also be seen.
- MRI usually shows an intermediate- to low-signal-intensity lesion with small foci of hyperintensity (intratumoral hemorrhage) on T1-WI and most exhibit very high T2-WI signal. After gadolinium administration, they usually show heterogeneous enhancement with a honeycomb appearance.

Chondrosarcomas are malignant tumors that arise from cartilage, usually located off the midline, preferentially at the petroclival junction. The off-midline location is helpful in discriminating these tumors from chordomas, which are usually midline. Local extension (intracranially, into the cavernous sinuses, paranasal sinuses, or infratemporal fossa) is common:

- CT demonstrates a destructive soft tissue mass that may contain rings and arcs of calcification, representing calcified chondroid matrix.
- MR shows high T2-WI signal intensity and heterogeneous enhancement after gadolinium administration.

Supra- and infrahyoid neck

Anatomic considerations

Excluding the sinonasal cavities, the mucosal-lined tissues of the upper aerodigestive tract can be divided into the oral cavity, pharynx (oropharynx, nasopharynx, hypopharynx), and larynx. These divisions help us to accurately determine and describe the spread of the superficial mucosa-based lesions, namely, squamous cell carcinoma.

The *oral cavity* extends from the lips posteriorly to a ring of structures that include circumvallate papillae of the tongue, anterior tonsillar pillars, and soft palate. It includes the buccal mucosa, alveolar ridges, oral tongue, floor of mouth, retromolar trigone, and hard palate.

The *oropharynx* is situated directly posterior to the oral cavity and includes the posterior third of the tongue (base of tongue), valleculae, palatine tonsils and tonsillar fossa, soft palate, and uvula.

The *nasopharynx* lies above the oropharynx and extends from the base of the skull to the superior surface of the soft palate. The boundaries include the posterosuperior wall; the lateral wall, also known as the fossa of Rosenmüller; and the anteroinferior wall, which is the superior surface of the soft palate. Laterally, there is a cartilaginous opening of the eustachian tube known as torus tubarius.

The *hypopharynx* includes the piriform sinuses laterally, postcricoid region inferiorly, and pharyngeal wall posteriorly.

The *larynx* is responsible for maintaining and protecting the airway and allowing phonation. It is traditionally separated into the supraglottis, glottis, and subglottis. The supraglottis extends from the base of tongue to the apex of the laryngeal ventricle and contains the epiglottis, aryepiglottic folds, false vocal cords, and arytenoid cartilages. The glottis consists of the soft tissues of the true vocal cord. The subglottis is the portion of the larynx extending from the inferior surface of the true vocal cord to the inferior margin of the cricoid cartilage, which demarcates the beginning of the trachea.

Suprahyoid neck

For submucosal lesions, a more practical approach to anatomy and differential diagnosis is to use a spatial approach in which layers of deep cervical fascia divide the head and neck into multiple fascia-enclosed spaces. These spaces are easily identified on axial CT and MR images (Figure 8.19).

A systematic approach to evaluating head and neck pathology is to determine which space the lesion is located within, what the

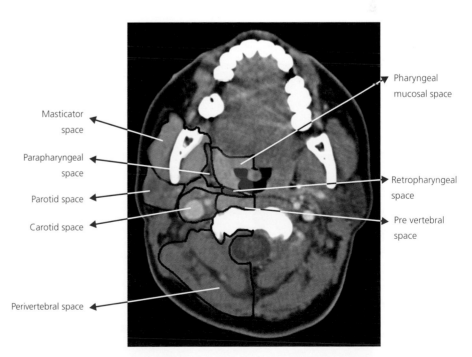

Figure 8.19 Axial CT shows normal spaces of suprahyoid neck.

Pharyngeal mucosal space

Masticator space

Parapharyngeal space

Parotid space

Carotid space

Retropharyngeal space

Pre vertebral space

Perivertebral space

normal contents of the space are, if the pathology arises from one of these components, and if there are specific radiologic findings that correlate with the clinical information and allow one to limit the differential diagnosis.

The suprahyoid neck is the region extending from the skull base to the hyoid bone. It is divided into seven major anatomical spaces by layers of cervical fascia:
1 *Pharyngeal mucosal space*—essentially the mucosal-lined tissues of the aerodigestive tract described earlier.
2 *Parapharyngeal space*—central, primarily fat-containing space around which the other deep neck spaces are located. It contains fat, lymphatics, nerves, and minor salivary glands.
3 *Carotid space*—includes the ICA, internal jugular vein, cranial nerves IX through XII, sympathetic plexus, and lymph nodes of deep cervical chain.
4 *Parotid space*—includes the parotid gland, facial nerve, retromandibular vein, external carotid branches, and intraparotid lymph nodes.
5 *Masticator space*—contains the muscles of mastication, the ascending ramus of the mandible, and the V3 branch of the trigeminal nerve.
6 *Retropharyngeal space*—predominantly includes fat and lymph nodes.
7 *Perivertebral space*—includes longus colli/capitis muscle complex, paraspinal musculature, vertebral body, and posterior triangle of the neck.

Differential diagnosis of suprahyoid masses can be easily formulated if the anatomic components of the each space are known and if one can localize a mass to the correct space.

The parapharyngeal space is the central space surrounded by the masticator space anteriorly, carotid space posteriorly, parotid space laterally, and superficial mucosal space medially. Deviation of the fat in the parapharyngeal space can help localize large masses to one of these four spaces. The parapharyngeal space fat is deviated posteromedially by large lesions in masticator space. A mass in the parotid space will deviate it medially, while a carotid space mass will deviate it anteriorly. Submucosal extension of a superficial mucosal mass will deviate the fat laterally. Furthermore, a mass arising either from the pharyngeal mucosal space or the retropharyngeal space displaces the prevertebral muscle complex posteriorly. If the muscle complex is elevated anteriorly off of the spine, then the lesion is suspected to arise from the perivertebral space.

Infrahyoid neck
The infrahyoid neck is the region of the neck extending from the hyoid bone to the cervicothoracic junction. The infrahyoid region is subdivided into five major spaces by the different layers of deep cervical fascia that are continuous with those in the suprahyoid neck. A few spaces also extend into the superior mediastinum (Figure 8.20).
Spaces of the infrahyoid neck include:
- *Visceral space*—located centrally and contains viscera including the larynx, thyroid, hypopharynx and cervical esophagus
- *Carotid space*—continuation of the suprahyoid carotid space, located lateral to the visceral compartment on either side, and contains the ICA, internal jugular vein, and several neural structures
- *Retropharyngeal space*—fat-only containing small space that is continuous with the suprahyoid retropharyngeal space superiorly and the middle mediastinum inferiorly
- *Posterior cervical space*—located posterolateral to the carotid space on either side and contains fat, lymph nodes, and neural elements
- *Perivertebral space*—a large space that includes the vertebral body and the pre- and paravertebral muscles

Pharyngeal mucosal space

Head and neck squamous cell carcinoma
Nasopharyngeal carcinoma
A variant of squamous cell carcinoma that occurs in the nasopharynx is referred to as nasopharyngeal carcinoma. Unlike mucosal squamous cell carcinoma associated with smoking and alcohol abuse, nasopharyngeal carcinoma is most commonly found in patients of Asian ethnicity and is believed to be associated with Epstein–Barr virus infection.

Early diagnostic criteria for nasopharyngeal malignancy are (Figure 8.21):
- Asymmetry of nasopharyngeal mucosa
- Mastoid opacification or nonresolving otitis media suggesting eustachian tube dysfunction as a result of infiltration
- Positive lymph nodes on ipsilateral side (seen in 80–90% of patients)

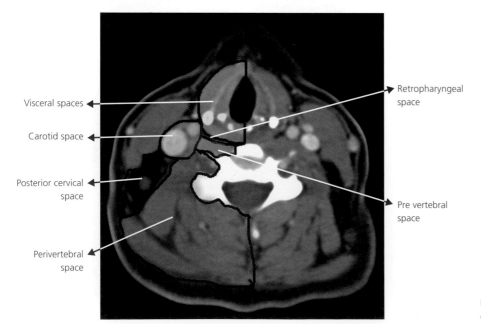

Visceral spaces

Carotid space

Posterior cervical space

Perivertebral space

Retropharyngeal space

Pre vertebral space

Figure 8.20 Axial CT shows normal spaces of infrahyoid neck.

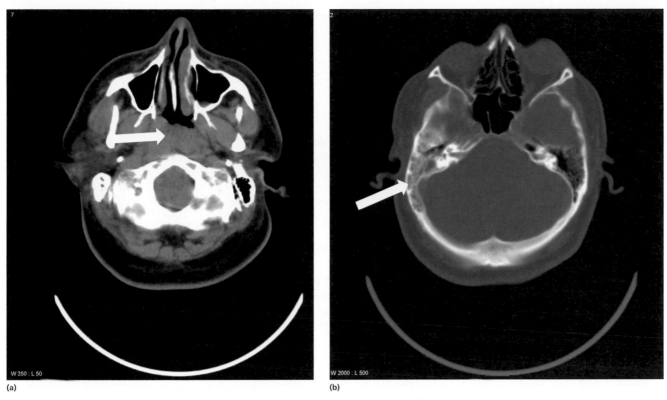

(a)   (b)

Figure 8.21 Nasopharyngeal carcinoma. Axial contrast-enhanced CT (a and b) images show NPC centered in nasopharynx and involving posterior wall (arrow) (a) with associated right mastoid effusion (b) (arrow).

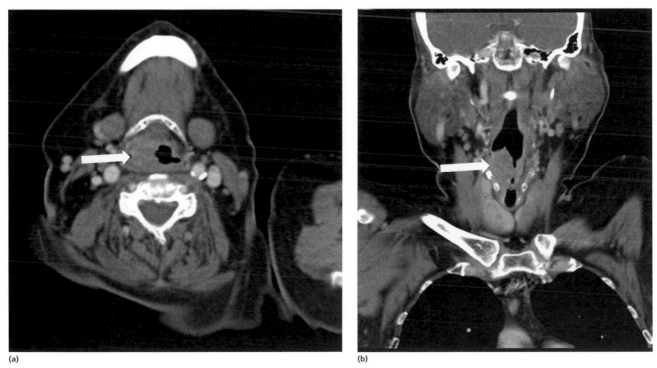

(a)   (b)

Figure 8.22 Laryngeal carcinoma. Axial (a) and coronal (b) contrast-enhanced CT show mass centered in the glottis region (arrows).

Laryngeal squamous cell carcinoma

The anterior portion of the true vocal cord in the glottis region is the most common site of laryngeal carcinomas. It may involve the contralateral true vocal cord by invading the anterior commissure located anteriorly. Recurrent laryngeal nerve paralysis resulting in hoarseness, cricoarytenoid joint arthritis, and vocalis muscle invasion are some of the associated complications (Figure 8.22).

- Obliteration of surrounding fat spaces
- Thickening of the anterior commissure
- Cartilage invasion

- Adenopathy
- Greater than 2 mm soft tissue indicating tumor spread to contra-lateral side of cord

Mobility of cords can be determined by fluoroscopy. CT has a high sensitivity and negative predictive value for detection of cartilage invasion using the following criteria: sclerosis, erosion, lysis, and extralaryngeal spread. MRI is superior to CT for specific tissue characterization, which helps in determining involvement of the laryngeal ventricle and transglottic spread. Midsagittal images are helpful for demonstrating the relationship between the tumor and the anterior commissure and thus play a major role in disease staging.

Carotid space

Paragangliomas

Paragangliomas are benign vascular tumors that arise from the neural crest cells of the sympathetic nervous system. These tumors are named on the location and the nerves of their origin and include glomus jugulare (jugular ganglion of vagus nerve at the skull base), glomus vagale (ganglion of vagus nerve below skull base), and carotid body tumor (carotid body at carotid bifurcation).

Paragangliomas are multiple in 3–5% of patients, and 20–30% of patients may have a positive family history:

- Painless slowly growing tumor that can be pulsatile with an associate bruit.
- On CT, they appear as an intensely enhancing lesion in carotid space.
- MRI shows intense enhancement with frequent multiple flow voids.
- Dense blush is a characteristic imaging finding seen in the capillary phase of angiography suggesting its highly vascular nature.

Schwannomas

Schwannomas are encapsulated benign tumors that arise from nerve sheath coverings within the carotid space. They do not infiltrate the substance of the nerve fibers. They do enhance, but unlike paragangliomas, they are not particularly hypervascular. Flow voids are not present. It is often impossible to differentiate schwannomas and paragangliomas based on imaging findings (Figure 8.23).

Metastatic nodal disease

Enlarged and pathologic-appearing nodes are seen in both metastatic disease and infection and cannot be differentiated on imaging. However, clinical presentation helps to distinguish both entities easily. Papillary thyroid cancer and squamous cell carcinoma are the most common causes of metastatic nodal disease are:

Imaging criteria for metastatic nodal disease

- Nodal architecture: any lymph node regardless of size that exhibits central low density (necrosis or cystic degeneration) with peripheral enhancement is pathologic until proven otherwise.
- Extracapsular spread: infiltration of adjacent tissues is highly suggestive of malignancy.
- On FDG PET, metastatic nodes are typically very FDG avid. A lymph node regardless of its size is considered malignant if it appears hot on PET scan.

- Nodal size: though nodal size itself is a less reliable indicator of malignancy, lymph nodes are considered pathologic in size if their long-axis measurement is greater than 1 cm, except for submental, submandibular, and jugulodigastric nodes that must measure 1.5 cm to be considered pathologic.
- Nodal shape: an enlarged lymph node that fails to maintain normal reniform configuration and becomes rounded in shape is suggestive of malignancy.

Non–Hodgkin lymphoma

Non-Hodgkin lymphoma should be highly suspected in an age group of 20–40-year-old patients presenting with a neck mass or bulky lymphadenopathy associated with other systemic manifestations like mediastinal or supraclavicular adenopathy and splenomegaly.

Parotid space

Pleomorphic adenomas

Pleomorphic adenomas are slow-growing, encapsulated tumors that account for 80% of benign parotid neoplasms. They may also arise from the submandibular and sublingual glands or from minor salivary glands scattered throughout the mucosa of the aerodigestive tract:

- They are most commonly located in superficial posterior gland.
- Ultrasound shows a well-circumscribed hypoechoic lesion.
- A calcified parotid mass with moderate and heterogeneous enhancement on CT is highly suggestive of pleomorphic adenoma.
- On MR, pleomorphic adenoma is hypointense on T1-WI and hyperintense on T2-WI with moderate enhancement on postcontrast T1-WI. Five percent of adenomas show malignant transformation.

Imaging findings suggestive of malignancy are irregular margins, heterogeneous signal with invasion of adjacent soft tissue spaces, and associated lymphadenopathy.

Warthin's tumor

They are the second most common benign parotid tumor and are the most common bilateral or multifocal benign parotid tumor. It typically occurs in the elderly:

- Seen as a well-defined, ovoid, hyperechoic mass on ultrasound.
- On CT, cystic changes appear as intralesional lower attenuation within the parotid with a focal tumor nodule.
- MRI shows low to intermediate signal on T1-WI and variable signal on T2-WI usually with no contrast enhancement.

Masticator space

The most frequently found pathology is odontogenic abscess. Primary tumors are commonly of benign nature and often of a neural or vascular origin. Adjacent lesions with secondary invasion into masticator space are often found, especially from the pharynx.

Retropharyngeal space

Retropharyngeal abscess

Common causes of retropharyngeal abscess are spread of infection to retropharyngeal lymph nodes from dental disease, pharyngitis, and vertebral osteomyelitis and also due to penetrating trauma caused by fish bones, endoscopy, and intubation (Figure 8.24).

- Widened retropharyngeal space with posterior displacement of prevertebral muscles.

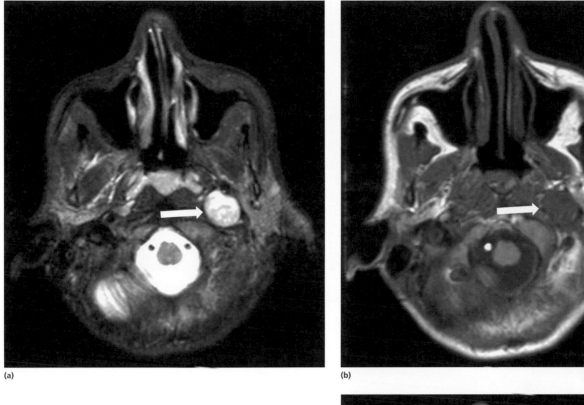

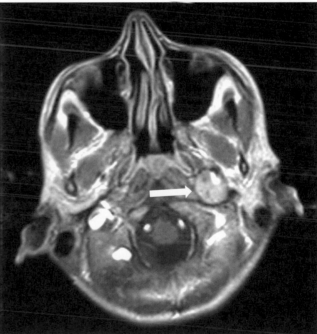

Figure 8.23 Schwannoma. Multiple axial MRI demonstrating a schwannoma in the left carotid space. The mass is hypointense on the precontrast T1-weighted image (a) and slightly hyperintense on the T2-weighted image (b). It also demonstrated enhancement on the arterial-phase postcontrast T1 image (c) (arrows).

- The infection may spread to the neighboring spaces and mediastinum.
- CT shows necrotic tissue and edema as fluid-dense areas often mixed with gas, with characteristic peripheral enhancement.
- On MR, it is isointense to muscle on T1-WI and hyperintense on T2-WI with rim enhancement and necrotic center on postgadolinium images.

Visceral space

Laryngocele

Laryngocele is defined as an abnormal saccular dilatation of the laryngeal ventricle. It may be congenital or acquired, most commonly seen in glass blowers or patients with chronic obstructive pulmonary disease (COPD). Sometimes, it extends through

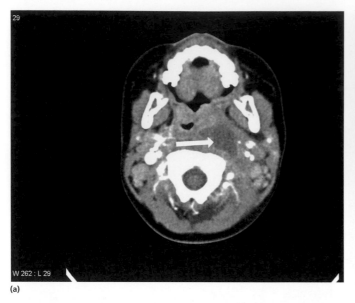

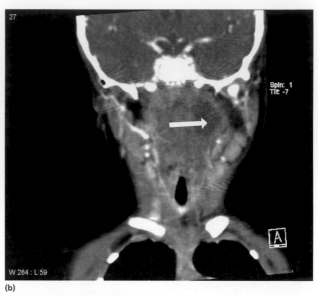

Figure 8.24 Retropharyngeal abscess. Axial (a) and coronal contrast CT (b) scan demonstrates a left-sided retropharyngeal abscess (arrow).

the thyrohyoid membrane and presents as a lump into the neck. On imaging studies, it appears as a sharply defined cystic lesion with enhancing boundaries.

Parathyroid adenoma

Adenomas are often single and may consist of pure or mixed cell types, with the most common variant composed mainly of chief cells:
- US is the first imaging modality and shows a hypoechoic lesion.
- If US is negative, further evaluation with CT or MRI may be helpful. Adenomas are hypervascular lesions adjacent to thyroid lobes or rarely in ectopic locations with variable contrast enhancement and early washout.
- Parathyroid scintigraphy shows an increased uptake with agents such as technetium (Tc)-99m sestamibi (MIBI).
- Angiography is usually done for patients with negative neck explorations and persistent symptoms.

Thyroglossal duct cyst

Thyroglossal duct cysts are the most common congenital neck cysts representing 70% of congenital neck lesions.

The cysts can occur anywhere along the course of the thyroglossal duct, although infrahyoid location is the most common (65%) (Figure 8.25).
- It is seen as thin-walled anechoic lesion on ultrasound, which moves simultaneously with extrusion of the tongue.
- On CT, it appears as thin-walled, smooth, and well-defined homogeneously attenuating lesions within 2 cm of the anterior midline.
- MRI shows low signal on T1-WI and high signal on T2-WI with no enhancement in uncomplicated cysts.
- Thickening and enhancement of wall indicate infection. In infection, they are seen as complex heterogeneous masses with internal fluid debris and associated inflammatory changes.

Thyroid masses

Ultrasound is the first imaging modality used to evaluate all patients with palpable thyroid nodules or masses.

Ultrasound helps to accurately locate and confirm the presence of a mass, distinguishes cystic from solid lesions, and determines if

a nodule is solitary or part of a multinodular gland, demonstrates any associated lymphadenopathy in the paratracheal region, and guides fine needle aspiration (FNA). It is often used in the follow-up of patients with multinodular goiter to evaluate nodule growth and consistency.

Certain ultrasonographic features have been identified that may suggest an increased risk for malignancy such as hypoechogenicity, the presence of microcalcifications, increased central blood flow, or irregular borders. However, in the absence of the aforementioned features, malignancy cannot be excluded definitively.

CT Scanning and MRI scanning are not routinely performed to evaluate the thyroid nodules because of their high cost, but these imaging modalities are highly valuable in determining the substernal extension and effect on surrounding structures particularly in large goiters with obstructive symptoms. Contrast-enhanced CT is limitedly used in patients to confirm the associated lymphadenopathy found on physical examination or ultrasound and in patients in whom FNA is positive for papillary thyroid carcinoma.

The major role of thyroid scintigraphy is to determine the functional status of a suspected autonomously functioning thyroid nodule.

Posterior cervical space

Lymph node metastases, lymphoma, schwannoma and neurofibromas arising from accessory nerve, lipoma, and lymphangioma arising from the primitive embryonic lymph sacs are some of the pathologies found.

Perivertebral space

Osteomyelitis, primary bone tumor or metastasis arising from vertebra, myositis, sarcoma, benign fibrous tumor, and vertebral artery aneurysm are some of the common pathology found in this space.

Osteomyelitis of vertebra

Vertebral osteomyelitis should be considered in all patients experiencing unremitting and/or focal vertebral pain that is not relieved by lying down, particularly if accompanied by fever or paravertebral symptoms indicating a psoas or other paraspinal extension.

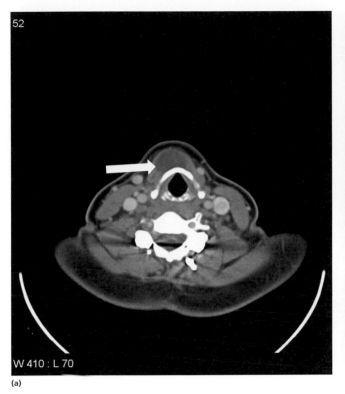

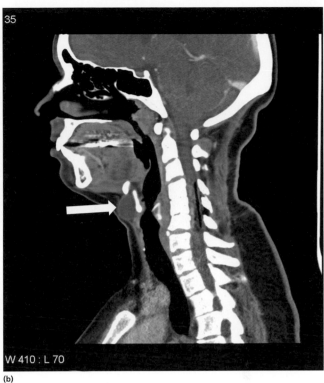

Figure 8.25 Thyroglossal cyst. Axial (a) and sagittal (b) contrast-enhanced CT show a cyst appearing thin-walled, smooth, and well-defined homogeneously hypodense lesion in the anterior midline of the neck (arrows).

Radiography should be ordered for all patients with suspected vertebral osteomyelitis. The earliest signs are loss of definition of a vertebral end plate and narrowing of the associated disc space. If radiography is not diagnostic and the patient has pain that is unremitting or if patient is febrile, other imaging should be considered.

MRI is the most sensitive imaging modality early in the course of infection. The acute-phase osteomyelitis presents as bone marrow edema appearing low signal intensity on T1-WI and high signal intensity on T2-WI.

Contrast MRI scans usually show diffuse enhancement in infected bone and discs and help to evaluate and establish the paraspinal soft tissue and epidural extent of disease. However, MRI is not completely specific, and the diagnosis can be confused with, for example, tumor, spondylosis, compression fracture, or postradiation changes.

If MRI is contraindicated, CT is useful as a sensitive modality for detecting erosions of bone and disc and is more sensitive than radiography in this respect.

Other common head and neck lesions

Second branchial cleft cyst

Embryologic cysts derived from second branchial apparatus typically present as a rounded cystic mass just below the angle of mandible, anterior to the sternocleidomastoid (Figure 8.26):
- On CT, it appears as sharply circumscribed, thin-walled cyst in classic location (anterior triangle or angle of mandible). Notch

sign is pathognomonic where the cyst wall extends between the ICA and ECA just above the carotid bifurcation.
- On ultrasound, it is seen as sharply demarcated cyst with variable echogenicity and shows posterior acoustic enhancement in 70% of the cases.
- On MRI, signal varies on T1-WI based on the protein content and may rarely show peripheral enhancement on postgadolinium images.

Cystic hygroma

Cystic hygroma is a type of congenital lymphatic malformation most commonly seen in the pediatric age group. It is an endothelial-lined cavernous lymphatic space arising from the expansion of embryonic lymph lakes that fails to develop normal lymphatic drainage.

They are usually well-circumscribed, uni- or multilocular fluid-containing lesions. They may show variable density/intensity, with a combination of fluid, soft tissue, and fat.

Less frequently, cystic hygromas may also show an infiltrative appearance:
- Most commonly located in the posterior cervical space.
- On prenatal ultrasound, they may present as a nuchal cyst and may show septations +/− evidence of fetal anasarca or fetal hydrops.
- CT shows a hypoattenuating ill-defined cystic mass.
- On MRI, these lesions are predominantly hypointense on T1-WI (unless hemorrhagic components are present) and predominantly hyperintense on T2-WI with no enhancement or occasional faint rim enhancement after gadolinium administration.

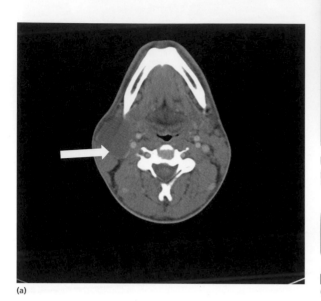

(a)

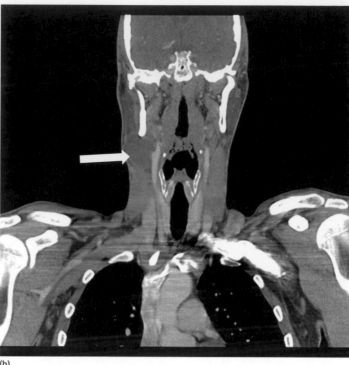

(b)

Figure 8.26 Second brachial cleft cyst. Axial (a) and coronal (b) contrast-enhanced CT show a cystic lesion appearing as sharply circumscribed and thin walled in classic location (anterior triangle or angle of mandible) on the right (arrows).

Suggested reading

Aribandi, M., McCoy, V. & Bazan, C., III (2007) Imaging features of invasive and noninvasive fungal sinusitis: a review. *Radiographics*, **27**, 1283–1296.

Brant, W.B. & Helms, C.A. (2012) *Fundamentals of Diagnostic Radiology*, 4th edn. Lippincott Williams & Wilkins, Philadelphia, PA.

Capps, E.F., Kinsella, J.J., Gupta, M. *et al.* (2010) Emergency imaging assessment of acute, non-traumatic conditions of the head and neck. *Radiographics*, **30**, 1335–1352.

Dwivedi, A. & Singh, K. (2010) CT of the paranasl sinuses: normal anatomy, variants and pathology. *Journal of Optoelectronics and Biomedical Materials*, **2** (I4), 281–289.

Fatterpekar, G.M., Doshi, A.H., Dugar, M. *et al.* (2006) Role of 3D CT in the evaluation of the temporal bone. *Radiographics*, **26**, S117–S132.

LeBedis, C.A. & Sakai, O. (2008) Nontraumatic orbital conditions: diagnosis with CT and MR imaging in the emergent setting. *Radiographics*, **28**, 1741–1753.

Tailor, D.T., Gupta, D., Dalley, R.W. *et al.* (2013) Orbital neoplasms in adults: clinical, radiologic, and pathologic review. *Radiographics*, **33**, 1739–1758.

Winegar, B.A., Murillo, H. & Tantiwongkosi, B. (2013) Spectrum of critical imaging findings in complex facial skeletal trauma. *Radiographics*, **33**, 3–19.

CHAPTER 9

Musculoskeletal imaging

Daniel B. Nissman[1], Frank W. Shields IV[2], and Matthew S. Chin[2]

[1]Musculoskeletal Imaging, Department of Radiology, University of North Carolina, Chapel Hill, USA
[2]Department of Radiology, University of North Carolina, Chapel Hill, USA

Musculoskeletal imaging concerns itself with imaging of bones, joints, muscles, and peripheral nerves. This chapter will discuss the role of the different imaging modalities in the evaluation of the musculoskeletal system, the normal appearance of musculoskeletal-specific structures, and the critical concepts in the analysis of musculoskeletal examinations. Brief overviews of trauma, arthritis, tumors, and interventional procedures will follow.

Imaging modalities

Radiography

Radiographs of biological tissues result in four densities: air, fat, soft tissue, and bone. The variation in soft tissue density between that of water, blood, muscle, and other organs is so small that these cannot be differentiated on a radiograph. Many structures in the extremities are bordered by fat, allowing one to identify normal contours. Radiography is particularly suited to imaging bones for two reasons: the very large difference in density between the bone and soft tissue and their high spatial resolution. Radiographs are the mainstay for the imaging of the arthritides, the initial assessment of bone tumors, the evaluation of orthopedic instrumentation, and, of course, trauma. Due to the relatively low cost of radiographs and wide availability, radiographs serve as the initial diagnostic study for all musculoskeletal complaints.

Limitations of radiography include limited ability to evaluate complex three-dimensional structures (such as the cervical spine, the sacroiliac joints, and the complex fractures), limited ability to penetrate large volumes of tissue, and quite limited ability to evaluate soft tissue pathology.

Routine diagnostic radiographic examinations have at least two (anteroposterior and lateral) and often more projections that are tailored to the body part in question. The tangential patellar view (or "sunrise view") of the knee, the mortise view of the ankle, and the outlet view of the shoulder are examples.

By convention, dense structures (such as bone) are bright on radiographs, whereas less dense structures (such as air) are dark.

Fluoroscopy

Fluoroscopy is a real time radiographic imaging method using X-rays. The primary use of fluoroscopy in musculoskeletal radiology is to guide needles for joint injections/aspirations and bone biopsies. Fluoroscopy is often used intraoperatively to guide and/or evaluate the placement of orthopedic instrumentation. The primary limitation of fluoroscopy is the use of ionizing radiation.

By convention, fluoroscopic images are displayed such that dense structures are dark compared to less dense structures, which are bright—the inverse of the radiographic convention.

Computed tomography

Compared to radiography, in which all soft tissue regardless of whether it is muscle, tendon, blood, or water looks the same, computed tomography (CT) is able to detect much greater variations in soft tissue density, which leads to much greater contrast resolution. Different soft tissue types can often be differentiated, such as tendon versus muscle. The difference in density between blood products and simple fluid can also be detected. With intravenous contrast, abscesses can be detected and intramuscular masses can also be detected. Finally, the acquisition of the images is rapid, taking no more than several seconds for a focused examination, such as the shoulder. An entire body can be scanned in the setting of trauma in around a minute.

Cross-sectional imaging is particularly important for the evaluation of skeletal trauma, both for identification and characterization. Fractures of the pelvis and cervical spine may be difficult to see on radiographs, and the ability to review axial, coronal, and sagittal cross-sectional images is essential to make an accurate diagnosis. Characterization of complex fractures is much easier on CT and guides surgical management. Examples include acetabular fractures, tibial plateau fractures, and some ankle fractures. CT is often obtained to evaluate for intra-articular bone fragments following reduction of a joint dislocation when there is an associated fracture. Except in the setting of extremity infection and rare instances of soft tissue tumors, intravenous contrast is not routinely used in musculoskeletal imaging.

Critical Observations in Radiology for Medical Students, First Edition. Katherine R. Birchard, Kiran Reddy Busireddy, and Richard C. Semelka.
© 2015 John Wiley & Sons, Ltd. Published 2015 by John Wiley & Sons, Ltd.
Companion website: www.wiley.com/go/birchard

Limitations of CT include insufficient soft contrast for the specific characterization of many abnormalities, metal artifact, and radiation exposure. Metal artifact results in streaks of apparent high or low density due to the interaction between the reconstruction algorithm and the marked disparity in density between metal and adjacent tissue, including the bone.

Magnetic resonance imaging

Magnetic resonance imaging (MRI) is the standard imaging modality for internal derangement of joints, bone marrow imaging, and tumor imaging. The primary reason for MRI's importance in musculoskeletal imaging is its unparalleled soft tissue contrast. Like CT, MRI has the ability to evaluate complex three-dimensional structures, such as the sacroiliac joints, though CT retains an edge in evaluating bone anatomy and mineralized tissue (such as mineralized tumor matrix).

Differentiating normal from abnormal tissues in musculoskeletal MRI is achieved by exploiting the concept that pathology, due to its association with free water, is bright on T2-weighted images and dark on T1-weighted images. Fat, on the other hand, is bright on both T1- and T2-weighted images. To make pathology stand out from fat, T2-weighted images are fat suppressed (bright pathology on a dark background), whereas T1-weighted images are not (dark pathology on a bright background) (Figure 9.1).

A few specific situations in musculoskeletal MRI involve the use of contrast material. For questions regarding infection or evaluation of tumors, intravenous contrast is used. MRI performed with intra-articular contrast is referred to as MR arthrography.

MRI has a number of limitations. First, due to its dependence on a uniform magnetic field, anything that distorts the magnetic field will affect the image. The most important situation that affects MR image formation is the presence of indwelling metal, such as a hip prosthesis. Although usually minor, motion artifact caused by patient movement may also be problematic on MRI.

All musculoskeletal MRI examinations involve a combination of T1- and T2-weighted sequences, often in more than one plane. Specific details and combinations may differ depending on the body part or clinical question. The vast majority of musculoskeletal examinations are for internal derangements, and routine protocols have been developed for every joint; these protocols do not employ intravenous or intra-articular contrast. For cases involving the administration of intravenous contrast, the routine protocols are often pared down to allow for the additional sequences needed to evaluate for tissue enhancement while still imaging the area in a reasonable amount of time.

Ultrasonography

Ultrasonography (US) is a real-time imaging modality based on the use of high-frequency sound waves and processing their reflections. The high resolution achievable with modern ultrasound equipment allows excellent characterization of tendons, ligaments, and nerves. Achievable resolution is directly proportional to the frequency of the sound wave—high resolutions require the use of high frequencies. Unfortunately, the depth of tissue penetration decreases with increasing frequency. As a result, high-resolution ultrasound excels in the evaluation of superficial structures, such as the rotator cuff of the shoulder. Another clinical advantage of ultrasound in comparison to the other modalities discussed here is the ability to perform dynamic evaluation of joints. Stress imaging, which can also be performed with fluoroscopy, can easily be performed with ultrasound without the radiation exposure. The real-time nature of sonography also lends itself well to guidance for percutaneous procedures. Additional advantages are low relative cost and portability.

The normal soft tissues of the musculoskeletal system have readily identifiable echotextures. Muscle in the short axis has a "starry sky" appearance, tendons and ligaments in the long axis have a fibrillar appearance, and nerves in the long axis have a fascicular appearance. Simple fluid, for example, joint fluid, is anechoic. Figure 9.2 shows the normal sonographic appearance of the patellar tendon and bony attachments and a subdeltoid fluid collection before and after aspiration.

Limitations of US include limited depth of penetration, inability to image through bone, anisotropy, and operator dependence. As discussed previously, high-resolution imaging is best reserved for superficial structures. The deeper a structure is from the skin surface at a particular frequency, the less signal is received back at the transducer to form images. This is a particular problem for deep tendons, such as the iliopsoas tendon, and in obese individuals at all sites. An oft-cited limitation of musculoskeletal sonography is operator dependence.

Sonography lends itself best to targeted examinations, such as the rotator cuff or lateral ankle. Most regions have a set of well-defined structures that need to be evaluated. For example, the rotator cuff examination includes evaluation of the long head of biceps tendon, the rotator cuff muscle bulk, and the acromioclavicular joint. The lateral ankle examination includes evaluation of the peroneus tendons, the lateral ankle ligaments, and the sinus tarsi.

Radionuclide imaging

Radionuclide imaging is a metabolic imaging modality wherein a tissue-specific radiotracer is injected and images are acquired after the radiotracer has had time to accumulate in the target tissue.

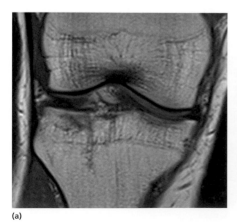

(a)

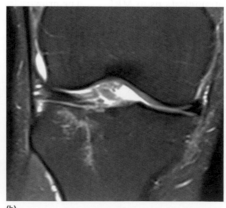

(b)

Figure 9.1 MRI of a lateral tibial plateau contusion/microfracture. Coronal T1-weighted (a) and fat-suppressed T2-weighted (b) images of the right knee demonstrate a reticular linear pattern of decreased signal in the lateral tibial plateau on the T1-weighted image in a background of bright normal fat and the corresponding high signal on the T2-weighted fat-suppressed image on a background of low-signal-intensity fat.

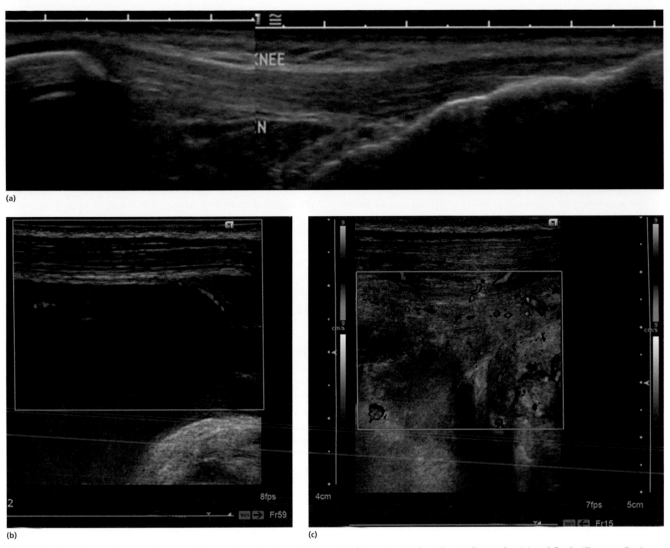

Figure 9.2 Examples of ultrasound images. Ultrasound excels at imaging superficial structures such as the patellar tendon (a) and fluid collections (b, c). The image in (a) was stitched together to show the entirety of the patellar tendon from its attachment on the patella (left side of the image) and the tibial tubercle (right side of the image). Note the fibrillar pattern of the patellar tendon and the bright reflections at the superficial surfaces of the bones. The images in (b) and (c) are of a very large and inflamed subdeltoid bursa before (b) and after (c) percutaneous aspiration. Note the large relatively anechoic region that represents fluid in (b). The fluid has been completely aspirated in image (c) but demonstrating marked regional soft tissue hypervascularity as illustrated by the color Doppler signal. This signal was less intense on the preaspiration image likely due to compression of the vessels by the fluid collection.

Radionuclide imaging for the musculoskeletal system is reserved for two general situations: evaluation for osseous metastatic disease and as a substitute for MRI when contraindications to MRI exist. The two most common radionuclide examinations are the technetium-99 m methylene diphosphonate (MDP) "bone scan" and fluorodeoxyglucose (FDG) positron emission tomography (PET). In both cases, a radiotracer is injected intravenously and the patient is imaged at a later time, 3 h for the "bone scan" and on the order of an hour for PET/CT. The bone scan radiotracer is taken up by areas of elevated bone turnover, such as might be seen in metastatic disease, fractures, or degenerative diseases. The PET radiotracer FDG is taken up by areas of elevated glucose metabolism. As such, both of these processes are sensitive, but not particularly specific. Both imaging studies represent metabolic activity and need to be correlated with anatomic imaging. Bone scans need to be interpreted in conjunction with contemporary radiographs or other anatomic cross-sectional imaging modality (CT or MRI).

Today, PET images are routinely acquired with CT images in the same scan to provide anatomic localization.

The primary limitations of radionuclide bone scan and PET/CT are low spatial resolution and whole-body radiation dose. Spatial resolution for the bone scan is on the order of 10 mm, which can make lesion localization difficult. The low-resolution and nonspecific nature of the bone scan eventually led to its replacement by MRI for all indications except whole-body assessment for metastatic disease. PET/CT is reserved for metastatic disease assessment, especially when nonosseous metastases are common, the bone scan is equivocal, or the process is normally "cold" on bone scan.

Appearance of normal tissues

In this section, the normal appearances of bone, muscle, tendon, ligament, articular cartilage, fibrocartilage, and peripheral nerve will be discussed. Knowledge of the normal appearance is essential to identifying pathology.

Bone

Bone is a complex tissue composed of both mineralized and nonmineralized components. The nonmineralized component is composed of extracellular matrix, osteoid, and a variety of cells, mainly osteoblasts and osteoclasts. Osteoblasts and osteoclasts are cells responsible for bone deposition and resorption, respectively. The general architecture of bones is a dense outer layer, the cortex, and a less dense inner layer, the medullary cavity. The nonmineralized spaces in the medullary cavity are bordered by thin spicules of bone called trabeculae. These spaces are filled with hematopoietic marrow early in life and are near completely replaced by fat in adulthood. Bone constantly undergoes remodeling in response to its load environment. Blood supply reaches the medullary cavity via nutrient foramina that penetrate the cortex.

The periosteum is a connective tissue layer that invests bones and is rich with blood vessels, nerves, as well as osteoblasts and osteoclasts. This layer plays an essential role in fracture healing but also can be stimulated by inflammatory processes and tumors:

- Imaging methods based on X-rays exploit the relative difference in density between the cortex and medullary cavity. The edges of the bone always appear much denser than the central portion because the medullary cavity is confined to the center of the bone. The inner and outer layers of the cortex are always smooth with abrupt transitions in density between both the external soft tissues and the medullary cavity of bone.
- The fine network of trabecular bone is often able to be visualized on radiographs and to varying degrees on CT.
- On MRI, mineralized tissue appears dark, regardless of its nature. As cortical bone represents highly mineralized tissue, cortical bone is uniformly dark on both T1-weighted and T2-weighted images. In adults, the medullary cavity is filled with fat and is therefore bright on both T1-weighted and T2-weighted images. Hematopoietic marrow appears somewhat darker than normal fat, but never darker than skeletal muscle. The trabecular bone can occasionally be seen, particularly in the periphery of the marrow cavity. Certain sequences make the trabecular structure more apparent but potentially at the expense of soft tissue information.
- As the soft tissue–bone interface represents a large change in acoustic properties, the vast majority of sound is reflected back to the transducer. Bone, therefore, appears as a bright line on sonographic images with minimal, if any, detail beyond the bone surface. Normal periosteum is not visible on any imaging modality.

Muscle

Muscle is composed of a relatively uniform population of myocytes, which are organized into fibers and fascicles, which are collections of fibers; a small amount of fat may occasionally interdigitate between the muscle fascicles. Muscles are covered in a thin connective tissue layer known as fascia.

The transmission of the contractile forces to the tendon and ultimately to the bone occurs initially at the myotendinous junction. This junction may be centrally located in the muscle or may even be at the periphery of the muscle, such as might be seen in the gastrocnemius and soleus attachments to the Achilles tendon or the rectus femoris muscle:

- The modalities most suited to imaging muscle are MRI and ultrasound.
- On MRI, muscle is of a uniform brightness "intermediate" between fat and bone. Small penetrating vessels can often be seen. For the evaluation of bone marrow abnormalities and soft tissue masses, the intensity of muscle serves as an internal referent, abnormalities being isointense, hyperintense, or hypointense to muscle. Subtle

pathologic findings are often evident on fluid-sensitive sequences when they are not seen on other sequences or modalities.
- In cross section, muscle has a "starry sky" appearance on sonographic images. All the tiny fascial septa investing the muscular subunits create acoustic reflectors that are easily seen on ultrasound. In the long axis, muscle has a characteristic striated appearance.
- Muscle appears to be of generally uniform density on CT occasionally with wisps of interdigitating fat. Muscle has a density between that of proteinaceous fluid and blood with considerable overlap. With the addition of intravenous contrast, penetrating vessels can be identified.
- On radiographs, muscle looks like any other soft tissue structure, including fluid and blood. Muscles are identified by their silhouette against the very low-density subcutaneous adipose tissues.

Tendon

Tendons are a connective tissue that efficiently transmit the contractile forces generated by muscle to bone. They are composed of a highly ordered array of collagen fibrils, noncollagenous matrix, and a few cells. At the muscular end of the tendon, they interface with muscle tissue at the myotendinous junction. At the bone end of the tendon, they interface with bone at the enthesis. The enthesis represents a very short, but very strong, interface between tendon and bone:

- Tendons are best imaged using sonography and MRI (Figure 9.3).
- Sonographically, tendons have a highly ordered fibrillar appearance. Bright lines are thought to represent collagen fibers, and dark lines likely represent noncollagenous matrix. In cross section, tendons appear to have bright speckles on a relatively hypoechoic background. The sound beam must strike tendon at exactly 90° or the reflected sound waves are directed away from the transducer resulting in artifactually low signal, a property known as anisotropy.
- On MRI, tendons are, in general, uniformly dark on both T1-weighted and T2-weighted images.
- Tendons are only visible in a few places in the body on radiography. The patellar tendon and Achilles tendon are profiled both anteriorly and posteriorly by fat, allowing the soft tissue density of the tendon to stand out.
- Tendons on CT are denser than muscle and are often readily visualized. For both radiography and CT, the density of associated pathology is usually similar enough to the density of the tendon that a specific determination of the abnormality is not possible.
- The normal peritendinous tissues are, in general, not visible on any imaging modality.

Ligament

Ligaments connect bone to bone at joints and provide stability at the joints. Ligaments are very similar structurally to tendons, though they are much thinner than tendons. The ligament–bone interface is called the enthesis, similar to the tendon–bone interface. Due to their association with joints, ligaments may represent focal areas of thickening within a joint capsule, such as the inferior glenohumeral ligament of the shoulder or the medial patellofemoral ligament of the knee. The joint capsule can be considered a specialized form of ligament but is lined internally by synovial tissue:

- Ligaments are best evaluated by MRI and sonography (Figure 9.4).
- On MRI, ligaments appear either as dense, linear bands of hypointensity on both T1-weighted and T2-weighted images or, if the ligament is thin enough, as a striated band of tissue. All major ligaments at the joints are readily appreciated on MRI.

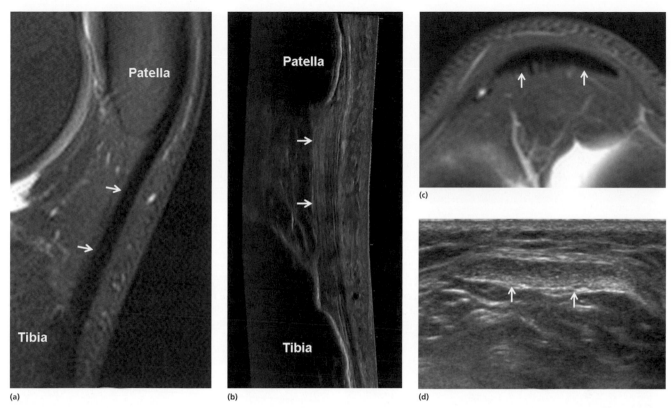

Figure 9.3 Normal patellar tendon. Longitudinal MRI (a) and US (b) and short-axis MRI (c) and US (d) images of the patellar tendon. *White arrows* point to the posterior border of the tendon. The MR images demonstrate a well-defined uniformly hypointense/dark linear band coursing from the patella to the tibia.

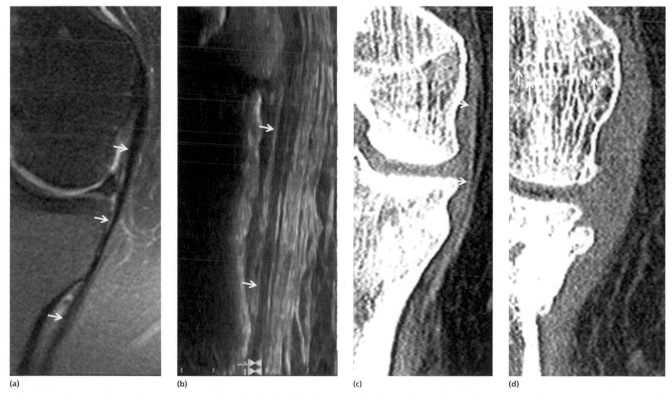

Figure 9.4 Normal medial collateral ligament. Coronal T2-weighted fat-suppressed MRI (a), long-axis medial collateral ligament US (b), and coronal CT (c) images show a normal medial collateral ligament. The *arrows* show the deep border of the ligament on these images. On MRI, the ligament is a thin uniformly dark band of tissue. On US, the ligament is thin with a barely discernible fibrillar structure. On CT, the ligament is slightly more dense than surrounding tissue. The ligament in (d) is no longer distinct due to surrounding fluid and soft tissue edema secondary to trauma (note the fractured tibial plateau); the status of the ligament cannot be determined in this case.

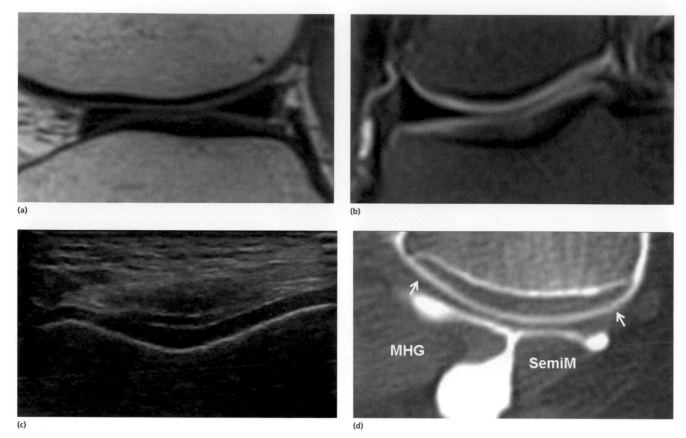

Figure 9.5 Normal knee articular cartilage. Sagittal PD-weighted MRI (a), coronal T2-weighted fat-suppressed MRI (b), US (c), and CT arthrogram (d) images of normal articular cartilage. In all cases, the cartilage is smooth and of nearly uniform thickness. The bright surface on CT is due to contrast (*arrows*) covering the articular surface. A popliteal cyst shows the medial head of the gastrocnemius tendon and muscle (*MHG*) and semimembranosus tendon (*SemiM*).

- Sonographically, ligaments have a similar striated/fibrillar appearance as tendons and also exhibit anisotropy. All superficial ligaments are readily evaluated sonographically, but deep ligaments, such as the anterior cruciate ligament (ACL), cannot be seen. Normal joint capsules are easily seen on both MRI and ultrasound.
- Large dense ligaments, such as the posterior cruciate ligament, can be seen on CT and have a similar density to tendons. Ligaments are otherwise not routinely visible on either CT or radiography.

Articular (hyaline) cartilage

Hyaline cartilage provides some degree of shock absorption and a low-friction environment so that articulating bones may move without damage. At the bone–cartilage interface, there is a region of calcified cartilage before its transition to the mineralized subchondral bone. The transition between the mineralized cartilage and nonmineralized cartilage is known as the tide mark:

- Articular cartilage is best imaged by MRI.
- Normal cartilage has a smooth surface and a layered appearance on T2-weighted, including proton density (PD), images.
- Articular cartilage is superficial enough to be evaluated sonographically in a few locations such as the femoral trochlea and the anterior talar dome. Normal cartilage appears uniformly anechoic. Articular cartilage has soft tissue density on radiographs and on CT. On routine radiographs, cartilage can be inferred on weight-bearing radiographs by the fact that the bones do not touch, but otherwise appear lucent.

- On CT, there is insufficient contrast difference between synovial fluid and cartilage to adequately assess the cartilage. Visualization of cartilage on radiography and CT requires intra-articular contrast, either air or iodinated contrast, to make out the cartilage interface. Figure 9.5 shows examples of the normal appearance of hyaline cartilage on MRI, US, and CT arthrography. ("Hyaline" refers to the glass-like appearance of thinly sectioned cartilage at histopathology, not its radiographic appearance.)

Fibrocartilage

A number of fibrocartilage structures exist in the body, including the knee menisci, the glenoid and acetabular labrums, the triangular fibrocartilage of the wrist, and the discs within the pubic symphysis and temporomandibular joints. The knee menisci and the glenoid and acetabular labrums represent dense connective tissue structures formed into either a complete ring in the case of the glenoid labrum or incomplete rings in the cases of the menisci and acetabular labrum. These rings serve to deepen the socket in which the ball, femoral condyle in the case of the knee, sits thus decreasing unwanted motion (subluxations) at these joints. In addition to helping to stabilize the joint, the knee menisci help to distribute load across the entire joint as the actual contact point between the femoral condyle and tibial plateau is quite small. The triangular fibrocartilage of the wrist serves predominantly as a load distributor:

- MRI is the preferred method for evaluation of the knee menisci as well as both the glenoid and acetabular labrums (Figure 9.6).

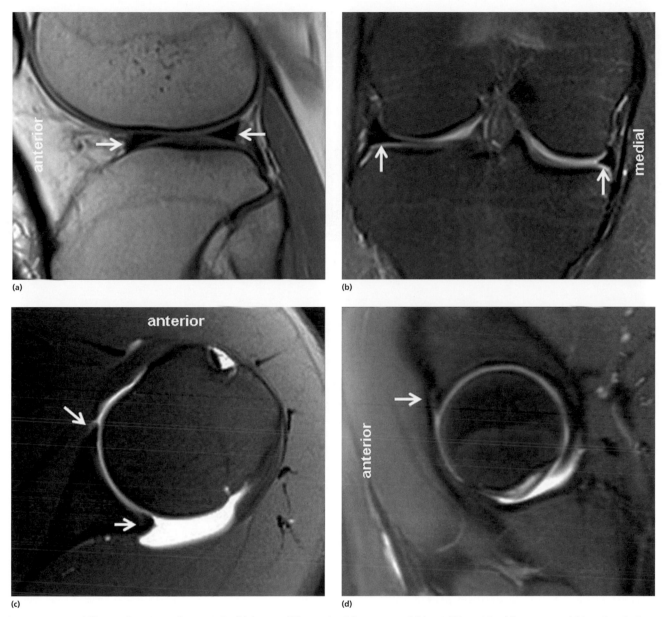

Figure 9.6 Normal fibrocartilage. Sagittal PD-weighted (a), coronal T2-weighted fat-suppressed (b), axial T1-weighted fat-suppressed (c), and sagittal T1-weighted fat-suppressed arthrogram (d) MR images of fibrocartilage. The knee menisci (a and b) and the glenoid (c) and acetabular (d) labrums normally have a well-defined triangular appearance (*arrows*). The sagittal image in (a) demonstrates the normal appearance of the anterior and posterior horn of the lateral meniscus. The coronal image in (b) demonstrates the normal appearance of the medial and lateral meniscal body. The axial image in (c) shows the normal appearance of the anterior and posterior glenoid labrum at the equator of the glenoid. The sagittal image of the hip in (d) shows the normal anterior acetabular labrum.

These structures normally have very distinct margins and are quite dark on both T1-weighted and T2-weighted images.

- The morphology is best depicted in the knee where the menisci appear as hypointense triangles at the periphery of the medial and lateral tibial plateau; the base of the triangle is oriented toward the periphery, and the apex of the triangle is oriented toward the inside of the joint. The glenoid and acetabular labrums have a similar appearance but may be more rounded in appearance.

Peripheral nerve

The peripheral nerves represent bundles of axons, each surrounded by insulating Schwann cells, bundled together by connective tissue. Nerves are usually surrounded by fat, and they usually follow blood vessels destined for the same body region as part of a neurovascular bundle:

- The peripheral nerves are best imaged with US and MRI (Figure 9.7).
- The sonographic appearance of nerves is often described as "fascicular": hypoechoic tubes in a hyperechoic background. The hypoechoic tubes are generally uniform in size.
- The appearance on MRI is quite similar to the sonographic appearance: grouped hypointense lines surrounded by bright fat. The presence of surrounding fat is extremely useful for the identification of nerves, so nonfat-suppressed sequences are used when nerve anatomy is important to evaluate.

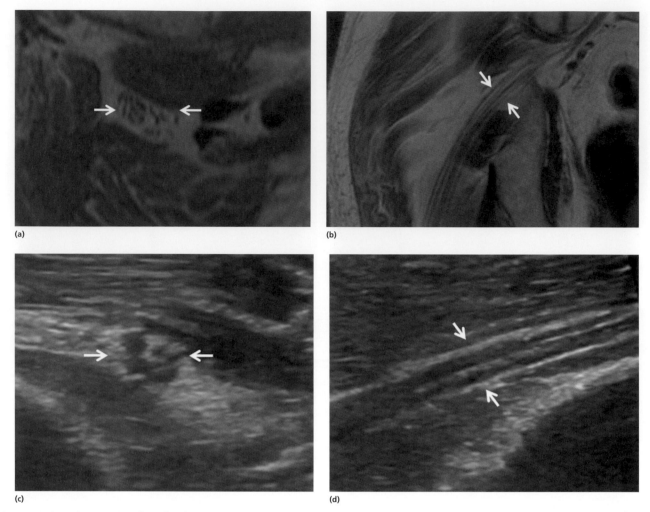

(a)

(b)

(c)

(d)

Figure 9.7 Normal appearance of peripheral nerve. Sciatic nerve on MRI: axial (a) and coronal (b) T1-weighted MRI of the sciatic nerve in the pelvis. The axial image is at the level of the common hamstring origin. The coronal image shows the course of the sciatic nerve as it exits the sciatic notch. Note the hypointense nerve fascicles surrounded by bright fat (*arrows*). Radial nerve in the arm on US: short-axis (c) and long-axis (d) US images of the radial nerve. Note the hypoechoic fascicles surrounded by hyperechoic tissue that is consistent with fat (*arrows*).

Critical concepts in musculoskeletal imaging

Several fundamental concepts are essential to keep in mind. First, some types of infection are emergency conditions that require immediate action. Second, normal radiographs do not exclude the diagnosis of fracture. Third, the distinction between bone-centered and joint-centered diseases will help to tailor the differential diagnosis for a finding. Fourth is the determination of whether a process is localized or systemic.

Infectious emergencies

Septic arthritis, gas gangrene, and necrotizing fasciitis are extremely destructive processes requiring emergent intervention. Recognizing these conditions is essential to preserve the function of joints (septic arthritis) and soft tissue (gas gangrene/necrotizing fasciitis).

Septic arthritis

As untreated infection of a joint can lead to rapid destruction of that joint, rapid establishment of a diagnosis is essential to preserve the articular cartilage. When an infected joint is suspected (severe joint pain, fever, elevated serum inflammatory markers), an aspiration will need to be performed to establish a definitive diagnosis:

- Often, the aspiration is performed by a musculoskeletal radiologist using fluoroscopic or ultrasound guidance.
- In cases of indeterminate clinical suspicion, an MRI or ultrasound may be obtained prior to aspiration to establish the presence of a joint effusion.

Aspirated fluid is sent for cell count and differential in addition to Gram stain and culture. Unfortunately, the Gram stain often shows no organisms and the culture may take too long to produce a result. The cell count with differential has excellent accuracy for diagnosing joint infection and has successfully guided management of suspected joint infections. In cases where minimal fluid is obtained, preference is often given to the cell count over the culture and Gram stain.

Figure 9.8 depicts septic arthritis and an example of the effect of delayed treatment on a joint.

Soft tissue infections requiring emergent intervention

Two types of soft tissue infections require emergent intervention to limit morbidity and prevent death: necrotizing fasciitis and gas gangrene. Both are associated with soft tissue gas, which are readily detectable on radiography and CT and play a central role in the diagnosis of these conditions. Necrotizing fasciitis is an infection of the

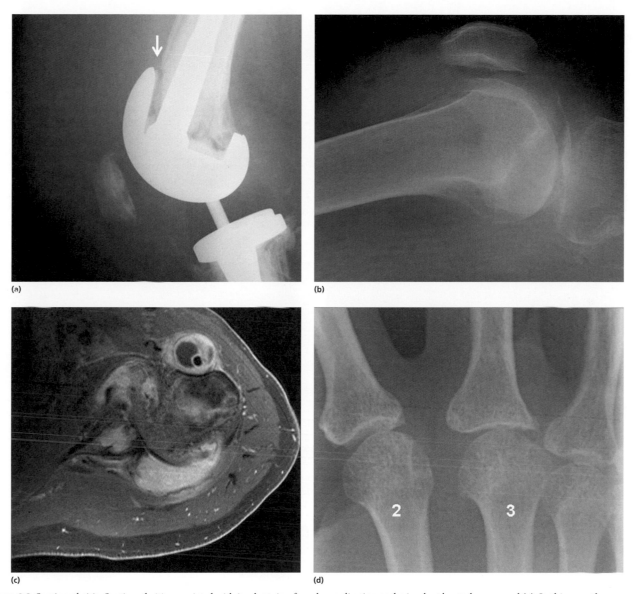

Figure 9.8 Septic arthritis. Septic arthritis associated with implants is a feared complication as the implant has to be removed (a). In this case, there are a large joint effusion, overlying soft tissue swelling, and, most importantly, erosion of the undersurface of the anterior femoral component (*arrow*). The presence of gas in a joint (b), such as in this knee, is due either to a recent surgical procedure, penetrating trauma, or gas-forming organism. On MRI, a large effusion with synovial hypertrophy and underlying bone marrow edema is concerning for infection as seen on this axial postcontrast T1-weighted fat-suppressed image (c). In (d), the patient had delayed diagnosis and treatment of third digit metacarpophalangeal joint septic arthritis that resulted in joint space loss (compared to the adjacent digits) and irregularity of the articular surface.

subcutaneous tissues and the superficial and deep fascia. Gas gangrene, also known as septic myonecrosis, is an infection of muscle. While both entities occur after a traumatic event causing a disruption of the skin, the injury may not be apparent in the case of necrotizing fasciitis. The vast majority of cases of necrotizing fasciitis occur in people who are overtly immunosuppressed or who have relative immunosuppression as might be seen in diabetes, chronic alcohol abuse, and malignancies. Necrotizing fasciitis has also occurred following surgical procedures, such as caesarean section, though this is rare. Gas gangrene is associated with direct inoculation of muscle through an open wound with soil.

Necrotizing fasciitis is usually polymicrobial, while gas gangrene is mostly associated with *Clostridium perfringens*, though it can be caused by any soil-based anaerobe. *Clostridium perfringens*, and other clostridial species, causes direct muscle injury through the production of exotoxins that destroy the muscle. Exotoxins play a role in tissue necrosis with infection by other organisms:

- The most specific imaging finding in these conditions is the presence of soft tissue gas. Large collections of gas are readily identifiable on radiographs, but tiny bubbles of gas may only be detectable on CT.
- Gas usually results in complete signal dropout on MRI; large collections are easily identifiable, but small bubbles may blend in with the surroundings, as fascia is often dark on all sequences as well.
- The gas in necrotizing fasciitis is usually located along the fascial planes, often adjacent to the superficial fascia. The gas in gas gangrene is intramuscular.

- While gas is best appreciated on radiographs and CT, the soft tissue findings of both necrotizing fasciitis and gas gangrene are best appreciated on MRI.
- CT is very insensitive to muscle pathology due to the considerable overlap in densities between normal and abnormal tissues.

  The main difference between the two entities is the epicenter of infection: the subcutaneous tissues and fascia for necrotizing fasciitis and a muscle for gas gangrene:

- Fascial edema is manifested by fluid-intensity brightness in the fascia on MRI and effacement of normal fat planes on CT.
- In necrotizing fasciitis, there is often adjacent muscle edema. In septic myositis/myonecrosis, infected tissue demonstrates high signal on T2-weighted images. Contrast-enhanced MRI will show marked enhancement of inflamed tissue (muscle and/or fascia). Complete lack of enhancement is consistent with necrotic tissue.
- Contrast-enhanced CT is often not helpful except to identify abscesses.
- Findings of cellulitis often accompany necrotizing fasciitis and gas gangrene and are characterized by increased soft tissue density (CT) or increased signal on T2-weighted images (MRI) within the subcutaneous tissues.
- On US, fascial planes may become hypoechoic and adjacent muscle may become hyperechoic, a nonspecific sign of muscle injury. Soft tissue gas is, however, readily identifiable sonographically as numerous hyperechoic foci with posterior often hyperechoic streaking oriented along a fascial plane.

Figure 9.9 demonstrates the appearance of soft tissue gas in the setting of necrotizing fasciitis and gas gangrene on US, CT, and MRI.

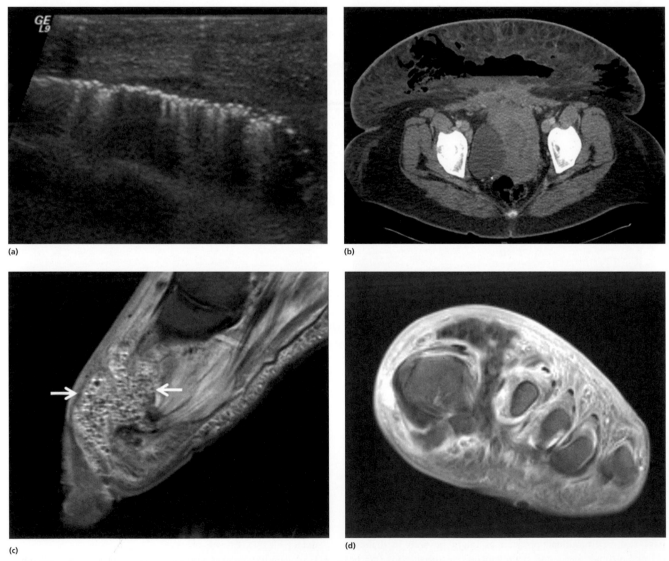

(a)   (b)

(c)   (d)

Figure 9.9 Soft tissue gas on US, CT, and MRI. On US, soft tissue gas appears like bright foci with the so-called "dirty" posterior acoustic shadowing as seen in this case of necrotizing fasciitis (a) where the gas bubbles are arrayed along the superficial fascia. On CT, gas is readily identifiable as completely black areas. In (b), there are large collections of gas in the subcutaneous tissues as well as a gas-containing abscess. On MRI, gas is represented by tiny round foci of little to no signal on all sequences. In the case shown here, the sagittal STIR image (c) depicts a collection (*arrows*) of bright material interspersed with innumerable tiny dark dots representing an abscess containing gas. From the same case as (c), the axial T1-weighted fat-suppressed image following the administration of contrast (d) shows a somewhat ill-defined low-signal region dissecting from the dorsum of the foot to the plantar aspect between the first and second metatarsals. The tiny foci of lower signal correspond to bubbles of gas.

Normal radiographs in the setting of trauma

A normal radiograph after trauma is due to one of two possibilities: the body part in question is normal, or the body part in question is fractured, but simply not detectable on the radiograph. There are two reasons for negative radiographs in the setting of a fractured bone: the fracture is nondisplaced or the fracture plane is not profiled in any of the obtained projections:

- When the fracture is still thought to be likely, appropriate management and repeat radiographs at least 14 days from the date of the injury can be obtained.
- Alternatively and depending on the clinical circumstances, an MRI can be obtained.

Fracture healing occurs in two phases: an osteoclastic phase and an osteoblastic phase. The osteoclastic phase is characterized by resorption of bone about the fracture site. In adults, the peak of osteoclastic activity occurs 2 weeks following injury:

- Imaging at this time or later would hopefully make the fracture visible as a new radiolucent line at the site of the fracture.
- The osteoblastic phase begins 1–2 weeks after the osteoclastic phase resulting in the formation of callus, which is visible radiographically (Figure 9.10). In children, this process is dramatically accelerated.
- CT may be helpful in the case where the fracture plane is not adequately profiled as can be observed on occasion in the acetabulum. The resolution of CT is less than that of radiography, so truly nondisplaced fractures will still not be seen on CT.
- MRI excels at the identification of fractures not because it is better at detecting the fracture line, but because it is able to visualize the marked surrounding reactive bone marrow edema. There is often a corresponding hypointense line on T1-weighted images that more closely corresponds to the fracture line; seeing this line surrounded by bone marrow edema is consistent with a fracture. If one does not see this line, contusion could also be entertained.

One scenario is worth specific mention. When a person over the age of 70 falls on their hip and radiographs are negative for a fracture, MRI should be obtained (Figure 9.11). The primary reason for this is that the morbidity and mortality following an undiagnosed and subsequently displaced hip fracture are extremely high. Rapid diagnosis and treatment are thought to mitigate against these dismal outcomes. In addition to the previously stated reasons why fractures may be occult on radiographs, people over the age of 70 often have osteopenic bones, making it even more difficult to identify trabecular disruption:

- These fractures are also often occult on CT.
- Unfortunately, the elderly are more likely to have contraindications to MRI (e.g., cardiac pacemakers, spinal cord stimulators, and the like), so CT is often the next step in these individuals.
- Alternatively, a radionuclide bone scan can be performed several days later (to allow the healing process to ramp up to a level that would be visible in the setting of osteopenic bones).

A radiographic sign of a nondisplaced, radio-occult fracture worth mentioning in this context is the presence of an effusion. Effusions are not well seen except in a few locations in the body, most notably the knee and the elbow. In the knee, a lipohemarthrosis indicates the presence of a fracture (Figure 9.12); fat can only enter a joint when there is an open path from the bone marrow into the joint. In the elbow, the elevation of the anterior and/or the posterior fat pad of the distal humerus is consistent with an effusion and, in the setting of trauma, most often indicates a radio-occult/nondisplaced radial head fracture.

Bone-centered versus joint-centered disease

Bone pathology adjacent to the joints may either be due to pathology originating within the joint itself or in the bone adjacent to the joint. Establishing whether the underlying process originates within the bone adjacent to the joint or from within the joint itself will help to focus the differential diagnosis.

The classic example of a bone-centered process that might be mistaken for a joint-centered process is osteonecrosis. Osteonecrosis often results in findings similar to osteoarthrosis (OA) as the disease progresses. Given that OA is far more common than osteonecrosis and given the overlap in imaging findings between these two entities in the later stages of disease, particularly radiographically, it would be easy to incorrectly assign the findings to OA. OA is characterized by a progression from cartilage destruction leading to loss of joint space, subchondral sclerosis, and subchondral cyst formation occurring generally equally on

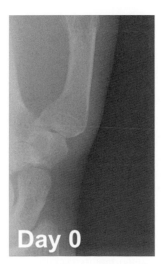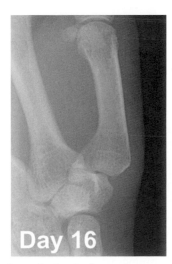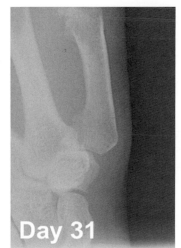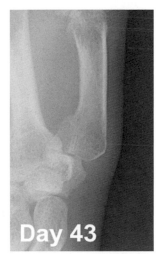

Figure 9.10 Time course of healing of a nondisplaced radio-occult intra-articular base of thumb metacarpal fracture. The initial radiograph (day 0) shows no evidence for fracture and was read as normal. Again, on the subsequently obtained radiograph (day 16), the fracture remains occult. Not until the next radiograph (day 31) is the presence of a fracture revealed by the presence of a small amount of callus along the ulnar aspect of the base of the metacarpal. The amount of fracture callus is noticeably increased on the final image in this series (day 43).

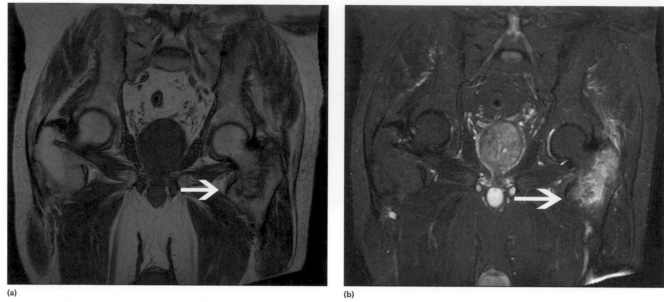

Figure 9.11 MRI of a nondisplaced intertrochanteric hip fracture. Coronal T1-weighted (a) and fat-suppressed T2-weighted (b) images demonstrate a nondisplaced left intertrochanteric femur fracture; the radiographs were negative for fracture. Note the well-defined hypointense curvilinear region through the intertrochanteric region of the left proximal femur that corresponds to the fracture itself (*arrow*). In (b), the reverse situation is true: the fracture and surrounding bone marrow edema are quite bright in comparison to the normal fat-suppressed bone marrow (*arrow*).

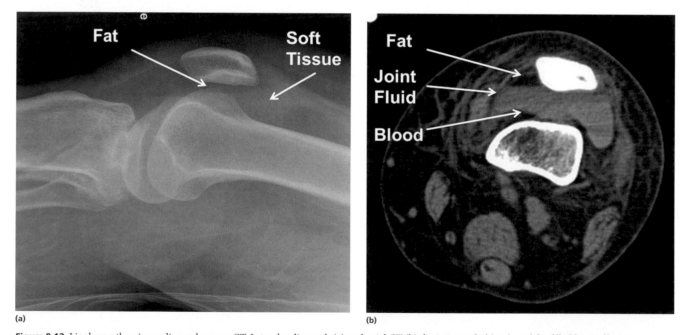

Figure 9.12 Lipohemarthrosis—radiograph versus CT. Lateral radiograph (a) and axial CT (b) depictions of a blood- and fat-filled knee effusion (lipohemarthrosis) following tibial plateau fracture. The distinction between the synovial fluid and blood cannot be made on a radiograph, but can be made on CT due to its higher contrast resolution.

both sides of the joint. Osteonecrosis is characterized by bone marrow infarction, followed by increased bone density/sclerosis. As the disease progresses, there is progressive involvement of the articular surface that eventually leads to subchondral fracture and articular surface collapse. Articular surface collapse results in an incongruent articular surface leading to cartilage destruction and, ultimately, the classic findings of OA. Even in this case, there is often greater involvement on the side of the joint in which the osteonecrosis manifested. Figure 9.13 illustrates the radiographic progression of femoral head osteonecrosis.

Localized versus systemic disease

The clinical implications of bone findings when found in multiple bones are often quite different than when found in a single bone. Syndromic and other systemic conditions are often, but not always, known at the time of the first identification of a multifocal/polyostotic bone lesion. It is therefore important to recognize that a polyostotic process is present. Similarly, implications for an arthrosis affecting a single joint (monoarticular) are quite different from one affecting many joints (polyarticular). Two examples will be illustrated here: fibrous dysplasia and periosteal reaction.

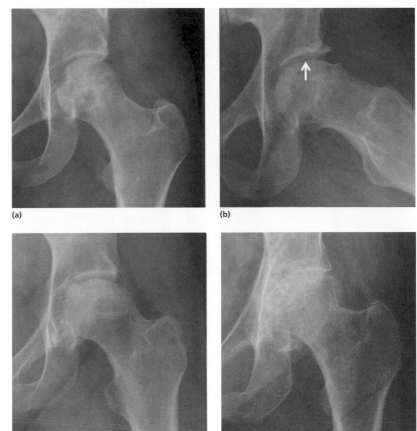

(a)

(b)

(c)

(d)

Figure 9.13 Progression of osteonecrosis of the femoral head. The earliest changes of osteonecrosis are not visible on radiographs, only MRI. The first radiographic manifestation is increased sclerosis within the femoral head (a). This is followed by the development of a nondisplaced subchondral fracture, often best seen on the frog leg lateral view of the hip (b). The subchondral fracture is characterized by a thin crescentic lucency just beneath the subchondral cortex (*arrow*). Articular surface collapse follows resulting in an incongruous articular surface (c). The final stage is characterized by secondary osteoarthrosis: joint space loss and subchondral sclerosis and cyst/geode formation on both sides of the joint (d).

A variety of bone tumors may have associations with syndromes or have other clinical implications, such as increased risk for malignancy, when found in more than one bone. A classic example is fibrous dysplasia. Polyostotic fibrous dysplasia is associated with the endocrine disorder McCune–Albright syndrome, whereas a solitary area of fibrous dysplasia will have only localized effects (Figure 9.14).

Periosteal reaction is a nonspecific finding that is typically a reaction to an inflammatory process. Cellulitis and stress fractures are commonly seen localized causes for periosteal reaction. Certain bone tumors are also associated with localized periosteal reaction. One systemic cause for a polyostotic periosteal reaction is an entity known as hypertrophic osteoarthropathy, which is often associated with pulmonary disease. The association with pulmonary malignancy is high; polyostotic periosteal reaction should always raise the possibility of lung cancer (Figure 9.15).

Musculoskeletal trauma

Musculoskeletal trauma is very common ranging from visually obvious fractures and dislocations resulting from high-energy impacts to more subtle soft tissue injuries. The vast majority of fractures and dislocations can be diagnosed radiographically, whereas soft tissue injuries often require MRI to make a definitive diagnosis.

Fractures and dislocations

Any bone in the body may be fractured and any joint may be dislocated:
- Radiographs are the initial and often only imaging modality needed for diagnosis.
- Occasionally, CT is needed to evaluate more complex structures.

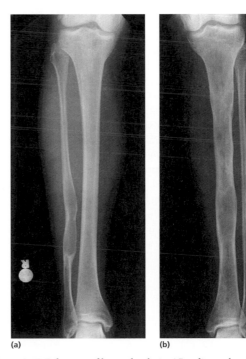

(a)

(b)

Figure 9.14 Polyostotic fibrous dysplasia. AP radiographs of the right (a) and left (b) legs demonstrate multiple lytic expansile lesions of the right fibula and left tibia. These lesions, characteristic of fibrous dysplasia, are characterized by an intramedullary location, expansion of the cortex with thinning of the cortex, and a vague internal density that has been described as appearing like "ground glass."

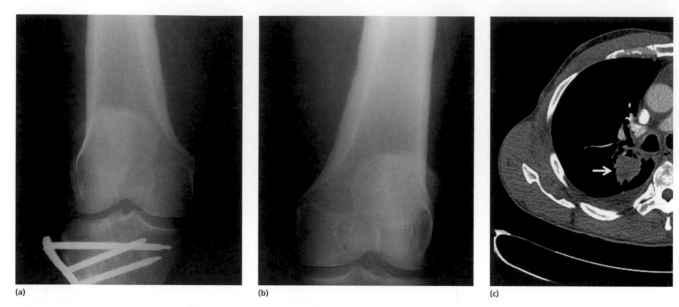

(a)   (b)   (c)

Figure 9.15 Hypertrophic osteoarthropathy. Radiographs of the right (a) and left (b) distal femurs demonstrate dense, thick periosteal new bone along both the medial and lateral aspects of the visualized distal femur. The axial CT image in (c), which is from the same patient, depicts a right upper lobe lung mass (*arrow*). The periosteal reaction in this patient is due to the paraneoplastic syndrome called "hypertrophic osteoarthropathy," which is secondary to the patient's lung cancer.

This section will discuss the identification of fractures and dislocations, stress fractures, and pathologic fractures.

Diagnosis of a fracture

The most obvious sign of a fracture is a lucent line separating the bone into two pieces. The greater the degree of displacement, the easier it is to recognize the fracture. For rapid trauma series, one view may be all that is obtained. Common signs of fracture are cortical step-offs and deformities, whereas an uncommon feature is a sclerotic line, resulting from overriding of the fracture margins. Figure 9.16 provides examples of these fracture signs.

Comminuted fractures are fractures in which more than one fracture line is present at the same location resulting in many pieces. A segmental fracture refers to long bone fractures with two separate fractures, such as one in the proximal shaft and one in the distal shaft. Intra-articular fractures have a fracture line extending to a joint; articular surface discontinuity may result in early posttraumatic OA. Depressed articular surface fragments are important to note as bone grafting may be needed to restore the articular surface; compressed bone does not spring back to its normal height. Open fractures, sometimes called compound fractures, are fractures where there is direct communication between the fracture site and the outside air; these fractures are at much greater risk for infectious complications. Figure 9.17 shows examples of these complicating fracture modifiers.

Fracture mimics

There are two main fracture mimics, nutrient foramina and accessory ossicles (Figure 9.18). Nutrient foramina are intracortical obliquely oriented channels that allow the bone's neurovascular bundle to access the internal structure of the bone. These foramina appear radiographically as linear lucencies in one cortex, unlike an actual fracture that should involve both cortices. Accessory ossicles represent either intratendinous ossifications or unfused secondary ossification centers and are mostly found about the foot and ankle.

Classic examples of intratendinous ossifications are os peroneus (within the peroneus longus tendon) and os navicularis (within the tibialis posterior tendon near its navicular attachment). The classic example of an unfused secondary ossification center is an os trigonum, an unfused posterior process of the talus. Os navicularis deserves special mention because there are 3 types, the type 2 variant of which may simulate a fracture and may result in chronic medial foot pain: type 1 is a round bone completely enveloped by the tibialis posterior tendon; type 2 is rounded proximally but squared off against the navicular proper, with intervening fibrous tissue; and type 3 results in a large projection off the navicular bone that has been called a cornuate navicular. The squared-off nature of the type 2 variant can result in a linear lucency through the medial navicular that may simulate a fracture.

Example: Ankle fractures

Ankle fractures are very common, the most common involving either the medial or lateral malleolus (Figure 9.19). There are, however, several other fractures about the foot and ankle that may simulate a typical medial or lateral malleolus fracture that should be considered. These include a base of fifth metatarsal fracture, anterior process of calcaneus fracture, lateral process of talus fracture, and a posterior malleolus fracture (Figure 9.20). Isolated medial and posterior malleolus fractures should prompt evaluation for a proximal fibular fracture due to the transmission of forces up the interosseous membrane.

Stress and insufficiency fractures

Stress and insufficiency fractures do not occur as a result of a single traumatic event. Instead, they are the result of repetitive stresses that overtime exceed the bone's ability to heal. Stress fractures occur as a result of abnormally high stresses in otherwise normal bone. Athletes are the most likely population to develop stress fractures, though military recruits have a high incidence as well—hence the name "march fracture" to describe a metatarsal stress fracture. Insufficiency

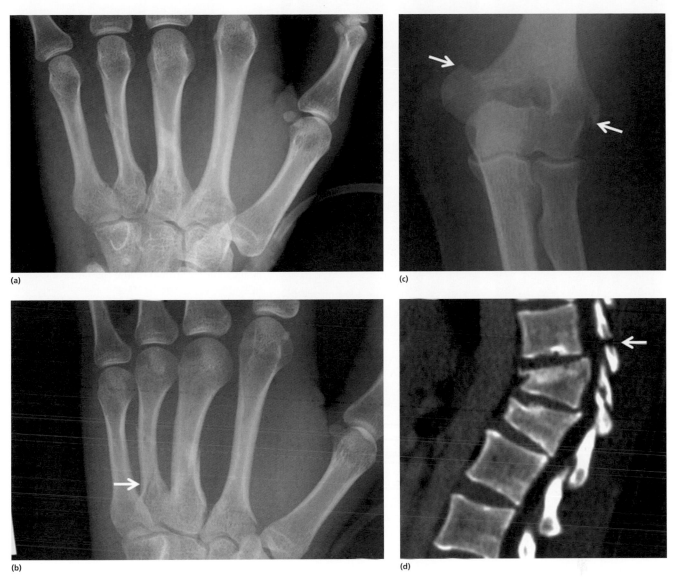

Figure 9.16 Signs of fracture. PA (a) and oblique (b) radiographs of the left hand demonstrate three different signs of fracture. A clear cortical discontinuity is present in the ulnar aspect of the fourth metacarpal on the PA view that persists on the oblique view. Also on the oblique view is a clear oblique lucent line at the proximal aspect of the metacarpal (*arrow*). On the PA view, an oblique dense band is present in the third metacarpal without an associated lucency or cortical discontinuity. On the oblique view, however, this band is seen to correspond to a fracture. On the oblique view of the elbow (c), there is a clear cortical discontinuity involving the lateral epicondyle, which is the lateral extension of a transverse supracondylar fracture. Once recognized as a fracture, subtle trabecular discontinuity can be seen along the fracture line (*arrows*). The sagittal CT image (d) depicts anterior wedge compression deformities consistent with compression fractures. This is an example of morphological change with any other signs of fracture. Note the facet fracture characterized by a lucency through the middle of the facet (*arrow*), the most obvious sign of fracture.

fractures occur as a result of normal stresses in abnormal bone. The most common stress fractures occur in the tibia, metatarsals (Figure 9.21), calcaneus, and femoral neck. Insufficiency fractures often occur in the lumbar spine, the sacrum, and the proximal femur and are usually the result of osteoporosis or osteomalacia.

Pathologic fractures

A focal bone lesion, benign or malignant, greatly weakens the bone, and a usually low-energy traumatic event results in fracture through this lesion (Figure 9.22). Recognizing the pathologic nature of a fracture is important as this may be the first clue that the patient has an underlying metabolic or malignant process. Sometimes, the only hint is a vague area of lucency about the fracture site that cannot be explained by the fracture itself.

Diagnosis of a dislocation

Diagnosis of a dislocation is based on the derangement of the normal relationships between joints:

- Findings can be subtle from widening of the normal joint space to mild incongruity at the joint (subluxation) to complete dissociation of the normal relationship (dislocation).

Common dislocations include the anteroinferior shoulder dislocation, the posterior hip dislocation, and dislocations of the joints of the fingers. All joint dislocations imply some degree of soft tissue damage ranging from disruption of the joint capsule to major ligament rupture and to vascular compromise. Some of these injuries may be inferred from the imaging, but often the dislocation has been at least partially reduced by the time they receive an imaging study. In dislocations where vascular compromise is a risk,

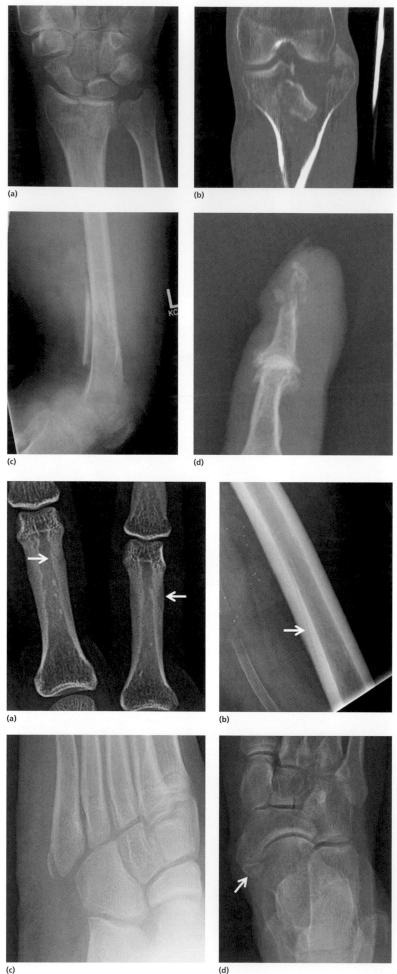

Figure 9.17 Modifiers of fracture severity. All fractures shown here are comminuted. (a) PA radiograph of the wrist demonstrates a minimally displaced distal radius fracture with extension into the radiocarpal joint. Intra-articular extension increases the likelihood of early posttraumatic osteoarthrosis. Also note the ulnar styloid tip fracture. (b) Coronal CT image of a lateral tibial plateau fracture with a large markedly depressed and rotated articular surface fragment. In order to restore the articular surface, bone graft or cement material will be needed. (c) Lateral radiograph of the femur demonstrates a comminuted fracture with extensive soft tissue gas both anterior and posterior to the fracture. This fracture is likely an open fracture. (d) Lateral radiograph of the distal finger demonstrates a comminuted fracture of distal tuft. The overlying finger nail appears elevated. Because of the involvement of the nail bed, even if not overtly elevated, fractures of the distal tuft are considered open fractures.

Figure 9.18 Fracture mimics. Coned PA radiograph of two proximal phalanges (a) shows the appearance of normal nutrient foramina (*arrows*). Lateral radiograph of the mid femur (b) shows the typical appearance of a nutrient foramen in this bone (*arrow*). Oblique radiograph of the foot (c) demonstrates an unfused base of fifth metatarsal apophysis. The dorsal–plantar view of the foot (d) demonstrates a type of os navicularis (*arrow*) that has a linear interface with the navicular bone. The linear squared-off nature and close apposition to the underlying navicular can be confused with a fracture. Note, however, that the cortex is rounded on both sides of the interface and that there is identifiable cortex at the interface; a fracture would not have cortex along the fracture line.

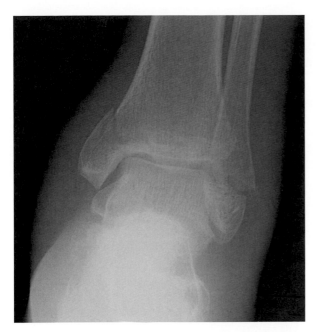

Figure 9.19 Bimalleolar ankle fracture. AP radiograph of the left ankle demonstrates an oblique medial malleolus fracture and a transverse lateral malleolus/distal fibular fracture, which was most likely the result of an inversion injury. Usually, the side with an oblique fracture is impacted (in this case by the talus), and the side with the transverse fracture is avulsed.

such as in posterior knee dislocations, a vascular study is often indicated to exclude this complication. MRI is usually obtained after major dislocations to assess the soft tissue injuries so that an appropriate surgical plan can be devised.

Not all subluxations and dislocations are the result of direct trauma. OA is a common cause of mild subluxations. More severe subluxations and even dislocations are seen in the later stages of the erosive inflammatory arthropathies, such as rheumatoid arthritis (RA).

Internal derangement of joints

Intra-articular and periarticular soft tissue damage may be the result of both acute trauma and degenerative processes:

- MRI or ultrasound can be used to assess for these types of injuries, with the role of ultrasound limited to the more superficial structures, such as ligaments and tendons.
- MR arthrography is a specialized form of MRI where a gadolinium-based contrast agent is injected directly into the joint of interest. This serves three purposes: first, it distends the joint separating structures that might otherwise be closely apposed to each other; second, small communications between the injected joint and other spaces can be identified, which might otherwise not be evident; and third, overt clefts in menisci and even bone can be identified.
- In patients who cannot have an MRI, an analogous CT arthrogram can be performed.

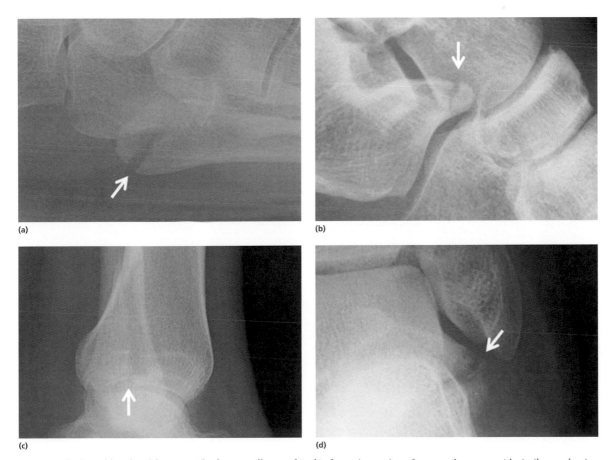

Figure 9.20 Nonmalleolar ankle-related fractures. The fractures illustrated in this figure (*arrows*) are fractures that occur with similar mechanisms as standard medial or lateral malleolar fractures or refer pain to the ankle and should be considered when the medial and lateral malleoli are intact. (a) Base of fifth metatarsal fracture. (b) Anterior process of calcaneus fracture. (c) Posterior malleolus fracture. The arrow points in the direction of the fracture line. Note the articular surface incongruity of the posterior tibiotalar (ankle) joint. (d) Lateral process of talus fracture.

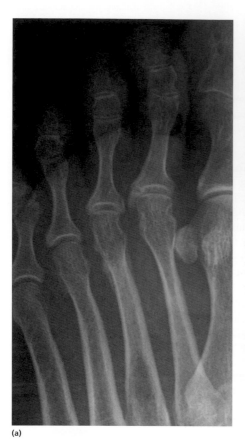
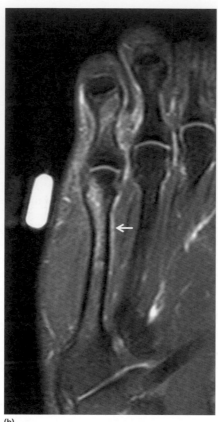

(a)   **(b)**

Figure 9.21 Metatarsal stress fractures. Dorsal–plantar radiograph of the foot (a) reveals periosteal new bone along the distal third metatarsal shaft, which is consistent with a stress fracture. In cases where the radiographs are normal and a stress fracture is still being considered, MRI can be obtained. Axial (long axis to the foot) T2-weighted fat-suppressed image of the lateral forefoot (b) reveals increased signal within the marrow of the distal fifth metatarsal shaft (compared to the fourth metatarsal) and periosteal edema (*arrow*). These findings are consistent with an early stress fracture.

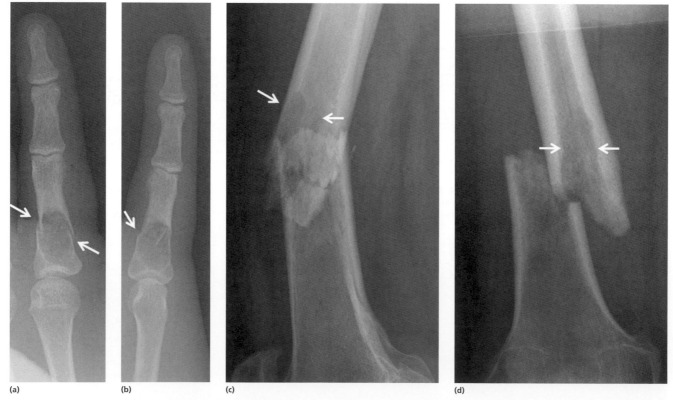

(a)   **(b)**   **(c)**   **(d)**

Figure 9.22 Examples of pathologic fractures. PA (a) and oblique (b) radiographs of the little finger reveal a lucent, slightly expansile lesion in the proximal phalangeal base. Through this lesion, consistent with an enchondroma, is a fracture that is identifiable by the cortical step-offs (*arrows*). Lateral (c) and AP (d) radiographs of the distal femur reveal a displaced fracture through a subtle lucent lesion (*arrows*), which turned out to be a myeloma deposit.

The focus of the section is to describe the general types of joint-related soft tissue pathologies that are encountered, with a discussion specific to tendons, ligaments, fibrocartilage, and articular (hyaline) cartilage.

Tendons

Tendon tears are characterized by overt gaps in the course of the tendon from muscle to bone or changes in the morphology of the tendon. For superficial tendons, MRI and sonography are equivalent in accuracy. MRI can provide a more global view of surrounding pathology. For cases where there is doubt about whether a tear is full thickness or partial thickness, dynamic examinations can easily be performed as part of a sonographic examination. Perhaps the most common tendon tear is a rotator cuff tear (Figure 9.23):

- Several meta-analyses and systematic reviews of the accuracy of MRI and ultrasound for diagnosing rotator cuff tears have shown that both perform equally well for full-thickness tears and only moderately well for partial-thickness tears.

- MR arthrography has a slight edge on the nonarthrographic MRI and sonographic examinations for partial-thickness tears but involves a joint injection.

Tendinosis is a common disorder of tendons caused by overuse and age-related tendon degeneration. The first sign of tendinosis is enlargement of the tendon with an otherwise preserved structure. This is followed by progressive collagen fiber damage that ultimately leads to changes in macroscopic morphology including surface irregularity and internal clefts. Fiber disruption is readily seen sonographically:

- The morphologic changes are apparent on both MRI and sonography. Tendinosis is often a precursor to tendon tear, especially in the rotator cuff.

Tenosynovitis is an inflammation of the tendon sheath, which is often caused by chronic friction. People with an inflammatory arthritis are also prone to developing this condition. Tenosynovitis is characterized by an effusion with one or more of the following signs of synovial inflammation: hyperemia, fibrin deposition, and/or thickening of the synovial lining of the sheath (Figure 9.24).

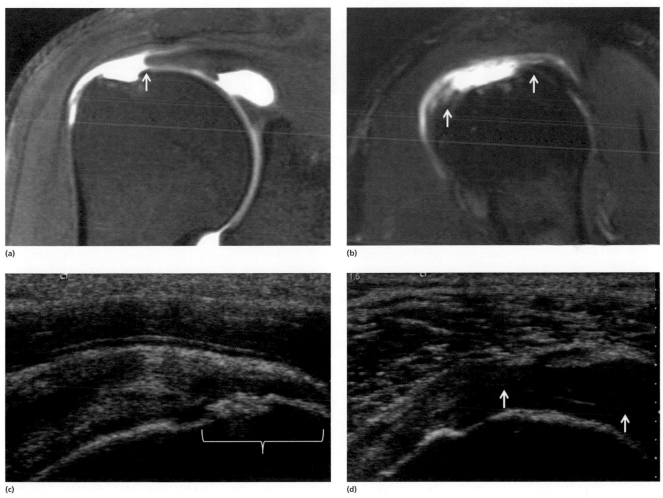

(a) (b) (c) (d)

Figure 9.23 MRI and US of a full-thickness partial-width superior rotator cuff tear. Oblique coronal T1-weighted fat-suppressed MR arthrogram image (a) and oblique sagittal T2-weighted fat-suppressed MR arthrogram image (b) demonstrate a full-thickness fluid-filled defect in the mid superior rotator cuff (supraspinatus–infraspinatus junction) at the insertion. *Arrow* in (a) points to the retracted tendon. On the oblique sagittal image (b), intact tendon is present both anterior and posterior to this defect (*arrows*), making this a partial-width tear. Long-axis (c) and short-axis (d) US images of the superior rotator cuff reveal a full-thickness nearly anechoic defect at the insertion in the long axis (*bracket*) and a full-thickness partial-width anechoic defect near the supraspinatus–infraspinatus junction. *Arrows* point to intact tendon on either side of the anechoic defect.

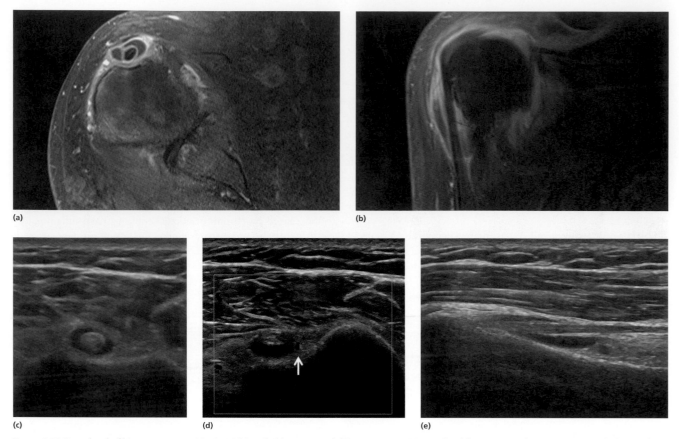

Figure 9.24 Long head of biceps tenosynovitis. Axial (a) and oblique sagittal (b) postcontrast T1-weighted fat-suppressed MR images reveal a bicipital tendon sheath effusion with enhancing synovial lining consistent with tenosynovitis. Then the tendon is normal in appearance. Short-axis (c), short-axis with color Doppler (d), and long-axis (e) US images demonstrate a bicipital tendon sheath effusion surrounding a normal tendon (note the fibrillar echotexture on the long-axis view). The presence of detectable blood flow by color Doppler is consistent with hyperemia (*arrow*). The effusion with the presence of hyperemia is consistent with tenosynovitis.

An effusion in the absence of the other findings is most likely reactive:

- Both MRI and sonography can adequately characterize tenosynovial inflammation by demonstrating the effusion, identifying hyperemia (enhancement of the synovium on MRI and color Doppler flow on sonography), and identifying material within the sheath. Thickening of the sheath is not always apparent due to reactive inflammatory changes external to the sheath.

Ligaments

Ligament tears are quite common in the lower extremity. The anterior talofibular ligament is likely the most frequently torn ligament in the body but is rarely a source of long-term ankle instability. Tears of the ACL of the knee can cause sufficient instability that ultimately leads to early knee OA. Tears of the other ligaments of the knee are also associated with knee instability, though not to the degree arising from an ACL tear. Ligament tears of any joint are for the most part due to direct trauma, though coexistent inflammatory arthritis can greatly weaken ligaments, increasing their susceptibility to tears:

- Ligaments are linear well-defined structures on imaging; any departure from this appearance is consistent with a tear (Figure 9.25).

- Sonography is suited to evaluation of the lateral ankle ligaments and the collateral ligaments of the elbow, knee, and fingers—any superficial ligament. The scapholunate ligament can be evaluated as well by experienced sonographers. MRI remains the gold standard for evaluation of the cruciate ligaments of the knee.

Fibrocartilage

Evaluation for knee meniscal tears is one of the most frequent, if not the most frequent, reasons a knee MRI is ordered. The knee menisci are quite large in comparison to the glenoid and acetabular labrums and are relatively easy to evaluate on MRI; all of these structures are triangular in shape. Any alteration of this morphology is consistent with a tear. For the menisci, tears are usually characterized by fluid-filled intrameniscal clefts, possibly with a displaced fragment. For both the glenoid and acetabular labrums, tears may also be manifested by intrameniscal clefts but are more frequently characterized by clefts at the attachment site of the labrum to bone and/or cartilage or abnormal morphology.

Three main types of knee meniscal tears are horizontal, vertical, and radial tears. Both horizontal and vertical tears are types of longitudinal tears. While all of these tears compromise the function of the meniscus to some degree, a full-thickness radial tear

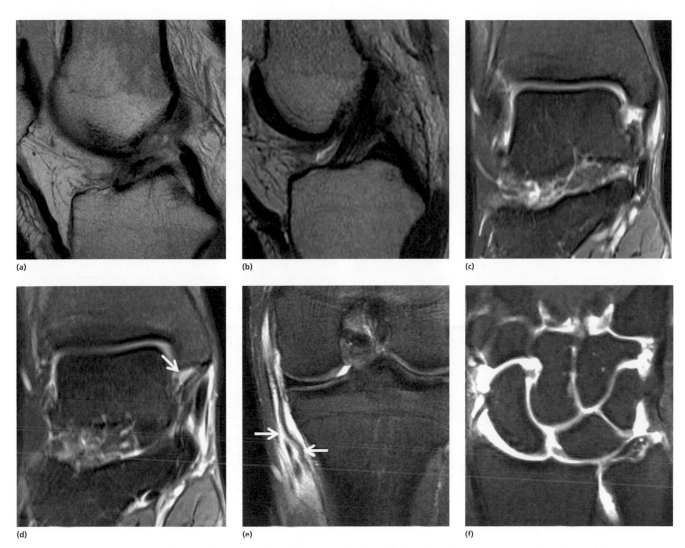

Figure 9.25 Ligament tears. Sagittal T2-weighted images through the intercondylar notch of the knee demonstrate a torn (a) and intact (b) anterior cruciate ligament (ACL). The intact ACL is taut, has a fibrillar but otherwise uniformly dark appearance, and parallels the roof of the intercondylar notch. The torn ACL has an abnormal course of the identifiable tendon, is curved consistent with laxity, and has marked elevated signal in the proximal portion of the tendon. Coronal T2-weighted fat-suppressed images through the talar dome, the medial malleolus, and the deep and superficial fibers of the deltoid ligament demonstrate torn (c) and intact (d) deep fibers of the deltoid ligament. The deep fibers course from the medial malleolus to the medial talus (*arrow* in (d)). In (c), the expected location of the deep fibers is replaced by fluid consistent with a tear. Coronal T2-weighted fat-suppressed image of the knee (e) demonstrates a torn medial collateral ligament (MCL). Like all ligaments, the MCL should be taut; this MCL is wavy (*arrows*) consistent with a complete tear. Coronal T1-weighted fat-suppressed MR arthrogram image of the wrist (f) demonstrates bright fluid filling both the radiocarpal and midcarpal joints. The scapholunate ligament is completely torn (*arrow*).

essentially inactivates the meniscus by interruption of the longitudinal collagen fiber network that provides the tensile ("hoop") strength of the meniscus:

- Knee meniscal tears are readily seen on conventional MRI (Figure 9.26).
- The diagnosis of labral tears is complicated by the presence of adjacent structures that may obscure a tear or mimic a tear.
- The anterior inferior glenohumeral ligament of the shoulder often abuts the anteroinferior labrum, and the hip joint capsule often lies directly on top of the acetabular labrum. To mitigate this effect, MR arthrography is performed to distend the joint and lift these adjacent structures off the labrum.

- If the patient cannot have an MRI, CT arthrography can be performed.

Figure 9.27 shows examples of glenoid and acetabular labral tears as well as a triangular fibrocartilage tear.

Articular cartilage

The majority of cartilage disease is degenerative in nature, whether due to abnormal stresses or due to instability as might be seen with knee meniscal and ACL tears (Figure 9.28). Acute trauma also produces cartilage disease due to direct cartilage impact or focal shear (Figure 9.29). Degenerative cartilage disease is characterized by more diffuse thinning of the cartilage, whereas traumatic cartilage

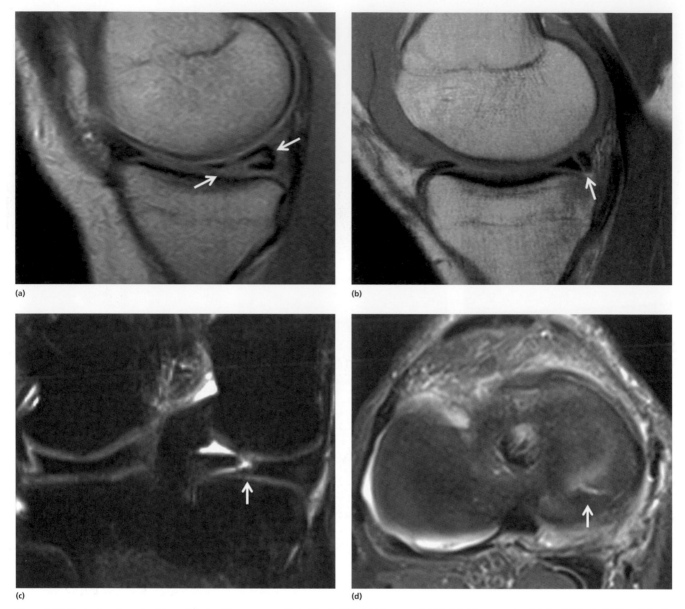

(a)

(b)

(c)

(d)

Figure 9.26 Examples of meniscal tears. Meniscal tears are manifested by fluid-bright (or near fluid-bright) intrameniscal clefts. (a) Sagittal PD-weighted MR image through the medial tibiofemoral compartment of the knee demonstrates a posterior horn medial meniscus horizontal tear (*arrows*). (b) Sagittal PD-weighted MR image through the medial tibiofemoral compartment of the knee demonstrates a posterior horn medial meniscus vertical tear (*arrow*). (c) Coronal T2-weighted fat-suppressed MR image through the posterior horns of both menisci demonstrates a posterior horn medial meniscus radial (*arrow*). (d) Axial T2-weighted fat-suppressed MR image through the plane of the tibiofemoral joint reveals a partial-thickness radial tear of the posterior horn of the medial meniscus that turns into a longitudinal vertical tear (*arrow*). This configuration is known as a parrot-beak tear and is at particular risk for tear propagation resulting in a displaced fragment.

defects are often focal full-thickness defects with well-defined margins. Alternatively, acute traumatic events may result in cartilage delamination where a cleft parallel to the articular surface develops, often at the cartilage–bone interface. The treatment for degenerative cartilage disease is mainly supportive, but when symptoms become intolerable, joint replacement is often performed. Focal traumatic cartilage defects may be treated via a number of surgical methods including microfracture and cartilage transplantation; sheared cartilage generally cannot be reattached.

Loose chondral bodies, resulting from trauma or degenerative breakdown of the cartilage, may be present. The posttraumatic chondral body is often easy to recognize as its shape matches the defect at the donor site. Degenerative loose bodies often begin as small fragments of cartilage that grow slowly over time due to diffusion of nutrients through the synovial fluid; ultimately, they ossify, hence the term osteochondral body. Loose bodies often migrate into a recess, such as the suprapatellar recess or the posterior tibiofemoral joint at the intercondylar notch. Occasionally, however, they may become interposed between two articular surfaces resulting in a block to flexion or extension of the knee:

- The standard for imaging articular cartilage is MRI.

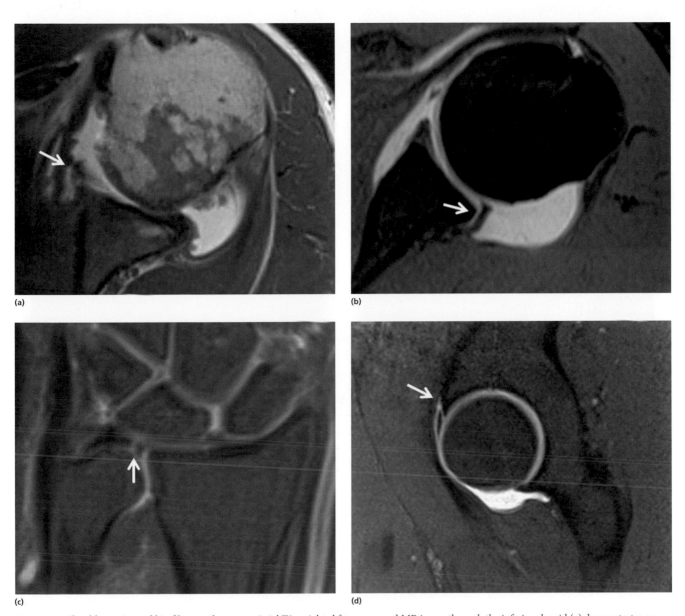

(a)

(b)

(c)

(d)

Figure 9.27 Shoulder, wrist, and hip fibrocartilage tears. Axial T2-weighted fat-suppressed MR image through the inferior glenoid (a) demonstrates an abnormal-appearing anteroinferior labrum (*long arrow*), especially when compared to the posterior labrum (*short arrow*) with a cleft between the labrum and the glenoid consistent with a tear. Axial T1-weighted fat-suppressed MR image through the mid glenoid (b) demonstrates a tear of the posterior labrum (arrow), with associated periosteal stripping. Note the normal anterior labrum. Coronal T2-weighted fat-suppressed MR image of the wrist (c) reveals a full-thickness cleft in the membranous portion of the triangular fibrocartilage (arrow). Sagittal T2-weighted fat-suppressed MR image of the hip (d) reveals a cleft at the chondrolabral junction of the anterior labrum consistent with a tear (arrow).

- Focal intrasubstance signal changes herald the onset of early chondrosis, which are followed by actual loss of cartilage beginning at the articular surface and progressing toward the subchondral bone.
- Occasionally, blistering of the cartilage surface will be observed. Fissuring is also a common finding in the diseased state. Elevated bone marrow signal deep to the cartilage abnormality may reflect more acute and symptomatic disease.
- CT arthrography is a reasonable alternative to cartilage assessment in the patient who has contraindications to MRI, with the limitation that the subchondral bone marrow cannot be assessed.

Arthritis

The most common disease of the joints is degenerative joint disease or osteoarthrosis (OA). The inflammatory/erosive diseases of the joints are sufficiently common as a group to warrant discussion as well. While OA is characterized by cartilage loss and reactive bone changes with variable but usually minor associated synovial inflammation, the inflammatory arthritides are characterized by inflammation of the synovium and adjacent soft tissue structures with relatively minor cartilage and bone changes, especially early in the disease. The erosive diseases will ultimately erode the bone supporting the cartilage leading to cartilage loss as a secondary effect.

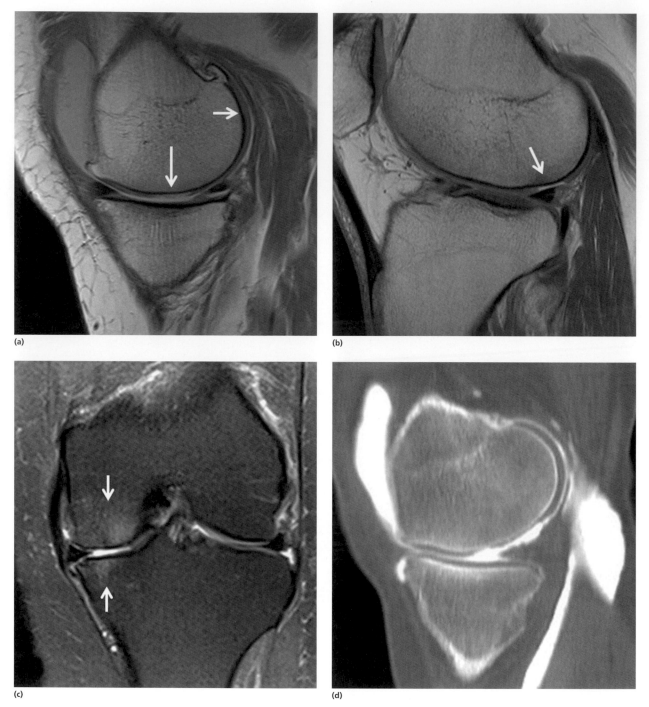

(a)

(b)

(c)

(d)

Figure 9.28 Degenerative articular cartilage derangements. Sagittal PD-weighted MR image through the medial tibiofemoral compartment of the knee (a) demonstrates region of full-thickness cartilage loss in the central weight-bearing region of the femoral condyle (*long arrow*) and diffuse full-thickness thinning of the central tibial plateau. Note the thickness of the non-weight-bearing region cartilage (*short arrow*); this can be used as an internal reference for the normal thickness of the cartilage for this person. Sagittal PD-weighted MR image through the lateral tibiofemoral compartment of the knee (b) demonstrates a more focal region of full-thickness cartilage loss in the posterior weight-bearing region of the femoral condyle where it overlies the posterior horn of the lateral meniscus (*arrow*). Coronal T2-weighted fat-suppressed MR image through the bodies of both menisci (c) reveals full-thickness cartilage loss in the medial tibiofemoral compartment with underlying bone marrow signal changes; the bone marrow signal changes (*arrows*) are often associated with symptoms. Sagittal CT arthrogram image through the medial tibiofemoral compartment of the knee (d) reveals full-thickness irregular cartilage loss of the posterior weight-bearing region consistent with cartilage degeneration.

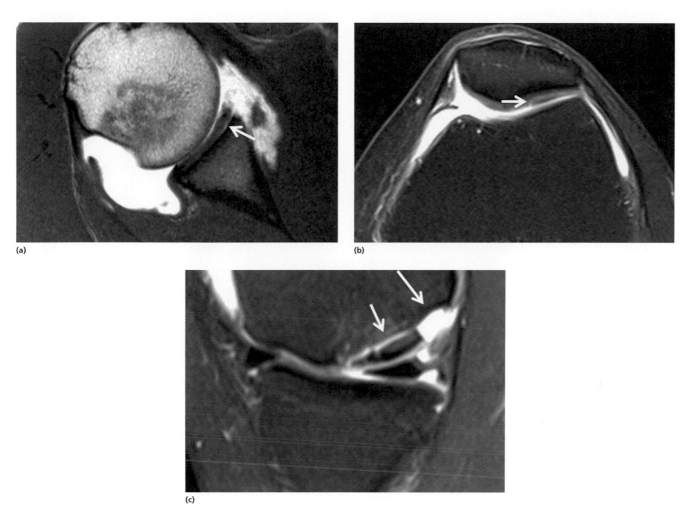

(a)

(b)

(c)

Figure 9.29 Acute/subacute articular cartilage derangements. Axial T2-weighted fat-suppressed MR arthrogram image of the shoulder through the glenoid (a) reveals a large delaminating cartilage lesion of the anterior glenoid (*arrow*) following direct trauma to the shoulder; high signal in the humeral head is likely related to a contusion. Axial T2-weighted fat-suppressed image of the knee through the patella (b) reveals an intrasubstance cartilage delaminating lesion (arrow). Sagittal T2-weighted fat-suppressed image through the medial tibiofemoral compartment of the knee (c) reveals a large osteochondral lesion with an *in situ* fragment (*short arrow*) and a fluid-filled void (*long arrow*) where another osteochondral fragment used to be located following a knee injury. The displaced fragment may cause mechanical symptoms of locking if interposed in a joint.

The term "arthritis" literally means joint inflammation. This accurately describes the situation in diseases such as RA, psoriatic arthritis, and systemic lupus erythematosus. Degenerative joint disease is commonly termed "osteoarthritis," though it in fact often has minimal associated inflammation. As a result, a more accurate term for "osteoarthritis" is "osteoarthrosis":

- Imaging evaluation of arthritis is predominantly based on radiographs. The standard hand radiographic series for arthritis is a PA radiograph of both hands and a slightly oblique view that is known as the Norgaard (or "ball catcher") view; the patient is asked to position their hands as if they were going to catch a ball. Some institutions also acquire a true lateral radiograph.
- Advanced imaging modalities such as MRI and ultrasound are reserved for indeterminate cases usually to document synovitis but also subradiographic erosions. Tendon disease is a common feature of the inflammatory arthritides; MRI or sonography is needed to assess these structures.
- Imaging features that help to characterize the arthritides include periarticular bone density, distribution (symmetric vs. asymmetric, proximal, or distal hand involvement), and the presence of bone production. Soft tissue calcifications can also be helpful in certain situations.

The following is a brief discussion of OA, RA, the seronegative spondyloarthropathies, and gout, focusing on radiographic imaging findings.

OA

OA is characterized by loss of cartilage, reactive subchondral bone remodeling, osteophyte formation, and normal bone density. The most common sites are the distal interphalangeal joints of the hands, the hips, the knees, and the great toe metatarsophalangeal joint. The presence of osteophyte formation separates this entity from the other arthritides:

- On radiographs, the presence of cartilage can only be inferred by the separation of the two articulating bones by a radiolucent space (Figure 9.30). Osteophytes are projections of bone at the peripheral edges of the affected joint that appear to broaden the articular surface as a whole.

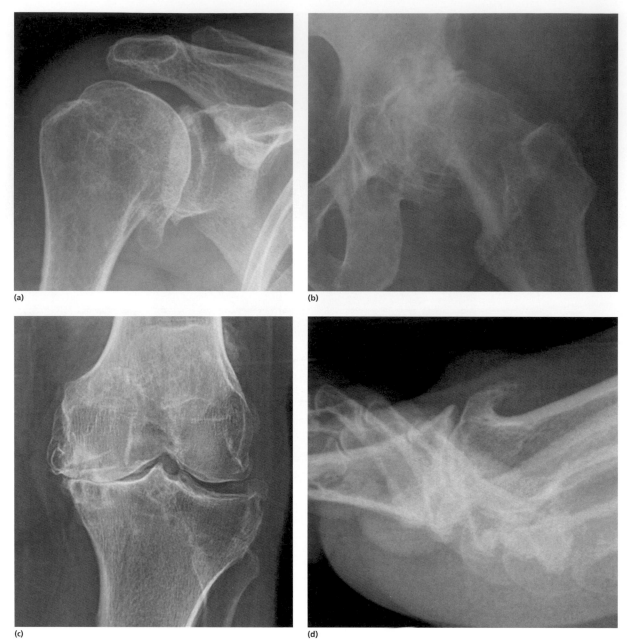

Figure 9.30 Examples of conventional osteoarthrosis. Radiographic examples of severe glenohumeral (a), hip (b), knee (c), and great toe metatarso-phalangeal (d) osteoarthrosis. The common theme is joint space loss, osteophyte formation, and subchondral cyst/geode formation. Joint space loss and osteophytes are usually predominant in the glenohumeral joint and great toe metatarsophalangeal joint. Subchondral cysts are more frequently observed in the hip and knee. In the hip, note that the femoral head–neck junction is convex rather than concave; when the hip is flexed, the acetabulum will contact the femoral neck earlier than normal, which is a process known as femoral acetabular impingement, a cause of early-onset osteoarthrosis.

- Subchondral sclerosis represents increased density within the subchondral bone. "Cystic" spaces ("cyst" is a misnomer, since there is no epithelial lining), also termed "geodes," often form in the subchondral bone as well due to inspissation of fluid through damaged bone over time.
- Radiographs are not sensitive for cartilage damage as there can be marked cartilage damage with a normal-appearing joint space; all that is needed is a pillar of normal thickness of cartilage to give the illusion of a normal joint.

- MRI may be considered to evaluate the extent of cartilage damage and to evaluate the status of the supporting soft tissue structures, such as the menisci and ligaments of the knee. Meniscal and ligament tears contribute to cartilage degeneration by creating microinstability in the tibiofemoral joints of the knee.

A variant of OA is known as "erosive OA," which essentially only affects the hands of postmenopausal women (Figure 9.31):

- In this variant, erosions form in the central articular aspect of the articular surface, usually at the distal interphalangeal joints

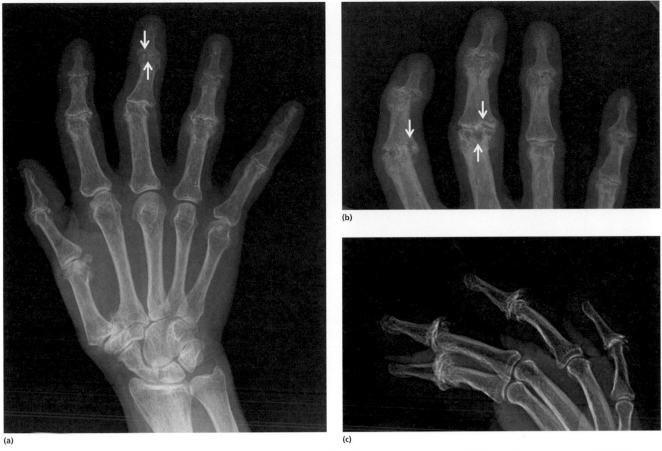

(a)   (b)   (c)

Figure 9.31 Erosive osteoarthrosis. PA radiograph of the right hand (a) reveals diffuse interphalangeal joint (DIP), thumb carpometacarpal (CMC) joint, and scaphotrapezial joint space loss and osteophyte formation. Central erosions are noted about the third DIP joint (*arrows*). Mild ulnar angulation of the third proximal interphalangeal joint (PIP) is also present. The pattern of DIP joint osteoarthrosis with central erosions and osteoarthrosis of the basal joints of the thumb is consistent with erosive osteoarthrosis. Coned PA radiograph of the distal aspects of the second through fifth digits of the right hand (b) in a different patient shows diffuse DIP and PIP joint space loss, osteophyte formation, and numerous central erosions (arrows). The classic appearance of a joint affected by erosive OA is the "gull-wing" appearance, formed by osteophyte formation in combination with central erosions, which is best illustrated by the appearance of the subchondral bone of the distal phalanx at the fourth DIP. Coned lateral radiograph of the fingers of the right hand (c) in a third patient with erosive OA shows large osteophytes that can form in this and conventional OA.

followed by the proximal interphalangeal joints. In combination with osteophyte formation at these joints, a "gull-wing" deformity is created. The thumb carpometacarpal joint and the scaphotrapezial joint are also usually affected, though without obvious focal erosions.

As OA is very common, it may coexist with the other arthritides later in life.

RA

RA is an autoimmune symmetric inflammatory/erosive arthritis characterized by periarticular osteopenia and marginal erosions. The hands and feet are most commonly affected, but any joint in the body may be involved (Figure 9.32). Periarticular osteopenia is due to hyperemia related to adjacent inflammation that leads to increased bone resorption. Synovial inflammation leads to the formation of a pannus that erodes into the bones at joints at the margins of the articular cartilage, hence the term "marginal" erosions. In advanced disease, the entire articular cartilage is completely eroded and bones can become fused together (ankylosis),

which is common in the carpus. In the hands, it affects predominantly the carpus and metacarpophalangeal joints. One of the most sensitive sites for early erosive involvement in the hand is the ulnar styloid. Distention of the metacarpophalangeal joint capsules due to synovial hypertrophy is a feature of active disease. In the feet, erosions commonly occur at the metatarsal heads and posterior calcaneus, but the most specific site for RA in the foot is the fifth metatarsal head. The presence of erosions is important to document as this usually necessitates giving the patient high-potency disease-modifying antirheumatic drugs:

- On imaging, active erosions are characterized by concavities in the normal contour of the bone without an identifiable cortex at its base. Often, however, erosions are not well profiled on radiographs and appear as round lucencies. Lucencies, unfortunately, are a nonspecific finding that may represent subchondral cysts related to OA or vascular channels (as may be seen in the carpus). Overt erosions are clearly helpful, but numerous lucencies in the typical pattern of involvement still remain highly suggestive of RA.

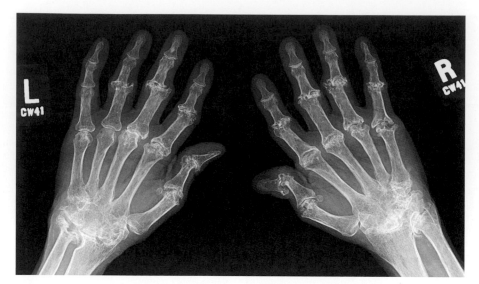

Figure 9.32 Rheumatoid arthritis in the hands. PA radiographs of both hands demonstrate complete loss of the intercarpal joint spaces with ankylosis of the radius and lunate on the right and near ankylosis of this joint on the left. Erosive changes at the distal radioulnar joints and ulnar styloids are present bilaterally. Marked erosive disease of the MCPs and proximal interphalangeal (PIP) joints is present. One of the hallmarks of an erosive inflammatory arthropathy is uniform joint space loss, which is best illustrated at the right second and third MCP joints. As the disease process affects ligaments as well, subluxations of joints are common (right thumb interphalangeal joint, left third and fourth PIP joints).

- On cross-sectional imaging, erosions must be documented in two planes. Active erosions appear bright on contrast-enhanced MRI and exhibit hyperemia on sonographic evaluation.
- Inactive erosions have a thin sclerotic rim at the base of the erosion. On MRI, there will be no associated enhancement and no demonstrable hyperemia will be seen sonographically.
- Tenosynovitis and bursitis are common features of RA (and the other inflammatory arthritides). These entities are often not appreciable radiographically unless very severe resulting in soft tissue contour abnormalities.
- MRI and sonography are the mainstay for evaluation of these entities. The use of contrast with MRI is helpful to document synovial inflammation as reactive effusions may appear identical to the inflamed counterpart.

Seronegative spondyloarthropathy

The seronegative spondyloarthropathies are a diverse group of auto immune inflammatory/erosive arthritides that have in common a negative rheumatoid factor. These entities include psoriatic arthritis, reactive arthritis, ankylosing spondylitis (AS), and inflammatory bowel disease (IBD)-related spondyloarthropathy. All four of these entities are associated with sacroiliitis and enthesitis. While AS and IBD-related spondyloarthropathy are associated with erosive joint disease (usually the hip), they are predominantly associated with enthesitis of the spine. On the other hand, psoriatic and reactive arthritides are particularly associated with periarticular erosive disease.

This section will focus on sacroiliitis and psoriatic arthritis

Sacroiliitis

The sacroiliac joints are a complex irregular joint that distribute load from the axial skeleton to the pelvis. The joint is oblique such that the anterior portion is more lateral than the posterior portion. Only the anterior aspect of the joint is synovial. Synovitis, therefore, will only affect this part of the joint. The other portions of the joint

are held together by strong ligaments, which can be involved with enthesitis. Sacroiliitis in AS and IBD-related spondyloarthropathy is generally symmetric, while sacroiliitis associated with psoriatic and reactive arthritides is generally asymmetric. The end point for AS and IBD-related spondyloarthropathy is sacroiliac joint ankylosis:

- Radiographs are the initial imaging study in suspected sacroiliitis. The typical radiographic series for evaluation of the sacroiliac joints is an AP view of the sacroiliac joints with tube tilted cranially to accommodate the oblique orientation of the sacrum supplemented by bilateral oblique views to profile the joints. Erosions, areas of narrowing, and subchondral sclerosis are all features of sacroiliitis.
- In cases when radiographs are normal, but clinical suspicion remains high, MRI may be obtained to document sacroiliac joint synovitis in the absence of radiographic findings.

Figure 9.33 shows cases of symmetric and asymmetric sacroiliitis on radiographs and an example of sacroiliitis on MRI.

Unilateral sacroiliitis, one completely normal and one abnormal joint, is infection until proven otherwise, particularly if the abnormal joint is very abnormal.

Psoriatic arthritis

Psoriatic arthritis, which is associated with the skin condition psoriasis, is an asymmetric erosive arthropathy associated with marginal erosions and bone production. The distribution is quite different from that of RA in that it typically involves the metacarpophalangeal joints and interphalangeal joints of one or more fingers. The erosions of psoriatic arthritis are associated with "fluffy periostitis," fine wisps of bone production about the erosions. Enthesitis plays a much bigger role in psoriatic arthritis than in RA. Any ligament or tendon attachment may become ossified as a result of chronic inflammation; periarticular enthesophytes are common in psoriatic arthritis. Enthesis ossification is not a feature of RA.

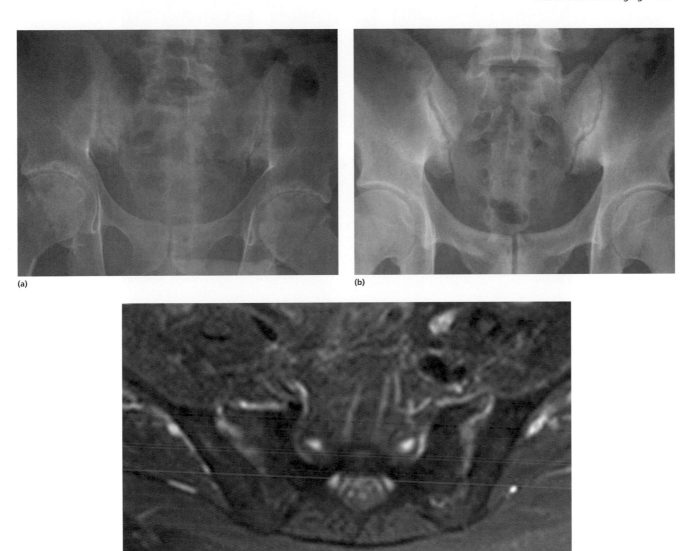

(a)

(b)

(c)

Figure 9.33 Examples of sacroiliitis. (a) Ferguson view of the sacrum reveals bilateral symmetric sacroiliac joint space loss, irregularity of the subchondral bone, and increased sclerosis in a patient with inflammatory bowel disease-related spondyloarthropathy. Note also the narrowed hip joint spaces and pitting of the femoral heads and acetabulum characteristic of erosive involvement of the hip joints in this disease process. (b) Ferguson view of the sacrum reveals bilateral asymmetric, right greater than left, sacroiliac joint space loss; irregularity of the subchondral bone; and increased sclerosis in a patient with psoriatic arthritis. (c) Axial T2-weighted fat-suppressed MR image through the sacroiliac joints reveals fluid within the sacroiliac joints and bone marrow edema on either side of the joint consistent with sacroiliitis.

The radiographic findings include marginal erosions, fluffy periostitis, and enthesophytes in the classic distribution. Soft tissue inflammation is best characterized on MRI or ultrasound:

- The classic soft tissue feature of psoriatic arthritis is the "sausage digit," one uniformly swollen digit secondary to severe flexor tenosynovitis.

Reactive arthritis is a seronegative spondyloarthropathy that follows an enteric or urogenital infection. While reactive arthritis has lower limb predominant manifestations, the imaging appearance is identical to that of psoriatic arthritis.

Figure 9.34 shows examples of some of the radiographic features of psoriatic and reactive arthritides.

Gout

Gout is an inflammatory erosive disease due to deposition of monosodium urate crystals. In advanced stages of disease, coalescent deposits of monosodium urate crystals form called tophi. These tophi may result in periarticular erosions, sometimes quite dramatic in size. The classic site of involvement is the great toe metatarsophalangeal joint. The dorsal tarsometatarsal joints of the foot are commonly affected. Hand and foot involvement is often indistinguishable from RA:

- Radiographic manifestations of gout are marginal erosions (Figure 9.35). They may be characterized by an overhanging edge, a characteristic specific to gout.
- Soft tissue masses associated with the erosions are occasionally identifiable, which also assists in the diagnosis.
- In the absence of an identifiable overhanging edge or soft tissue mass, a serum uric acid level will be needed to establish (or exclude) the diagnosis.

Tumors

Tumors and tumorlike lesions of the musculoskeletal system are relatively uncommon.

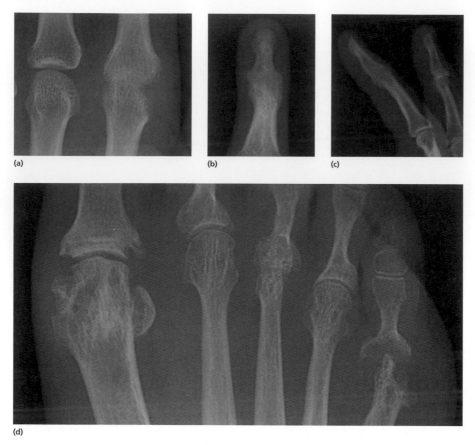

(a)   (b)   (c)

(d)

Figure 9.34 Psoriatic and reactive arthritides. Coned PA radiograph of the left second and third metacarpophalangeal (MCP) joints (a) reveals complete uniform joint space loss of the second MCP joint, a radial marginal erosion of the metacarpal head, and small enthesophyte of the distal radial joint capsule in the setting of normal bone density. The normal bone density and enthesophyte formation increase the likelihood that this patient has psoriatic arthritis based on the radiographs alone. PA (b) and lateral (c) radiographs of a right-hand finger distal interphalangeal joint reveal complete ankylosis of this joint. Ankylosis of an interphalangeal joint is characteristic of a seronegative spondyloarthropathy. Coned dorsal–plantar view of the right metatarsophalangeal (MTP) joints (d) has several findings characteristic of a seronegative spondyloarthropathy: marginal erosions are present involving the great and little toe MTP heads. Bulky capsular enthesophytes are present on the distal aspect of the great toe MTP joint. Uniform joint space loss is present clearly involving the third and fourth digit MTP joints. The little toe MTP joint demonstrates the classic "pencil-in-cup" deformity.

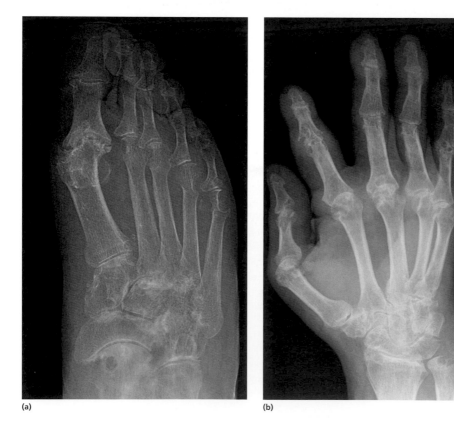

(a)   (b)

Figure 9.35 Gout. The dorsal–plantar radiograph of the right foot (a) and the oblique radiograph of the right hand (b) demonstrate numerous marginal erosions at the foot metatarsophalangeal and hand metacarpophalangeal joints. The classic radiographic finding of gout is an "overhanging edge" of an erosion (*arrows*).

The general approach to tumors and tumorlike lesions is based on whether they are bone centered or soft tissue centered. A general approach is presented for each of these broad categories, rather than an exhaustive list.

Bone tumors

Many benign and malignant bone lesion histologies have been described. In a few cases, one can predict the histology based on imaging alone. In nonspecific cases, which comprise the majority of cases, one can make general assessments regarding the relative indolence versus aggressivity of the lesion. Then using data on the age of the patient, where in a bone the lesion is located (medullary, cortical; metaphyseal, diaphyseal, and epiphyseal), the type of mineralized matrix, and morphologic details, a narrow differential can be generated. While there is a general trend for benign lesions appearing indolent and malignant lesions appearing aggressive, the association is not sufficient to base diagnosis on these features alone: indolent lesions may be benign or malignant, and aggressive lesions may be either benign or malignant. An example of indolent lesions that cannot be separated on the basis of imaging is an enchondroma and low-grade chondrosarcoma. An aggressive process such as an Ewing sarcoma or certain metastatic lesions can appear identical to an infection, a benign process. Regardless of the histologic origin, any lytic bone lesion may be at risk for pathologic fracture:

- The imaging workup of all bone lesions begins with radiographs.
- Indeterminate cases may require CT to document the type of tumor matrix, extent and configuration of ossification/mineralization, and possible coexistent pathologic fracture (Figure 9.36). CT, however, may occasionally lead to a definitive diagnosis, such as an osteoid osteoma.
- Unless the lesion is clearly benign on radiographs, such as a fibroxanthoma, MRI is obtained to assess both intramedullary and extraosseous extent. Unfortunately, MRI characteristics are for the most part nonspecific. Biopsy is always performed to establish a definitive diagnosis as the histology often dictates whether chemotherapy or radiation therapy is used prior to resection.

Once a definitive diagnosis of a primary bone sarcoma has been made, an evaluation for metastatic disease is performed:

- First, if not already available, an MRI of the entire involved bone is obtained to assess for local "skip" lesions.
- Second, a nuclear medicine bone scan is obtained to assess for skeletal metastasis.

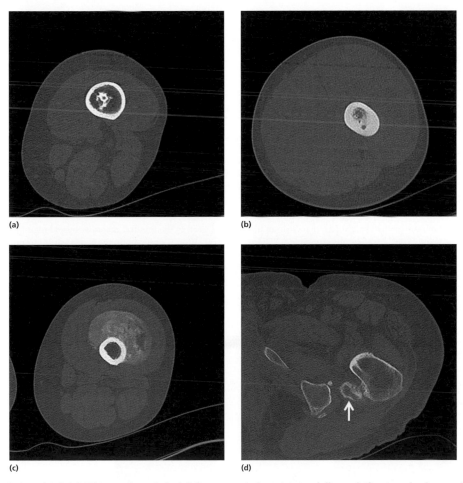

(a) (b) (c) (d)

Figure 9.36 CT of bone lesions. (a) Axial CT image through the left femur reveals dense intramedullary calcifications that have an "arc and whorl" appearance that is characteristic of low-grade chondroid lesions, enchondroma, and low-grade chondrosarcoma. (b) Osteoid osteoma: axial CT image through the left femur reveals focal cortical thickening of the posterolateral cortex with a focal round lucency not connected to a nutrient foramen. This is the classic appearance for a (c) parosteal osteosarcoma: axial CT image through the left femur reveals a well-defined mineralized mass abutting but otherwise completely external to the femur. (d) Myositis ossificans: axial CT image through the left hip reveals a corticated osseous body (*arrow*) interposed between the proximal femur and the ischium within the quadratus femoris muscle consistent with Myositis ossificans.

- Finally, a CT of the chest is obtained to evaluate for the presence of pulmonary metastases; all sarcoma metastases have a predilection for the lungs.

A short discussion of lesion descriptors follows: lesion margin, type of associated periosteal reaction, lesion density, and age.

Lesion margin

The margin of a lesion may be well defined with an abrupt transition from lesion to normal bone or may be ill defined with a gradual transition from clearly identifiable lesion to clearly identifiable normal bone (Figure 9.37). The spectrum from well defined to ill defined parallels the spectrum of indolence from indolent to aggressive. At the indolent end of the spectrum is a unicameral bone cyst, which has an abrupt transition and a sclerotic margin. At the aggressive end of the spectrum are osteosarcomas, lymphomas, and infection, which have quite ill-defined and gradual transitions to normal bone, an appearance sometimes termed "permeative."

A benign indolent lesion warranting special mention is the fibroxanthoma, which when small is called a fibrous cortical defect and when large a nonossifying fibroma (Figure 9.38). These are quite

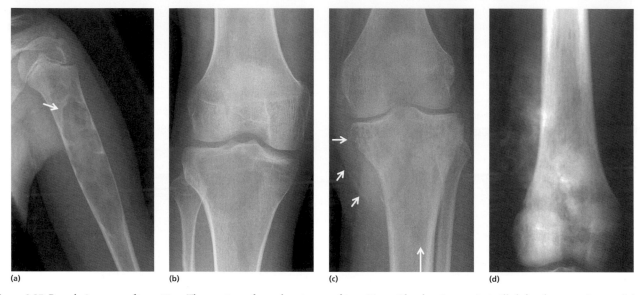

(a)　　　(b)　　　(c)　　　(d)

Figure 9.37 Bone lesion zone of transition. The spectrum from abrupt zone of transition with sclerotic margin to ill-defined permeative parallels the spectrum of lesion activity from indolent to aggressive. (a) Unicameral bone cyst—AP radiograph of the left humerus reveals a large medullary, slightly expansile mostly lucent lesion. The zone of transition is abrupt with sclerotic margin (*arrow*). (b) Giant cell tumor of bone—AP radiograph of the right knee demonstrates a lucent lesion in the proximal tibia that abuts the articular surface and without identifiable matrix. The zone of transition is abrupt but without a sclerotic margin. (c) Lymphoma—AP radiograph of the left knee demonstrates an ill-defined/permeative lesion in the proximal tibia with cortical breakthrough (*midlength arrow*) and likely associated soft tissue mass (*small arrows*). The zone of transition is gradual; the exact borders of the lesion are difficult to determine (*long arrow* is probable distal extent of the lesion). (d) Osteosarcoma—AP radiograph of the distal right femur reveals an ill-defined lesion in the femoral metadiaphyseal region with "cloud-like" regions of increased density and large extraosseous component. The zone of transition is quite gradual; the transition to normal bone is not likely represented on this image.

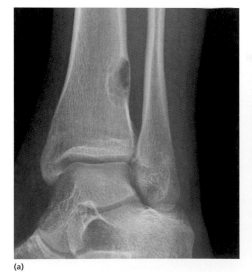

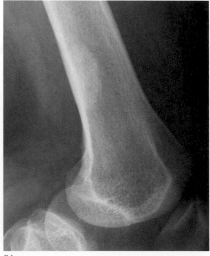

Figure 9.38 Nonossifying fibroma. (a) Mortise radiograph of the left ankle reveals a cortically based lucent lesion with sclerotic borders consistent with a nonossifying fibroma, a common benign bone lesion. (b) Lateral radiograph of the left distal femur reveals a well-defined cortically based somewhat ovoid sclerotic region consistent with an involuted nonossifying fibroma.

(a)　　　(b)

common and often occur in the metaphyseal regions of long bones. They are lytic, sometimes expansile lesions centered in the cortex with an abrupt zone of transition including a thin sclerotic margin. Over time, they involute leaving behind a well-defined region of relative sclerosis compared to the adjacent normal bone.

Periosteal reaction

Periosteal reaction is a feature of many processes in the body, benign and malignant. It is often reactive to adjacent inflammatory changes whether due to infection, trauma, a systemic process, or adjacent tumor. Some bone-centered tumors, however, are rapidly growing. When their soft tissue component extends beyond the cortex of the bone, the periosteum becomes involved. The periosteum responds to the injury by trying to lay down new bone. As the tumor continues to grow, it disrupts the periosteal new bone resulting in what is known as interrupted periosteal reaction (Figure 9.39). At the edges of the tumor, the periosteum appears elevated in a triangular fashion, the Codman triangle, with the apex of the triangle toward the edge of the mass and the base toward the center of the mass. Another potential appearance of a rapidly growing tumor is the "hair-on-end" or "sunburst" appearance, often observed with osteosarcoma, where mineralized new bone is deposited in streaks perpendicular to the long axis of the involved bone.

Dense and uninterrupted periosteal reaction is more likely a reactive process, whereas subtle and ill-defined periosteal reaction is more associated with an aggressive process. Bone lesions that may be associated with reactive periosteal reaction include eosinophilic granuloma and chondroblastoma. Pathologic fractures involving an indolent lesion may also result in periosteal reaction/callus formation as part of the healing process rather than direct periosteal irritation. Ewing sarcoma and osteosarcoma are the two primary bone tumors associated with particularly aggressive periosteal reaction. Infection can also be associated with ill-defined, interrupted periosteal reaction. An example of thick, uninterrupted periosteal reaction due to a systemic condition is illustrated in Figure 9.26.

A final type of periosteal reaction is multilayered, or "onion skin," periosteal reaction. Periosteal new bone is deposited in layers corresponding to alternating periods of increased and decreased activity. This type of periosteal reaction has been associated with Ewing sarcoma, infection/osteomyelitis, and osteosarcoma.

Lesion density

Lesions of bone are lytic (more lucent than adjacent normal bone), sclerotic (denser than adjacent normal bone), or of mixed density. The purely lytic lesions include bone cysts, certain fibro-osseous lesions, and multiple myeloma (Figure 9.40). The sclerotic lesions include osteomas and osteosarcomas as well as enostoses ("bone islands"). Mixed lesions generally are lytic with internal calcifications. Tumor matrix refers to the pattern of internal calcifications. There are three types: chondroid, osteoid, and ground glass. Chondroid matrix is described as "arcs and whorls" and represents calcium deposition between grapelike clusters of chondrocytes. Osteoid matrix is ill-defined increased density, due to mineralized osteoid, often superimposed on a background of normal bone density, which has been termed "cloud-like." Ground glass is a feature of fibrous dysplasia: diffuse variable intermediate density on a background of relative bone lucency, which is due to a relative increase in woven bone. While these types of matrix can help guide a differential diagnosis, it is not uncommon for the matrix to be relatively nonspecific and other features will be needed to narrow down the differential.

Metastatic disease is often lytic, but a few histologies are particularly associated with sclerotic lesions (Figure 9.41): prostate cancer in particular followed by bladder and gastric cancer. Breast cancer has a variable presentation having both lytic and sclerotic lesions.

Age

Certain bone lesions are more common in people less than the age of 30, which is likely due to rapid bone and cartilage turnover in the growing skeleton. Epiphyseal lesions such as chondroblastoma and eosinophilic granuloma occur much more frequently in the skeletally immature; chondroblastoma can occur up to the age of 25. Osteosarcoma is most common in the teen years (and most commonly in the distal femur) because of the rapid growth occurring during this time. The unicameral bone cyst and Ewing sarcoma both occur nearly exclusively in the pediatric age group. Metastatic

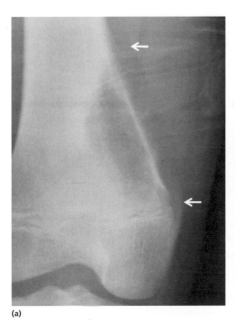
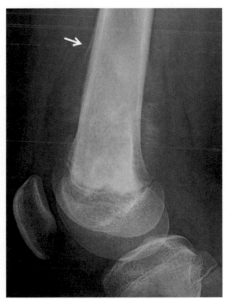

Figure 9.39 Aggressive periosteal reaction. (a) Coned AP radiograph of the right knee in a patient with Ewing sarcoma reveals a mostly lytic eccentrically located lesion in the medial distal femoral metaphysis. At the edges of the lesion are areas of mineralized periosteal elevation known as Codman triangles (*arrows*). (b) Coned lateral radiograph of the distal right femur in a different patient with osteosarcoma demonstrates an ill-defined intramedullary lesion, with predominate areas of sclerosis. In addition to a Codman triangle (*arrow*), there is hair-on-end periosteal bone, also known as "sunburst" periosteal reaction, which is a particular sign of an aggressive underlying bone-forming process.

(a)

(b)

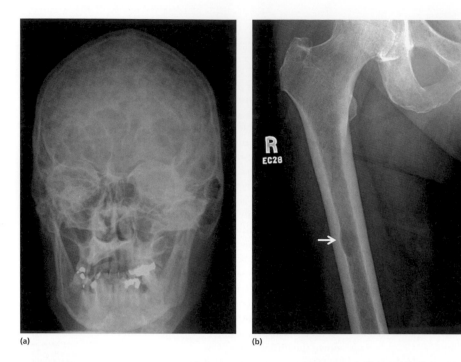

(a)   (b)

Figure 9.40 Multiple myeloma. The AP view of the skull (a) reveals numerous small well-defined lytic areas. The AP radiograph of the proximal right femur (b) demonstrates several lucent lesions. One of the defining characteristics of myeloma is endosteal scalloping (*arrow*), where the inner margin of the cortex is eroded.

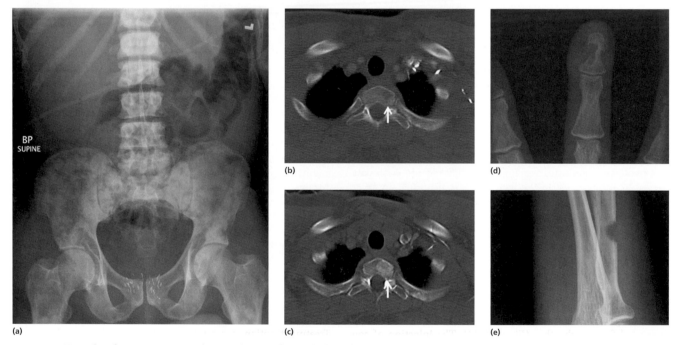

(a)   (b)   (d)   (c)   (e)

Figure 9.41 Examples of osseous metastatic disease. The AP radiograph of the abdomen (a) reveals numerous areas of increased density consistent with prostate cancer metastases. Axial CT image of the upper thoracic spine before (b) and after (c) treatment for breast cancer reveals a lytic lesion in the left aspect of the thoracic vertebral body on the pretreatment scan and a sclerotic lesion on the posttreatment scan (*arrow*) seen in breast cancer metastases. Metastases to the fingers are unusual. This coned PA radiograph of the long finger (d) reveals a lytic lesion destroying the radial aspect of the distal phalanx, which turned out to be due to metastatic lung cancer. The lytic lesion causing focal destruction of the lateral aspect of the proximal radius on this coned AP radiograph of the right forearm (e) is also due to metastatic lung cancer.

disease is highly unlikely unless there is a known malignancy such as a neuroblastoma. Multiple myeloma is incredibly rare before the age of 30. The giant cell tumor of bone starts in the metaphysis but crosses a closed physis into the epiphysis where it ultimately makes contact with the articular surface.

Chondrosarcoma, metastatic disease, and multiple myeloma are all more common later in life. Osteosarcoma has a minor second peak in

incidence in older patients, likely due to sarcomatous degeneration of Paget disease of bone or secondary to prior radiation therapy.

Soft tissue tumors

Many soft tissue masses and mass-like lesions occur. The two most common are lipomas and ganglion cysts, both benign entities. Both have clearly defined imaging characteristics and allow for a diagnosis to be made on the basis of imaging alone. Different mass histologies are common at different sites. For example, in the hands and feet, ganglion cysts and giant cell tumors of tendon sheath are common. If the mass is intra-articular, the differential changes to include pigmented villonodular synovitis and primary synovial osteochondromatosis. Elsewhere in the extremities, the most common lesions are sarcomas, nerve sheath tumors, and vascular lesions (Figure 9.42). Unless the mass has a preponderance of macroscopic fat suggesting a lipoid spectrum tumor, there are essentially no definitive imaging characteristics that can determine the histology of these masses. Biopsy of these lesions is essential for guiding subsequent treatment:

- Imaging evaluation of these lesions begins with radiographs to evaluate for underlying bone involvement.
- MRI evaluates the extent of the mass to document the normal soft tissue structures involved by the mass and whether the neurovascular bundle is involved.
- If the patient cannot get an MRI, either ultrasound or contrast-enhanced CT might be obtained instead. For some lesions, a complete assessment of the mass can be performed with US. Percutaneous biopsy for soft tissue masses is also usually ultrasound guided.
- For sarcomas, CT of the chest is obtained to evaluate for metastatic disease.

Figure 9.43 demonstrates neurovascular involvement by a large sarcoma and metastatic disease to the chest.

Musculoskeletal interventions

Musculoskeletal radiology employs the use of image-guided procedures for both diagnostic and therapeutic purposes. Diagnostic procedures include arthrography, aspirations, and percutaneous biopsy. Image-guided joint injection and CT-guided radiofrequency ablation have therapeutic benefits. Image-guided fluid aspiration can have both diagnostic and therapeutic benefits.

Arthrography

Conventional arthrography has largely been replaced with diagnostic MRI. The MR arthrogram involves injecting a contrast agent into a joint to make internal joint structures easier to see. For certain pathologies, such as shoulder and hip labral tears, augmenting a routine diagnostic MRI with the use of intra-articular contrast improves the diagnostic quality of MRI by distending the joint so that closely apposed structures are separated from each other (Figure 9.44). The injection of contrast also allows abnormal communications between normally separate compartments to be documented. In general, the guidance modality is fluoroscopy, but sonographic guidance can also be performed, especially in the setting of an iodinated contrast allergy.

Unlike the evaluation of glenoid and acetabular labral tears where the primary benefit of arthrography is joint distention, MRI arthrography of the wrist depends on documenting abnormal communications between normally water-tight compartments. If contrast fills a wrist compartment other than the compartment injected, a ligament tear is suspected. For example, if the radiocarpal joint is injected and contrast opacifies the midcarpal joint, there must be a scapholunate or lunotriquetral ligament tear allowing contrast to pass. This diagnosis is often made on fluoroscopy alone,

but subsequent MR imaging is used to better characterize the anatomy of the injury.

Biopsy

Bone biopsies are most readily performed using CT guidance. Bone biopsy can be performed on both lytic and blastic skeletal lesions to diagnose malignancy or to confirm osseous metastatic disease. Additionally, CT-guided biopsy is useful in the setting of osteomyelitis and discitis, where samples can be sent both to microbiology and pathology:

- CT allows for precise needle localization during biopsy of small lesions in precarious locations such as in the spine. CT-guided biopsy most often employs a coaxial technique using an outer penetration cannula, a drill (sometimes), and an inner cutting biopsy cannula.
- US may be used to perform biopsy of soft tissue masses and drainage of cystic lesions in the extremities. Ultrasound allows real-time visualization of the biopsy device within the mass as it takes the sample.

Joint injections

Fluoroscopy or ultrasound can be used to guide joint injections. Intra-articular corticosteroids are often administered as a treatment for synovitis associated with OA, RA, and juvenile idiopathic arthritis. Response to corticosteroid injection is variable, but it can improve clinical symptoms to delay joint replacement or arthrodesis in OA, as well as improve functional limitations of children and adults with inflammatory arthropathies.

Fluid aspiration

Aspiration of joint fluid with imaging guidance employs similar techniques to joint injection. This can be performed using fluoroscopy or ultrasound. A pitfall of using fluoroscopy for aspiration of a prosthetic hip is that the needle can sometimes be completely shadowed by the prosthesis itself, resulting in the lack of needle tip control throughout the procedure. In this setting, ultrasound has the advantage of visualizing the joint space directly so that the needle can be directed into it in real time, regardless of prosthesis or native joint. Ultrasound is also a useful tool for aspiration of fluid from cystic masses and tendon sheaths.

Radiofrequency ablation

Osteoid osteomas are solitary bone tumors most commonly found in older children and young adults, which produce a local inflammatory response that can be quite painful. These tumors are centered on a "central nidus" thought to be a vascular lesion. Treatment options for osteoid osteoma include watchful waiting with medical pain management, surgical resection, and radiofrequency ablation. Radiofrequency ablation is often more desirable than resection since no bone is removed and normal physical activity can be resumed shortly after the procedure, even if the tumor is located in a weight-bearing bone. A radiofrequency probe is advanced through the cannula and medullary tunnel of the needle introducer under CT guidance, and its tip is positioned precisely at the tumor nidus. The probe is heated using a radiofrequency generator to a temperature of 90–95°C for 6 min. Full relief of baseline pain is not immediate and may take many months. Follow-up imaging shows the central nidus replaced by sclerotic bone.

The technique of radiofrequency ablation can also be used to treat painful osseous metastatic lesions.

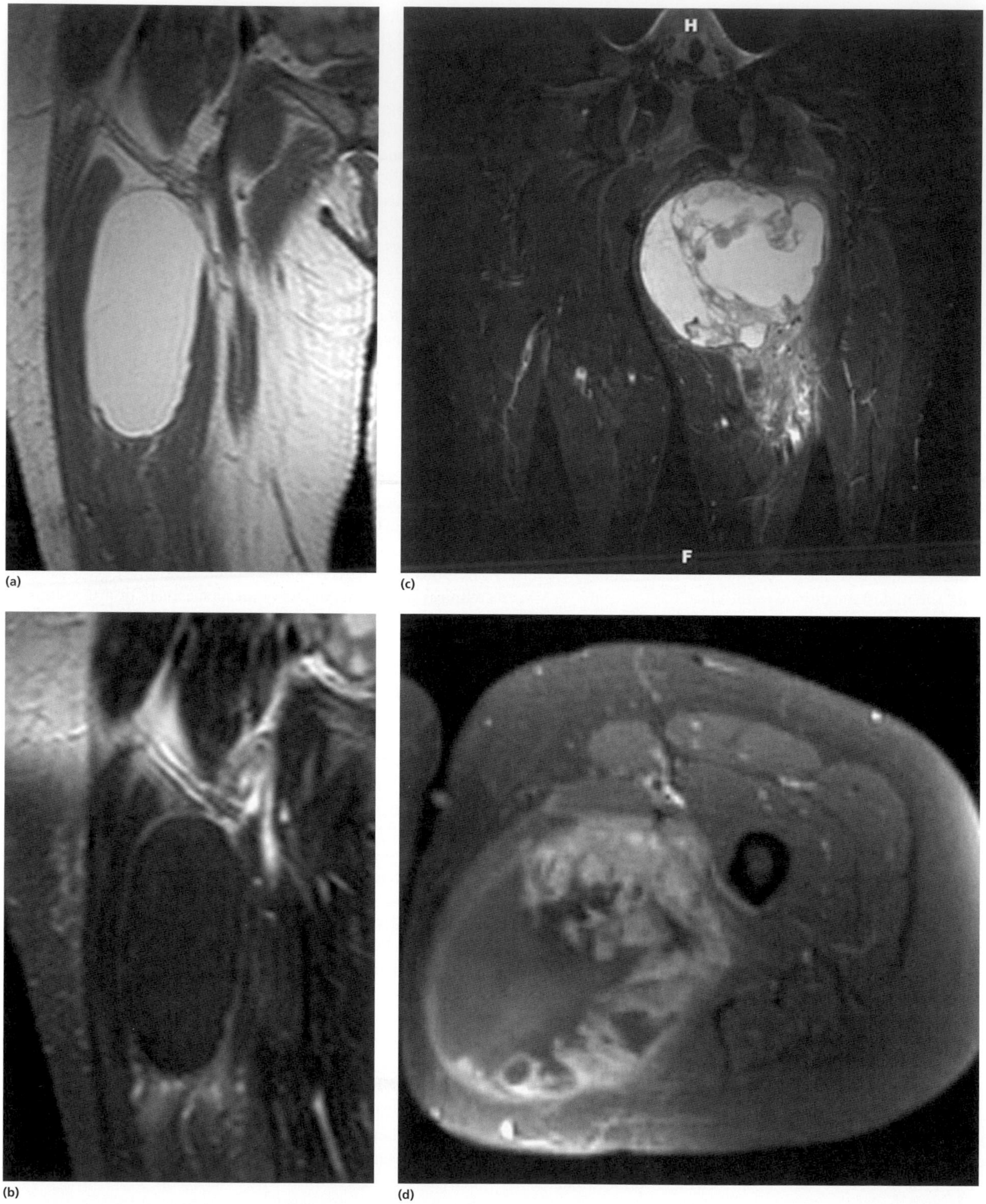

Figure 9.42 Examples of soft tissue masses. **Atypical lipomatous tumor**. Coronal T1-weighted (a) and coronal STIR (b) MR images of the right thigh reveal a large, well-circumscribed, homogeneously bright mass on the T1-weighted image and homogeneously dark on the STIR image within the anterior thigh consistent with a fat-only containing lesion. **Malignant peripheral nerve sheath tumor**. Coronal STIR MR images of both thighs (c) and axial postcontrast T1-weighted fat-suppressed MR image of the left thigh (d) reveal a very large heterogeneous-appearing mass in the medial thigh. The postcontrast image reveals peripheral nodularity, but the mass is predominantly fluid filled consistent with necrosis.

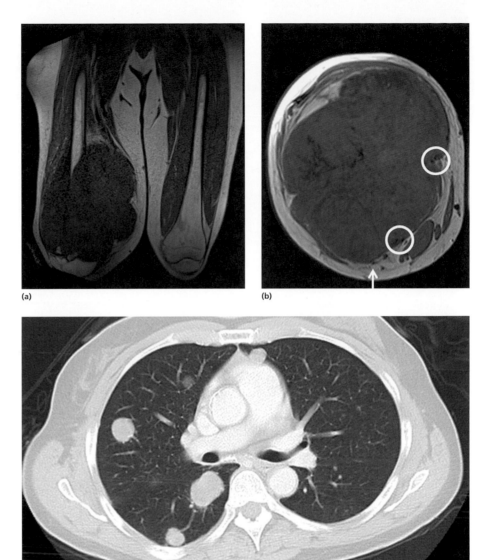

Figure 9.43 Soft tissue tumor. Coronal T1-weighted MR image of both thighs (a) and axial T1-weighted MR image through the distal right thigh (b) reveal a large soft tissue mass (sarcoma) near completely replacing the entire distal thigh; no identifiable bone is seen. The sciatic nerve (*arrow*) has been displaced posteriorly, and the vascular bundles are likely surrounded by tumor (circles). Axial CT image of the chest (c) reveals multiple large pulmonary nodules in the right lung consistent with, in this patient, metastatic leiomyosarcoma.

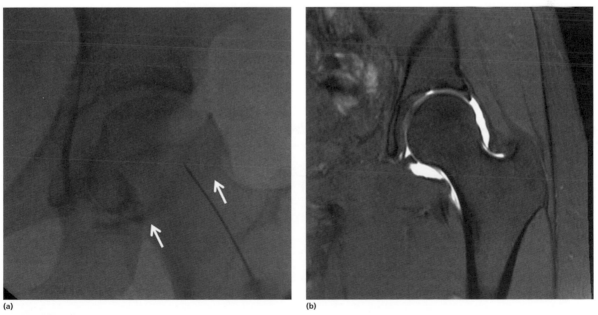

Figure 9.44 MR arthrography of the hip. (a) Fluoroscopic image from a left hip arthrogram injection from a lateral oblique approach. The collar of increased density (*arrows*) about the femoral head–neck junction represents injected contrast proving intra-articular position of the needle tip. (b) Coronal T1-weighted fat-suppressed MR image following left hip arthrogram injection in a different patient.

Suggested reading

Introductory texts in musculoskeletal imaging include:

Helms, C.A. (2013) *Fundamentals of Skeletal Radiology*, 4th edn. Saunders, Philadelphia, PA.

Manaster, B.J., May, D.A. & Disler, D.G. (2013) *Musculoskeletal Imaging: The Requisites*, 4th edn. Saunders, Philadelphia, PA.

Excellent focused texts on arthritis and musculoskeletal ultrasound are:

Brower, A.C. & Flemming, D.J. (2012) *Arthritis in Black and White: Expert Consult*, 3rd edn. Saunders, Philadelphia.

Jacobson, J.A. (2012) *Fundamentals of Musculoskeletal Ultrasound: Expert Consult*, 2nd edn. Saunders, Philadelphia.

Good comprehensive reference texts include:

Pope, T.L., Bloem, H.L., Beltran, J. *et al.* (2014) *Musculoskeletal Imaging*, 2nd edn. Saunders, Philadelphia.

Stoller, D.W. (2006) *Magnetic Resonance in Orthopaedics and Sports Medicine*, 3rd edn. Lippincott Williams & Wilkins, New York, NY.

Selected reference

de Jesus, J.O., Parker, L., Frangos, A.J. *et al.* (2009) Accuracy of MRI, MR arthrography, and ultrasound in the diagnosis of rotator cuff tears: a meta-analysis. *American Journal of Roentgenology*, **192**, 1701–7.

CHAPTER 10

Breast imaging

Susan Ormsbee Holley
Assistant Professor, Breast Imaging Section, Mallinckrodt Institute of Radiology, Washington University School of Medicine, St. Louis, MO, USA

Goal

Unlike other radiology specialties, breast imaging is predominantly performed in the screening setting—meaning that patients are asymptomatic and without known breast disease. The goal of screening is to detect breast cancer and, if present, to detect it as early as possible: this maximizes the patient's chances of survival and minimizes the morbidity of her treatment. To illustrate, a 5 mm cancer can be easily excised and is unlikely to have metastasized (spread to other sites in the body); by contrast, a 5 cm cancer requires much more extensive surgery, treatment with chemotherapy, and is more likely to have metastasized.

Breast cancer is the second leading cause of cancer death in women. Approximately one in eight women will develop breast cancer during their lifetime; the American Cancer Society estimates that about 230,000 new cases of invasive breast cancer will be diagnosed in 2014. The incidence of cancer increases with age and plateaus just before menopause. Men, too, can have breast cancer, but the incidence in men is significantly less than women (~2000 cases per year).

Current screening recommendations from the American Cancer Society state: "Women age 40 and older should have a mammogram every year and should continue to do so for as long as they are in good health." Some women are at a higher-than-average risk for breast cancer and may undergo more vigilant screening regimens (such as having screening breast magnetic resonance imaging exams plus mammograms, or starting screening earlier than age 40). There are various risk calculators that are employed by clinicians to determine a woman's lifetime risk for breast cancer and take into account family history, hormonal factors, and the like.

Controversy over the most appropriate screening regimens for breast cancer is a recurrent theme in the breast imaging world and often comes to the attention of the media. Recommendations for screening are made based on decades of data from various types of trials and studies (such as randomized controlled trials, case–control studies, longitudinal observational data, etc.). The vast majority of these trials demonstrate that screening mammography confers a survival benefit for women. Optimal screening intervals and appropriate ages to screen continue to be discussed in the context of evolving technology, ability to determine an individual woman's risk, and a woman's personal preferences for screening.

Anatomy

The female breast is a specialized glandular organ for lactation, located between the 2nd and 6th ribs, overlying the pectoralis muscle. During lactation, milk is produced in the terminal duct lobular units and is expressed through converging ducts to the nipple. Each breast typically has approximately 15–20 ductal systems (lobes), radially oriented around the nipple.

The breast is attached to the dermis by suspensory ligaments and is predominantly composed of fat and glandular tissue. The ratio of fat to glandular tissue is important to the radiologist, as the greater the proportion of glandular tissue, the more difficult it is to detect cancers.

Consider Figure 10.1, which depicts mammographic images from four different patients, illustrating the spectrum of breast parenchymal density. A tiny cancer would be much more easily overlooked in a heterogeneously or extremely dense breast, compared to a fatty breast. This is why every interpretation of a mammogram includes a statement describing the breast parenchymal density; this conveys the radiologist's assessment of her/his sensitivity for detecting cancer on a particular mammogram.

Imaging

Mammography

The primary tool used for breast cancer screening is mammography, which uses X-rays to image the breast tissue. A standard bilateral screening mammogram is shown in Figure 10.2.

This exam consists of two views of each breast, obtained from two different angles: one from above (craniocaudal view) and one from the side (mediolateral oblique view). The breasts are imaged while in gentle compression; this minimizes the overlapping/superimposition of tissue and allows for the best depiction of abnormal findings.

Critical Observations in Radiology for Medical Students, First Edition. Katherine R. Birchard, Kiran Reddy Busireddy, and Richard C. Semelka.
© 2015 John Wiley & Sons, Ltd. Published 2015 by John Wiley & Sons, Ltd.
Companion website: www.wiley.com/go/birchard

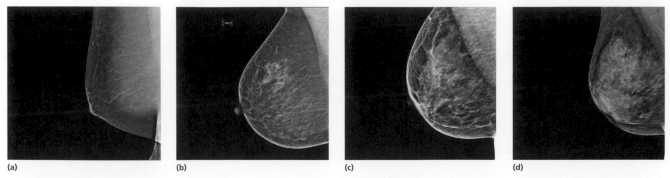

(a)   (b)   (c)   (d)

Figure 10.1 Images from four different women illustrate the variation in breast parenchymal density. Radiologists assign each mammogram one of four density classifications: (a) almost entirely fatty, (b) scattered areas of fibroglandular density, (c) heterogeneously dense, or (d) extremely dense. Density classifications reprinted with permission of the American College of Radiology (ACR). No other representation of this material is authorized without expressed, written permission from the ACR. Refer to the ACR website at www.acr.org/Quality-Safety/Resources/BIRADS for the most current and complete version of the BI-RADS® Atlas. © American College of Radiology.

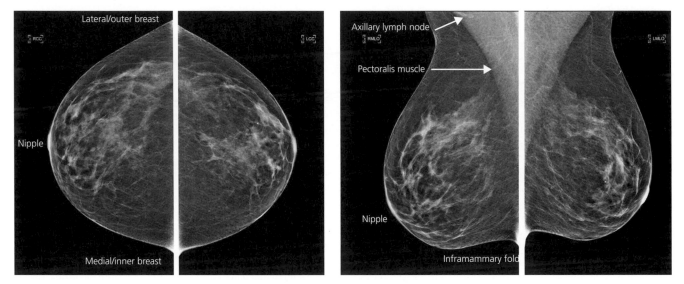

Figure 10.2 A screening mammogram. All mammographic images are labeled to include side, view, and the initials of the technologist who took the image. In clinical practice, patient and imaging institution information are also included on the image.

The mediolateral oblique view includes the breast tissue and axilla. The pectoralis muscle is visible, and axillary lymph nodes are often seen. Notice how the breast is positioned to include the inframammary fold. The craniocaudal view should include nearly as much tissue as the mediolateral oblique view. By convention, on the craniocaudal view, the lateral (outer) breast is at the top of the image, and the medial (inner) breast is at the bottom of the image. The nipple should be in profile on all views—otherwise, it can obscure underlying tissue or even simulate a mass.

As this description implies, imaging technique is extremely important in breast imaging—all of the breast parenchyma must be included, and it must be clearly depicted. Consider Figure 10.3 an example of a cancer that was nearly excluded from the image; if the technologist had been slightly less diligent, it wouldn't have been visible at all.

Ultrasound

A second important tool in breast imaging is ultrasound, which uses high-frequency sound waves to produce an image of the breast tissue. Typically, ultrasound is used to further characterize a finding

seen on mammogram. A handheld 15 MHz ultrasound probe is used to scan the breast in real time with the patient lying down (supine). Still images or video clips are recorded for interpretation.

A typical ultrasound image is shown in Figure 10.4. Simple fluid/water is shown as black (anechoic), fat/fibrous tissue are white (hyperechoic), and normal tissue is seen in shades of gray (hypo- to isoechoic). The skin at the interface of the transducer is depicted at the top of the screen, followed by the subcutaneous layer and breast parenchyma; at the bottom of the screen are the structures of the chest wall (ribs, muscle). Ducts and blood vessels can be seen traversing the parenchyma.

The location of a breast finding is routinely described using quadrants, clock positions, distance from the nipple, depth within the breast, or any combination of these. For example, a finding could be (exhaustively) described as residing within the upper outer quadrant of the right breast, at the 10:00 position, 5 cm from the nipple, at posterior depth. Notice the pictogram in the lower left corner of the image: it depicts which breast is being imaged. The smaller orange line shows were the transducer was positioned on the breast when the image was acquired.

Magnetic resonance imaging (MRI)

Contrast-enhanced breast MRI is routinely used to evaluate certain patients with breast cancer (very young women with dense tissue, women with invasive lobular carcinoma) and to screen women who are at a higher-than-average risk for having breast cancer. Figure 10.5 shows an MRI from a patient with breast cancer.

Breast MRI is more sensitive than specific, which makes it a very good tool for high-risk populations. The fact that it results in relatively more false-positive exams, however, renders it an inappropriate choice for screening the average-risk patient.

Digital tomosynthesis

Digital tomosynthesis is a relatively new technique that uses X-rays to image the breast. It differs from the standard mammogram in that images are obtained from multiple angles (the X-ray tube rotates in an arc over the breast) and are then reconstructed into "slices." This allows the imager to "scroll through" the breast tissue, evaluating thin planes of breast tissue in sequence. Trials and studies are being conducted to evaluate the role of digital tomosynthesis in clinical practice Figure 10.6 shows how tomosynthesis can make a cancer more conspicuous.

Screening process

When a breast radiologist evaluates a screening mammogram, she/he is looking for breast cancer. Entities from other etiologies—trauma, vascular, inflammatory, infectious, and so on—are occasionally diagnosed, but they make up a minority of cases. Ideally, a screening test would detect all the cancers (perfect sensitivity) and dismiss all the noncancers (perfect specificity), but no screening test for breast cancer is perfect. A breast radiologist must maximize her/his sensitivity and specificity, finding as many cancers as possible while recalling as few patients as possible.

A basic outline of a breast imaging program is illustrated in Figure 10.7. Tier A of the figure depicts the average-risk, asymptomatic woman in the outpatient setting obtaining a screening mammogram. Due to the volume of patients seen in a breast imaging center and the time needed to interpret the exam, screening mammograms are usually not read in real time. The results of the exam are sent to both the woman and her referring clinician a day or so after the exam was performed. Figure 10.8 shows a typical report for a normal exam.

You may have noticed that the exam is assigned a numeric category, which is a Breast Imaging Reporting and Data System (BI-RADS®) assessment. When interpreting a breast imaging study,

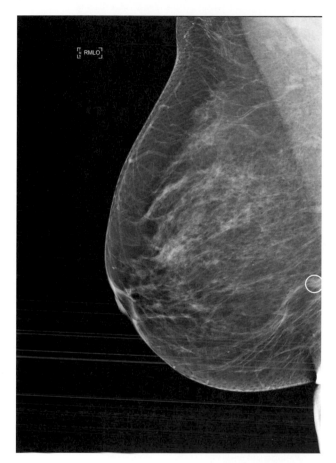

Figure 10.3 A tiny cancer in the posterior lower right breast, nearly excluded from the image. This case exemplifies how good technique leads to better cancer detection.

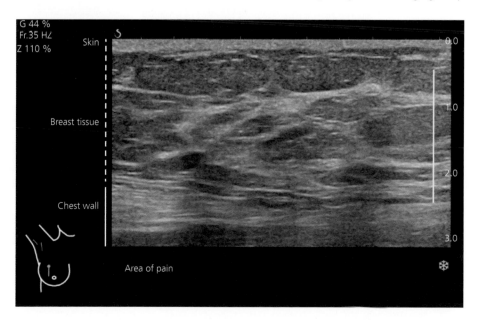

Figure 10.4 An image from a breast ultrasound exam depicting normal tissue.

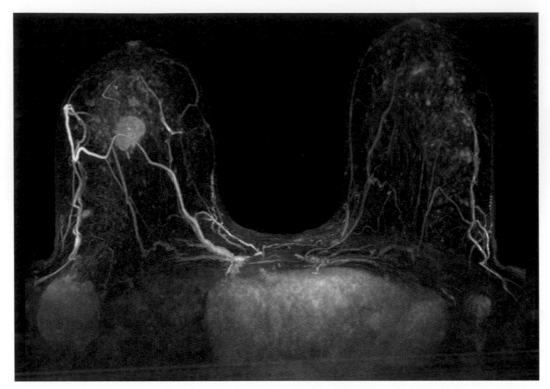

Figure 10.5 This is a maximum intensity projection (MIP) from a contrast-enhanced breast MRI exam. A MIP displays all the data acquired as a single volume, providing an overview of the imaged tissue. This patient has a cancer in her central right breast (depicted on the left side of the image) and a large axillary lymph node metastasis.

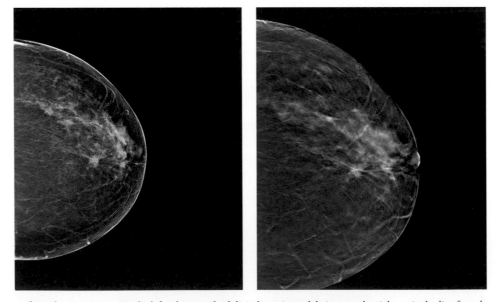

Figure 10.6 Two images from the same exam. On the left is her standard digital craniocaudal view; on the right, a single slice from her craniocaudal digital tomosynthesis sequence. There is an irregular mass in the central left breast, deep to the nipple; its irregular/stellate shape is more conspicuous on tomosynthesis.

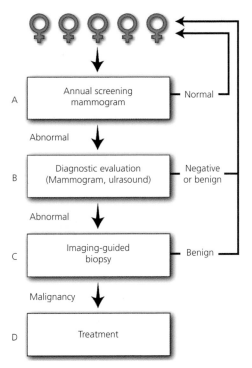

Figure 10.7 Schematic of a breast imaging program.

EXAMINATION: SCREENING MAMMOGRAM

TECHNIQUE: Bilateral full-field digital screening mammogram was performed. Views obtained: bilateral craniocaudal and bilateral mediolateral oblique.

FINDINGS: The present examination has been compared to prior screening mammograms dated 02/26/2013, 02/21/2012 and 02/15/2011.

There are scattered fibroglandular densities.

There is no suspicious abnormality in either breast.

IMPRESSION: Negative exam. Annual screening mammography is recommended.

OVERALL FINAL ASSESSMENT: BI-RADS® CATEGORY 1: Negative.

Figure 10.8 A typical report for a normal screening mammogram. Notice the breast density description.

radiologists use a standardized vocabulary and grading system called BI-RADS®. BI-RADS® was created in order to provide a clear, unambiguous way of reporting findings and, more importantly, conveying a recommendation regarding the findings—that is, recommending the appropriate next step for the patient. In this case, a normal mammogram is assigned a BI-RADS® 1: negative. This patient can be seen again next year for her annual screening mammogram.

Most women have normal mammograms (BI-RADS® 1). If the radiologist detects a possible abnormality, however, the patient will be asked to return for additional imaging Figure 10.9 shows a report from an abnormal screening exam. It was assigned a BI-RADS® 0, meaning that the radiologist needs more information in order to make a final recommendation. At the

EXAMINATION: SCREENING MAMMOGRAM

TECHNIQUE: Bilateral full-field digital screening mammogram was performed. Views obtained: bilateral craniocaudal and bilateral mediolateral oblique.

FINDINGS: The present examination has been compared to prior screening mammograms dated 5/6/2013 and 5/1/2012.

There are scattered fibroglandular densities.

There are new grouped calcifications in the upper outer right breast.

There is no suspicious abnormality in the left breast.

IMPRESSION: Calcifications in the right breast require additional evaluation. Additional views are recommended.

OVERALL FINAL ASSESSMENT: BI-RADS® CATEGORY 0: Incomplete: need additional imaging evaluation.

Figure 10.9 A typical report for an abnormal screening mammogram.

patient's return visit, the finding of concern will be evaluated in detail with additional mammographic images and/or a targeted ultrasound exam. These additional mammographic images can be obtained at different angles or projections, utilize different patient positioning, or focus narrowly on the finding with spot compression or spot magnified views. With this additional information, the radiologist must first decide whether the finding of concern is a distinct histologic entity or was simply a fluke of positioning. If it is a real finding, the radiologist must then decide if it is a benign/normal structure, or if it requires biopsy for definitive characterization.

Most women who return for additional imaging are subsequently dismissed as either having a negative exam (BI-RADS® 1) or benign findings (BI-RADS® 2). However, a fraction of patients will go on to biopsy (Figure 10.7, tier C). Occasionally, the patient requires a surgical excisional biopsy, but most cases are amenable to an imaging-guided needle biopsy performed by the radiologist. A breast biopsy can be performed using either ultrasound or mammographic guidance, meaning that the radiologist uses imaging to guide the position of the needle and take tissue samples. This brief outpatient procedure can provide the necessary diagnostic information for the patient, without her having to undergo surgery.

If the patient's biopsy demonstrates benign findings, then she may then return to having regular annual screening mammograms. If she is diagnosed with breast cancer, she goes on to treatment (Figure 10.7, tier D); the radiologist can further assist the oncologic team by evaluating for extent of disease, localizing the cancer for surgical excision, and subsequently monitoring the patient for any recurrent or new disease.

Detecting cancer

Breast cancer can present in various ways on a mammogram. The three most common manifestations are calcifications, masses, and architectural distortion. The following scenarios illustrate how patients may progress from screening to diagnostic evaluation, and then to biopsy if necessary. They also demonstrate radiologic features of a few common benign and malignant lesions.

Scenario 10.1 My patient had a screening mammogram, and the report says she needs additional imaging evaluation.

As you recall from Figure 10.7, screening mammograms that are interpreted as abnormal—that is, having a finding that requires additional evaluation—are assigned a BI-RADS® 0. This designation means that the patient returns to the imaging center for addition imaging in order to further characterize the finding in question.

The pertinent images from her screening mammogram are shown in Figure 10.10.

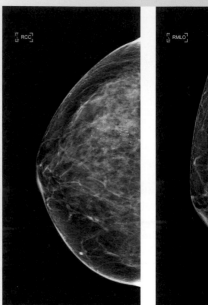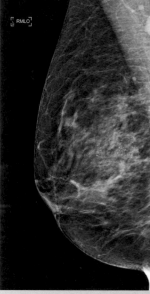

Figure 10.10 There are heterogeneous calcifications in the upper outer right breast. Most of them are at posterior depth, but there are a few similar appearing calcifications in the subareolar breast as well.

Calcifications can form in the breast tissue from many different processes, both benign and malignant. To discriminate between benign and malignant calcifications, the radiologist must assess both the morphology (shape) and distribution of the calcifications (see Table 10.1).

Table 10.1 BI-RADS® descriptors of calcifications on mammogram.

Morphology

Typically benign	*Suspicious*
Skin	Amorphous
Vascular	Coarse heterogeneous
Coarse or "popcorn-like"	Fine pleomorphic
Large rodlike	Fine linear or fine-linear branching
Round	
Rim	
Dystrophic	
Milk of calcium	
Suture	

Distribution
Diffuse
Regional
Grouped
Linear
Segmental

Reprinted with permission of the American College of Radiology (ACR). No other representation of this material is authorized without expressed, written permission from the ACR. Refer to the ACR website at www.acr.org/Quality-Safety/Resources/BIRADS for the most current and complete version of the BI-RADS® Atlas.
© American College of Radiology.

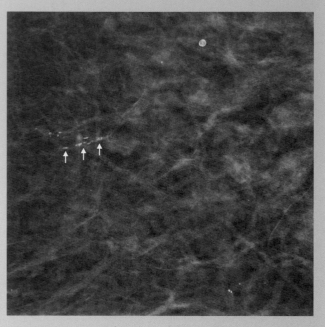

Figure 10.11 Spot magnification image from a different patient, showing calcifications of ductal carcinoma *in situ* (DCIS).

Some morphologies are definitely worrisome, such as "fine pleomorphic" or "fine-linear branching"—these shapes suggest that the calcifications conform to a duct and may represent ductal carcinoma *in situ* (DCIS). Similarly, the distribution of calcifications is also important in assessing their etiology. If calcifications appear to depict a duct or ductal system—that is, if they are "linear" or "segmental"—this also raises concern that the calcifications are a by-product of DCIS. Figure 10.11 depicts a different patient, with DCIS manifesting as fine pleomorphic calcifications in a linear distribution. Alternatively, there are some calcifications that are definitively benign (see Figure 10.12). These can be confidently dismissed on a screening mammogram.

The patient in our scenario returns to the breast imaging center for additional spot magnification views of the calcifications of concern (Figure 10.13).

These views confirm that the calcifications are linear and assume many different sizes and shapes (pleomorphic); importantly, they also appear to conform to a segmental distribution, suggesting that they reside within a ductal system. The radiologist decided that these calcifications were highly concerning for DCIS and recommended a biopsy for further evaluation. Thus, she assigned this patient a final BI-RADS® assessment of BI-RADS® 5: highly suspicious for malignancy.

A listing of all the BI-RADS® assessments are listed in Table 10.2. You are familiar with the BI-RADS® 1 and BI-RADS® 0 designations. A category BI-RADS® 4 or BI-RADS® 5 is assigned when the radiologist decides that an imaging finding is concerning enough to require tissue sampling to make the diagnosis.

In this case, the patient had these calcifications biopsied; the tiny tissue "cores" (from the core needle biopsy) are depicted in Figure 10.14. As you can see, the tissue cores represent a relatively small volume of tissue, which is usually more than enough to make the diagnosis. However, after the pathologist makes her/his diagnosis, the onus then falls upon the radiologist to decide whether the pathologist's diagnosis is *concordant* with the imaging findings—that is, whether the tissue diagnosis adequately explains the imaging findings.

At this point, the finer subdivisions of the BI-RADS® assessments are helpful to the radiologist in deciding whether a biopsy is concordant or not. As you have noticed, both BI-RADS® 4 and BI-RADS® 5 assessments will

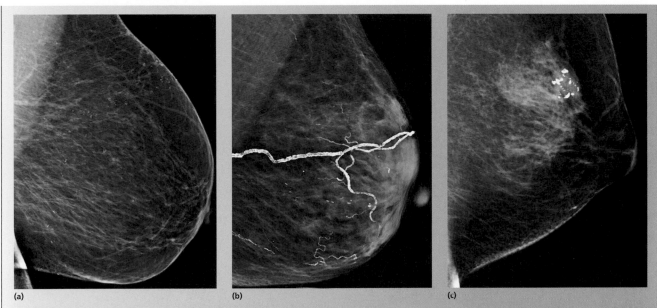

(a)   (b)   (c)

Figure 10.12 Various benign calcifications. (a) Skin calcifications, which are typically round and have lucent centers. Notice how they are seen in tangent within the skin, in both the upper and lower breast. (b) Vascular calcifications in both medium and small vessels. (c) Coarse, "popcorn" calcifications within an involuting fibroadenoma.

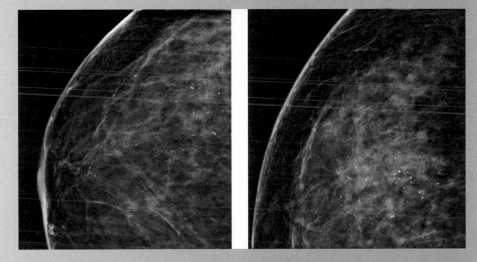

Figure 10.13 Spot magnification views in the craniocaudal and mediolateral projections. The magnification allows better definition of the calcifications and can depict calcifications too faint or tiny to be seen on the full views.

prompt a tissue biopsy. These two assessments both signify concern for malignancy, but this level of concern is subdivided into several levels—4A, 4B, 4C, and 5. These subdivisions signify to the radiologist how suspicious the finding is and what diagnoses she/he is willing to accept as an etiology for the finding. For example, this patient had calcifications that were deemed a BI-RADS® 5. This means that the radiologist is virtually certain that they represent malignancy. If the pathologist had reported that these calcifications were benign, the radiologist would be concerned that the pathology results did not explain the appearance of these highly suspicious calcifications, and would deem this a *discordant* result. A discordant biopsy prompts the radiologist to recommend that the patient undergo additional tissue sampling, usually via surgical excisional biopsy, in order to ensure the correct diagnosis.

One might ask: if you know the finding represents a cancer (BI-RADS® 5), why perform a needle biopsy instead of proceeding to treatment? The answer: treatment planning. Breast cancer can arise from different cell types and varies in aggressiveness and biomarker profile. Knowing the diagnosis prospectively allows the oncologic team to pursue the best treatment options for the patient. It also allows her physicians to assess

Table 10.2 BI-RADS® assessments.

Category 0: incomplete—need additional imaging evaluation and/or prior mammograms for comparison
Category 1: negative
Category 2: benign
Category 3: probably benign
Category 4: suspicious
   Category 4A: low suspicion for malignancy
   Category 4B: moderate suspicion for malignancy
   Category 4C: high suspicion for malignancy
Category 5: highly suggestive of malignancy
Category 6: known biopsy-proven malignancy

Reprinted with permission from the American College of Radiology (ACR). No other representation of this material is authorized without expressed written permission from the ACR. Refer to the ACR website at www.acr.org/Quality-Safety/Resources/BIRADS for the most current and complete version of the BI-RADS® Atlas. © American College of Radiology.

her prognosis. In this case, the patient's biopsy did indeed result in a diagnosis of DCIS, and she was referred on for treatment.

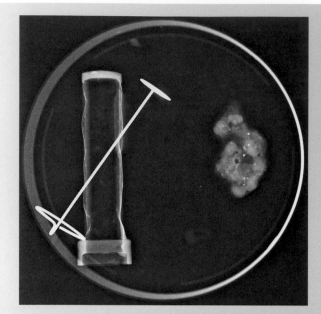

Figure 10.14 X-ray image of the specimen dish containing the tissue cores. The calcifications are within the biopsied tissue.

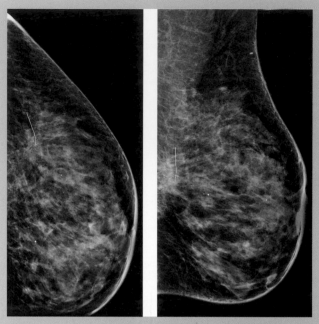

Figure 10.15 Mammogram from a patient who has undergone breast conservation therapy (BCT).

Most breast malignancies originate within the epithelium of the ducts; hence, most cancers are described as "invasive ductal carcinomas." However, other, less common histologic types of breast cancer are also seen, such as invasive lobular carcinoma, mixed ductal and lobular, medullary, mucinous, papillary, and tubular cancers. Entities such as primary breast lymphoma, metastases to breast, and sarcomas are also occasionally seen, but are far less common.

Depending on the extent of malignancy, patients may choose to pursue mastectomy (removal of the breast) or a partial mastectomy (excising the malignancy and some surrounding tissue). Figure 10.15 shows an example of a patient who has had a partial mastectomy. The combination of partial mastectomy and radiation therapy is called breast conservation therapy (BCT).

As you can see, BCT causes scarring, which results in architectural distortion. This means that the tissue is abnormally tethered, with a resulting focally stellate (distorted) appearance. In this case, the distortion is benign (we know it's from her surgery—note how the location of her scar is designated with a linear metallic marker placed on the skin). However, normal postoperative distortion can make detecting a new or recurrent malignancy very challenging.

Architectural distortion can arise from other processes, both benign (such as a radial scar) and malignant (invasive lobular carcinoma can present this way). Distortion can be difficult to discern on mammogram; digital tomosynthesis can often make distortion much more conspicuous. Often, sonographic correlates for architectural distortion are subtle, and biopsy is often performed using mammography to guide needle placement. Figure 10.16 shows an example of distortion that was very subtle on standard mammogram but much more conspicuous on tomosynthesis. Biopsy showed an invasive lobular carcinoma.

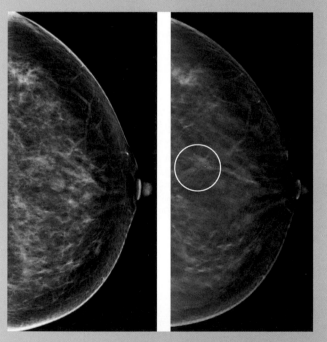

Figure 10.16 Two images from the same exam. On the left is her standard digital craniocaudal view; on the right, a single slice from her craniocaudal digital tomosynthesis sequence. There is an irregular mass in the deep central left breast; its irregular/stellate shape is more conspicuous on tomosynthesis.

Scenario 10.2 My patient, a 55-year-old woman, has a palpable lump in her breast.

This scenario raises a very important point: if your patient is symptomatic (has a palpable breast lump, nipple discharge, focal breast pain, skin thickening/redness), then she needs to have a diagnostic evaluation, *not* a screening mammogram.

Critical observation: A symptomatic patient should not undergo a screening mammogram, but instead should be referred for a diagnostic imaging evaluation.

There are two important reasons for this distinction. First, some cancers can be quite subtle or even occult on mammogram. If the radiologist is not directed to specifically evaluate the palpable area of concern with targeted imaging, a mammogram could be passed as normal and provide false reassurance to the patient and her clinician. Second, if the palpable area is a cancer, it expedites the patient's evaluation to be able to obtain all the imaging necessary in anticipation of biopsy. Figure 10.17 shows the patient's mammogram. These images demonstrate an obvious breast cancer: the patient's palpable lump corresponds to an irregular mass with spiculated margins. Again, BI-RADS® descriptors are used in order to characterize the findings; masses are described by their shape, margins, and density on mammogram (Table 10.3).

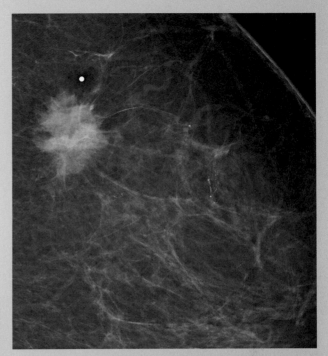

Figure 10.18 Spot magnification mammogram demonstrates an irregular, high-density mass with spiculated margins. (Did you notice the additional fine-linear calcifications?)

In this case, the mass is an irregular shape and has spiculated (stellate, jagged) margins; these depict the disorganized growth of the malignancy and the desmoplastic reaction of the surrounding tissue.

Density (i.e., how white an area is on an X-ray) is a surrogate for the amount of cellular material present; radiographically dense things (metal, calcifications, highly cellular cancers) appear whiter on X-rays, while less dense things (fat, air) appear blacker on X-ray. "Equal density," in breast imaging, refers to the density of normal glandular tissue. This patient has a high-density mass.

Additional spot magnification views of the mass are performed in order to better evaluate its margins and to evaluate for any additional subtle findings that could indicate more extensive disease (Figure 10.18).

After the mammographic evaluation is completed, a targeted ultrasound is also performed. In addition to the evaluation of the mass itself, this also allows the radiologist to perform a physical exam, to evaluate for extent of disease within the breast, and to evaluate the ipsilateral (same side) axilla for abnormal lymph nodes. Directed physical exam is important, as it allows the radiologist to assess not only the physical characteristics of the mass itself but also to assess for other features of malignancy, such as skin thickening and nipple changes (inversion, erythema or excoriation).

The sonographic features of a mass give the radiologist more information about the mass's characteristics—not only the shape and margins, but also its orientation within the surrounding breast tissue, its echo pattern (resultant "gray" color/pattern), and the posterior features of the mass (the character of the sound waves deep to the mass) (Table 10.4).

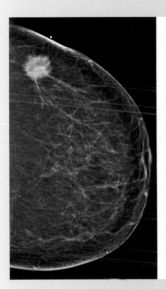 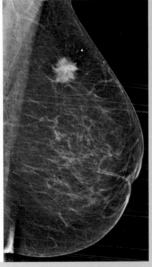

Figure 10.17 Diagnostic mammogram of a patient who presented a palpable lump. Notice the small metallic BB marker; this is placed on the breast where the patient feels the lump.

Table 10.3 BI-RADS® descriptors of masses on mammogram.

Shape	Margin	Density
Oval	Circumscribed	High density
Round	Obscured	Equal density
Irregular	Microlobulated	Low density
	Indistinct	Fat containing
	Spiculated	

Reprinted with permission from the American College of Radiology (ACR). No other representation of this material is authorized without expressed written permission from the ACR. Refer to the ACR website at www.acr.org/Quality-Safety/Resources/BIRADS for the most current and complete version of the BI-RADS® Atlas. © American College of Radiology.

Table 10.4 BI-RADS® descriptors of masses on ultrasound.

Shape	Orientation	Margins	Echo pattern	Posterior features
Oval	Parallel	(a) Circumscribed	Anechoic	None
Round	Not parallel	(b) Not circumscribed	Hyperechoic	Enhancement
Irregular		(i) Indistinct	Complex cystic and solid	Shadowing
		(ii) Angular	Hypoechoic	Combined pattern
		(iii) Microlobulated	Isoechoic	
		(iv) Spiculated	Heterogeneous	

Reprinted with permission from the American College of Radiology (ACR). No other representation of this material is authorized without expressed written permission from the ACR. Refer to the ACR website at www.acr.org/Quality-Safety/Resources/BIRADS for the most current and complete version of the BI-RADS® Atlas. © American College of Radiology.

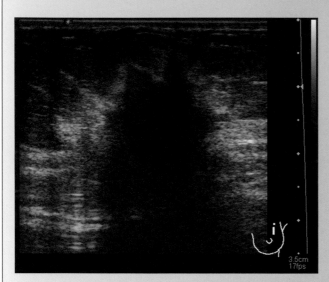

Figure 10.19 An image from the patient's ultrasound exam, depicting the palpable mass.

Sonogram of this patient's mass demonstrates many typical characteristics of malignancy: it is irregular in shape, is not parallel, has angular and indistinct margins with a hyperechoic rim, and demonstrates posterior acoustic shadowing (Figure 10.19).

Physical exam demonstrates that the mass is hard and irregular. If a cancer has invaded the underlying muscle, the mass may feel "fixed" in place.

Sonographic evaluation of this patient's axilla demonstrates that she has an abnormally enlarged axillary lymph node. The normally thin, uniform cortex of the node has a focal cortical bulge: this is concerning for a metastatic deposit (Figure 10.20).

In combination, the mammographic and sonographic features of a mass allow the radiologist to designate the level of suspicion for malignancy and make an appropriate recommendation. This patient's findings were highly suspicious, and the radiologist assigned a BI-RADS® 5. The patient underwent ultrasound-guided biopsy of the breast mass and the abnormal axillary lymph node, and was diagnosed with invasive ductal carcinoma with axillary metastasis. She also underwent biopsy of the linear calcifications elsewhere in the same breast, which showed DCIS. Given the extent of her disease, she underwent mastectomy and was referred on for additional oncologic treatment.

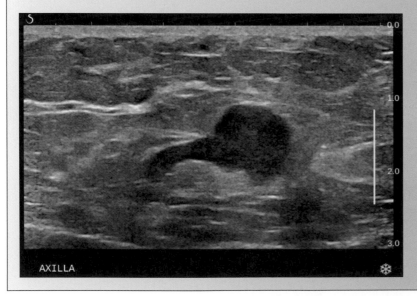

Figure 10.20 An image from the patient's ultrasound exam, depicting an abnormally enlarged axillary lymph node.

Scenario 10.3 My patient, a 25-year-old woman, has a palpable lump in her breast.

As in Scenario 10.2, this patient also has a palpable lump. However, since this patient is only 25 years old, she is much less likely to have a malignancy. We know that an ultrasound will be necessary to characterize her breast lump and is likely to be sufficient to decide upon an appropriate BI-RADS® assessment. Mammography is less likely to be informative, as she probably has very dense breast tissue because of her young age; doing a mammogram would probably be an unnecessary radiation exposure. Thus, we do not begin her workup with a mammogram, but instead with a targeted ultrasound exam.

An ultrasound of this patient's palpable lump demonstrates a mass (Figure 10.21).

Note how this mass differs from the previous case—it has a regular, oval shape; it has a circumscribed, defined margin; it shows no posterior acoustic shadowing; and it is parallel in orientation. On physical exam, this mass is slightly firm, but is smooth and mobile. These are all features of a benign mass, a fibroadenoma. Fibroadenomas are composed of fibrous and glandular elements and are common in younger women.

Even though this mass has benign imaging characteristics, biopsy is almost always recommended when a mass is palpable. A newly palpable mass suggests that it has been growing in size (such that the patient is now able to feel it); and although benign masses can grow, usually you'd rather biopsy a fibroadenoma than miss a cancer.

In expert hands, a classically benign-appearing palpable mass can be observed closely over time, rather than biopsied. In this situation, the mass can be assigned a BI-RADS® 3—designating a *probably* benign finding—and is evaluated every 6 months for 2 years total. If the mass remains unchanged over this time period, it is deemed benign and can be downgraded to a BI-RADS® 2. However, this management decision is the exception, rather than rule.

This scenario raises another critical point in breast imaging: when a patient presents with a palpable lump, you need to be absolutely sure that you are imaging the lump that she feels. Consider Figure 10.22, which shows mammogram images from a different patient presenting with a palpable mass.

In this case, the palpable mass was actually too deep/posterior to be included on the mammogram, although the skin BB marker is seen. However, there is a second mass in the vicinity—a small spiculated mass. Don't assume that the mass you see on mammogram is the mass that she feels!

An ultrasound exam shows clearly that the two masses are completely different in appearance, as well as location (Figure 10.23). At biopsy, the palpable mass was a papillary cancer, and the incidentally noted spiculated mass was an invasive ductal carcinoma.

Critical observation: Evaluate palpable masses with an extremely critical eye. Do your own exam to ensure that you are feeling (and imaging) what the patient and/or clinician felt.

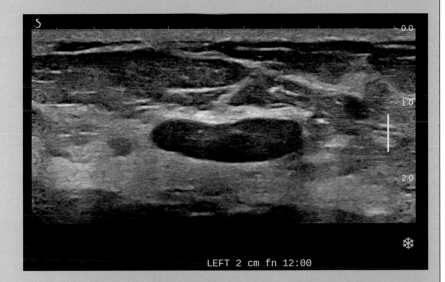

Figure 10.21 An image from the patient's ultrasound exam, depicting the palpable mass.

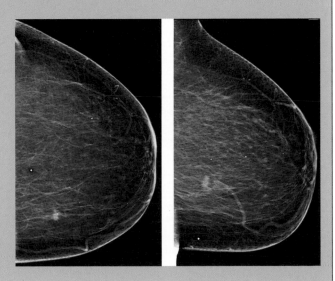

Figure 10.22 Mammogram of a patient who presented with a palpable mass in her inframammary fold. A small spiculated mass is seen within the inner breast, but does *not* correspond to the palpable mass!

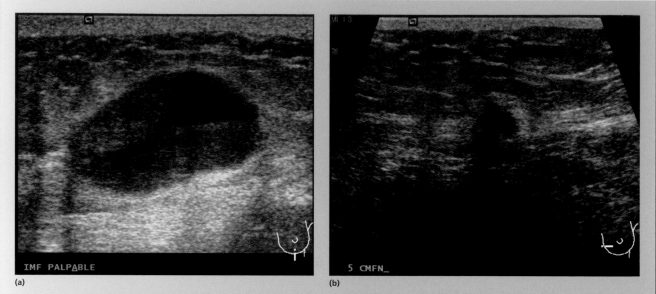

Figure 10.23 (a) The palpable lump is a complex solid and cystic mass in the inframammary fold, 6:00 position. (b) The small spiculated mass on mammogram corresponds to a hypoechoic mass with indistinct margins in the lower inner quadrant.

Summary

The goal of breast imaging is to detect breast cancer, diagnose it, and assist in its treatment. Radiologists depend on several different imaging modalities to evaluate the breast tissue, primarily mammography and ultrasound.

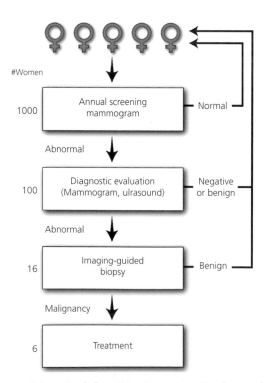

Figure 10.24 Schematic of a breast imaging program. Numbers on the left side of the diagram indicate an estimate of how many women are seen at each step, based on an initial screening pool of 1000 women.

Breast cancer can assume many different forms on imaging: it usually presents as calcifications, a mass, or architectural distortion. A standardized lexicon called BI-RADS® is used to describe the imaging findings and to recommend appropriate management of the finding.

Figure 10.24 again illustrates a typical screening program. To give you a sense of proportion, a typical breakdown of the number of women undergoing each step is now included.

The goal of a screening program is to be as sensitive and specific as possible—that is, to find cancers and to pass normal/benign findings. Good imaging technique is critical in order to obtain maximal sensitivity and specificity (remember how cancers can be excluded from the image?).

Screening mammography is an appropriate test for *asymptomatic* women. If your patient has a palpable lump or other breast symptom, then she should have a diagnostic imaging workup so that the radiologist can specifically evaluate the area of concern.

Screening mammography has been studied extensively and has been shown to benefit women by reducing breast cancer mortality. As our understanding of breast cancer continues to evolve, screening regimens can be refined to provide the greatest benefit for women's health.

Suggested reading

American Cancer Society. Learn about Breast cancer http://www.cancer.org/cancer/breastcancer/index.

American College of Radiology. BI-RADS Committee (2013) *BI-RADS® Atlas*, 5th edn. American College of Radiology, Reston, VA.

Appleton, C.M. & Wiele, K. (eds) (2011) *Breast Imaging Cases*. University Press, Oxford.

Gilda, C. (2008) *Breast Imaging Companion*, 3rd edn. Lippincott Williams & Wilkins, Philadelphia, PA.

CHAPTER 11

Pediatric imaging

Cassandra M. Sams

Department of Radiology, University of North Carolina, Chapel Hill, USA

Unlike other diagnostic imaging subspecialties, pediatric radiology is not limited to a single organ system or imaging modality. Instead, this subspecialty is based predominantly on age, with those patients under the age of 18 typically in the purview of the pediatric radiologist. The breadth and depth of imaging in this subspecialty makes it both challenging and exciting.

Another element of the complexity of pediatric radiology hearkens to the well-known saying that "children are not just little adults." To take that one step further, a neonate is not just a small child; an abdominal mass in a newborn infant has a different differential diagnosis than a 5-year-old with a similar presentation. Thus, pediatric radiology represents a complex interplay between a variety of organ systems, imaging modalities, and age-specific pathologies.

Role of imaging

As described previously, pediatric imaging uses all imaging modalities to evaluate all organ systems. Thus, a thorough discussion of what constitutes "normal" would be a lengthy discussion and would have considerable overlap with prior chapters. As such, the following discussion will be limited to relevant differences in imaging techniques and important considerations when imaging the pediatric population.

Emphasis will be placed on dose reduction strategies in this particularly radiosensitive population. While radiation is an important consideration when selecting the appropriate imaging test in all patients, it is even more important in the pediatric population due to both their heightened radiosensitivity and their anticipated longer life expectancy. Thus, imaging studies using ionizing radiation (radiographs, fluoroscopy, computed tomography (CT), and nuclear medicine studies) should be used judiciously. As a result, magnetic resonance imaging (MRI) and ultrasound (US) play an even more important role in the diagnosis and monitoring of diseases.

Radiography

Despite the increasing utilization of cross-sectional imaging, such as CT and MRI, radiographs continue to play an important role in the diagnostic workup. Although substantially smaller than the radiation risk of a CT, radiographs do require radiation for image formation and thus they should be used judiciously. An important consideration is that the more soft tissue that the X-ray must penetrate, the more radiation is required to create a diagnostic image, that is, a lateral chest radiograph requires more radiation than a frontal chest radiograph. Another consideration is that imaging findings of pathology may persist for some time despite clinical improvement. For example, a patient with pneumonia may improve within hours to days after receiving appropriate antibiotic therapy, but their chest radiographs will likely remain abnormal for weeks.

However, for certain indications, radiography is indispensible. For example, in the ICU setting, frequent radiographs are needed to assess the position of the various lines and tubes. With a patient presenting with an acute or surgical abdomen, an upright radiograph of the abdomen or chest is a quick and relatively reliable way to determine the presence of free air. Finally, with virtually any musculoskeletal (MSK) concern, a radiograph is the appropriate initial study to obtain.

Fluoroscopy

Fluoroscopy is the imaging modality that uses X-rays to capture real-time images. The indications for various fluoroscopic exams, particularly those involving the upper gastrointestinal (UGI) tract, can be extensive. Therefore, only a critical selection of these exams, and their respective indications, will be discussed briefly in the section GI. A *modified* barium swallow is an exam performed in conjunction with speech pathology whose primary purpose is to assess swallowing function and the presence of aspiration with a variety of tested liquid and solid food consistencies. A barium swallow is rarely used in the pediatric population and is limited to an evaluation of the esophagus. This is most frequently ordered in

Critical Observations in Radiology for Medical Students, First Edition. Katherine R. Birchard, Kiran Reddy Busireddy, and Richard C. Semelka.

the setting of esophageal stricture or rupture. A UGI is an examination of the esophagus, stomach, and duodenum using liquid contrast and most frequently dilute barium. One of the most frequent indications for a UGI in the pediatric population is to evaluate for the presence of malrotation. A small bowel follow-through (SBFT) can be ordered in conjunction with a UGI. This test can be useful to assess the transit time of the bowel as well as to evaluate for disease processes that preferentially affect the small bowel, such as Crohn's disease.

US

US uses sound waves and their differential rate of transmission through tissues to create images.

With their small sizes and typically slim body habitus, pediatric patients are ideal candidates for ultrasonography. In pediatrics, particularly neonates, it can be used to assess virtually any organ system, ranging from brain to chest and to abdomen. There is even an increasing usage of US for the assessment of bowel wall and MSK pathology.

Of course, there are limitations of US. Bone prevents the transmission of the US beam so, for example, while the brain can be evaluated through the anterior fontanel of a neonate, once this fontanel starts to close, US becomes progressively limited. Bowel gas also prevents the transmission of the US beam, so if a patient is particularly gassy (often from crying) or has eaten recently, their abdominal US may be of low yield. This explains why patients are required to be NPO for several hours prior to abdominal US if at all possible. Lastly, as the girth of the patient increases, image quality often declines.

CT

CT uses a rotating gantry to transmit and receive X-rays that are then reconstructed into the cross-sectional images.

In current practice, CTs are obtained almost exclusively using only a single phase, that is, the patient is scanned only once with *or* without contrast, due to radiation risk; multiphase CTs, or CTs with *and* without contrast, are very rarely used in the pediatric population. Thus, in the setting of trauma or other emergent situations, CT remains the primary choice for imaging. CT is also unparalleled in imaging ossified bone matrix, particularly in the evaluation of complex fractures and bone tumors.

MRI

MRI excels at soft tissue contrast; thus, pathology in the brain and solid organs is exquisitely depicted. Additionally, dynamic imaging performed by imaging the same body part at various time points after the administration of contrast can be performed as there is no radiation risk.

The intravenous (IV) contrast agent used with MRI is gadolinium, a rare earth metal. In the pediatric population, the length of the exam coupled with the need for the patient to remain motionless frequently requires the use of sedation. Recently, however, studies have demonstrated the deleterious effects of repeated use of sedation so there has been a push to create faster imaging sequences coupled with inventive methods of keeping children entertained and still in the magnet, such as the use of video goggles.

Nuclear medicine

Nuclear medicine represents a heterogeneous group of exams whose similarity relies on the use of radioactive materials (radiotracers) to obtain images as they decay. Nuclear medicine visualizes physiology in action. For example, a VQ scan shows how well lungs are ventilated and perfused and a DMSA scan shows how well the renal cortex is functioning. In general, nuclear medicine exams are used to answer a very specific question (e.g., does this patient have biliary atresia? or is this kidney obstructed?). The drawbacks to nuclear medicine are its use of ionizing radiation as the radiotracer decays and its generally poor image resolution. The patient also needs to stay still for prolonged periods of time so sedation is often necessary.

Imaging findings in critical disease processes

(a) Airway

1 *Acute epiglottitis* (Figure 11.1g)
  ◦ Thickened epiglottis "thumbprint sign" on lateral radiograph of neck.
  ◦ Supine imaging is contraindicated in the setting of acute epiglottitis.

2 *Croup* (Figure 11.1d–f)
  ◦ Steeple sign on frontal radiographs of the neck and chest, caused by subglottic edema
  ◦ Ballooning of the hypopharynx on the lateral radiograph

3 *Retropharyngeal abscess* (Figure 11.1h)
  ◦ Increased prevertebral soft tissue swelling on lateral chest radiograph
  ◦ CT with IV contrast to characterize the extent of abscess

4 *Foreign body aspiration* (Figure 11.2)
  ◦ Asymmetric inflation of the lungs on frontal radiographs.
  ◦ Decubitus views or chest fluoroscopy can be used to assess for the presence of hyperinflation.

(b) Chest

5 *Respiratory distress syndrome (RDS) (surfactant deficiency)*
  ◦ Low lung volumes (in the absence of positive pressure ventilation).
  ◦ Diffuse opacities, most frequently described as fine and/or granular.
  ◦ Be alert to complications of air leak/barotrauma in ventilated patients.

6 *Round pneumonia* (Figure 11.3)
  ◦ Rounded, well-defined opacity seen on frontal and lateral chest radiographs with clinical suspicion of pneumonia.
  ◦ If doubt exists as to the origin of this "mass," repeat radiographs in 4–6 weeks.

7 *Bronchiolitis*
  ◦ Chest radiographs important in excluding other causes of respiratory distress.
  ◦ Hyperinflation is the most sensitive finding in the setting of bronchiolitis.

(c) GI

8 *Hypertrophic pyloric stenosis (HPS)* (Figure 11.4)
  ◦ US is currently the imaging test of choice.
  ◦ Hypertrophied pylorus measuring greater than 3 in thickness and greater than 1.6 cm in length.
  ◦ Minimal gastric contents seen to pass through the pylorus.

9 *Intussusception* (Figure 11.5)
  ◦ Small bowel obstruction with right lower quadrant soft tissue lesion on radiographs.
  ◦ Targetoid appearance on US.
  ◦ Air-reduction enema should be performed by an experienced pediatric radiologist after consultation with a pediatric surgeon.

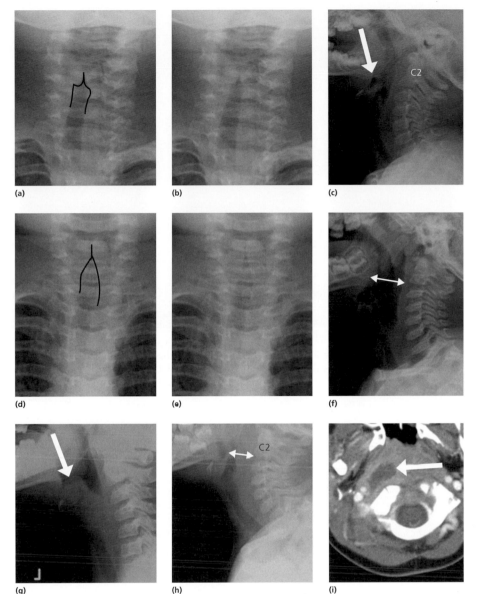

Figure 11.1 Normal frontal radiographs of the neck. Normal frontal radiographs of the neck show the normal "shoulders" of the airway (outlined in black on a) representing the vocal cords (a and b). Normal lateral radiograph of the neck. Note the arrow demonstrating the appropriate size of the epiglottis. Anterior to C2, the soft tissue is normal and thin (c). Abnormal frontal radiograph of the neck due to croup. The loss of the normal "shoulders" due to subglottic edema creates the "steeple sign" (outlined in black on d) (d and e). Abnormal lateral radiograph of the neck due to croup. The white arrow indicates "ballooning" or widening of the hypopharynx when compared to c (f). Abnormal lateral radiograph of the neck demonstrating marked thickening of the epiglottis, as indicated by the arrow, in the setting of epiglottitis (g). Abnormal lateral radiograph of the neck demonstrates thickening of the soft tissues anterior to C2 (h). Axial contrast-enhanced CT of the same child as in (h) showing a rim-enhancing fluid collection compatible with a retropharyngeal abscess (i).

○ Abdomen radiographs must be obtained prior to reduction to exclude bowel perforation with resultant free air.

10 *Malrotation with midgut volvulus* (Figure 11.6b and c)

○ Malrotation with volvulus is a pediatric emergency due to the risk of bowel ischemia.

○ UGI is the gold standard for the diagnosis of malrotation. Some institutions also use US, although this is controversial.

○ The normal duodenum has a C-shaped course in which it courses posteriorly with the duodenojejunal junction (DJJ) to the left of the midline at the level of the duodenal bulb.

11 *Necrotizing enterocolitis (NEC)* (Figure 11.7)

○ Bowel distension with lack of bowel motion between sequential radiographs

○ Pneumatosis in the bowel wall

○ Close inspection for evidence of portal venous gas and free air

12 *Appendicitis* (Figure 11.8)

○ US is a good first-line imaging choice for the evaluation of possible appendicitis in children.

○ Noncompressible appendix measuring greater than 6 mm, with secondary signs including appendicolith, wall thickening greater than 2 mm, periappendiceal free fluid, enlarged mesenteric lymph nodes, and inflammatory changes in the mesentery.

○ While US and CT are both excellent at visualizing periappendiceal abscesses, CT is more sensitive in the evaluation of free air.

○ MRI has been shown to be as sensitive and specific as CT and has the benefit of nonionizing radiation.

13 *Ingested foreign body*

○ Important to differentiate coins from disc batteries or magnets. While coins may pass without complication, batteries and magnets must be removed emergently due to risks of bowel wall injury (which can be life-threatening within hours of ingestion).

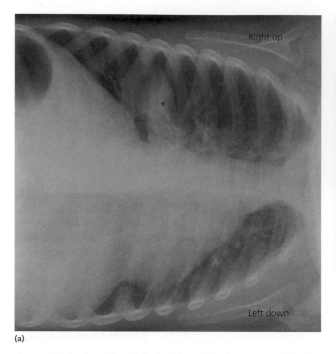

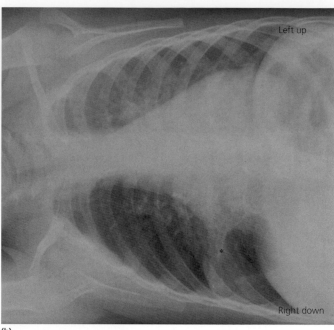

(a)   **(b)**

Figure 11.2 Aspirated foreign body. Bilateral decubitus views of the chest in a toddler who aspirated a peanut. Note how in (a) the left side is hazier than the right side due to the compressive effects of gravity (a). However, in (b), the right side remains radiolucent (dark) due to air trapping from a foreign body in the airway. The asterisk is indicating an area of persistent atelectasis (b).

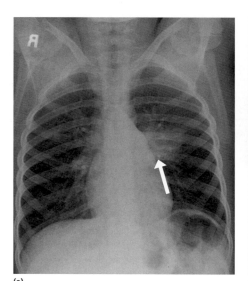

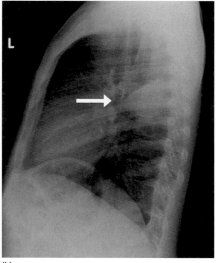

(a)   **(b)**

Figure 11.3 Round pneumonia versus posterior mediastinal mass. Frontal and lateral view of the chest in a young child presenting with fever and cough. The arrows indicate a rounded opacity in the posterior aspect of the left lower lobe. This is compatible with a round pneumonia in this clinical setting. However, in the absence of fever or cough, this may be concerning for a posterior mediastinal mass (a–b).

(d) Genitourinary (GU)

    14 *Ovarian and testicular torsion*
- US used in the diagnosis of both these entities.
- Asymmetrically enlarged or heterogeneous gonad.
- The presence of blood flow on US does not exclude the diagnosis of torsion.

    15 *Posterior urethral valves (PUV)* (Figure 11.9)
- Marked dilatation of the posterior urethra during the voiding portion of the voiding cystourethrogram (VCUG).
- Actual valve is thin and difficult to visualize.

(e) MSK

    16 *Slipped capital femoral epiphysis (SCFE)* (Figure 11.10)
- Two views (frontal and frog leg) should be ordered to evaluate for this condition.
- Initial imaging findings may be subtle with asymmetric widening of the physis.
- More advanced cases present with the femoral head slipping posteromedially off the metaphysis.
- Patient should be told not to weight bear and urgent consultation with orthopedics is required.

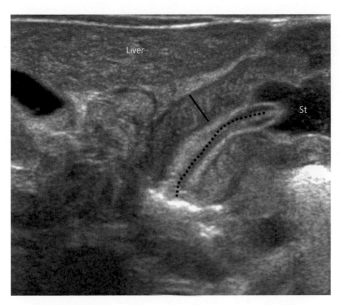

Figure 11.4 Hypertrophic pyloric. Grayscale ultrasound image of the epigastrium of a 6-week-old infant with hypertrophic pyloric stenosis. The liver is seen along the superior margin of the image, and ST indicates the stomach along the right aspect of the image. The dotted line indicates the length of the pyloric channel, and the solid line indicates the width of one wall of the pylorus. The pylorus is longer and thicker than normal.

17 *Developmental dysplasia of the hips (DDH)* (Figure 11.11)
  ° Initial US should be performed at approximately 6 weeks of age.
  ° After 6 months, radiographs are most useful.
  ° Imaging should demonstrate shallow acetabulum with possible subluxation/dislocation of femoral heads.
(f) MISC
18 *Umbilical catheters*
  ° Umbilical artery catheter (UAC) should terminate preferably between T6 and T10, although L3–L5 is also permissible.
  ° Umbilical venous catheter (UVC) should terminate at the inferior cavoatrial junction.

Congenital developmental diseases and anomalies

Chest
Congenital pulmonary airway malformation
A number of nonneoplastic masses can be present in the neonatal lung. Antenatally, the diagnosis can be suggested based on the presence of a mass lesion in the lung. These masses may shrink considerably in size while still in utero and not be apparent on postnatal radiographs. Thus, postnatal CTs are required for the evaluation of any antenatally suspected lung masses.

Congenital pulmonary airway malformation (CPAM) is a heterogeneous entity that has undergone a number of name changes in recent years. Based on the specific subtype, this may appear solid (due to the presence of numerous microcysts) or as a cystic lesion (due to the presence of macrocysts):
• At birth, the cystic lesions may appear solid on chest radiographs and chest CT due to the presence of retained fetal fluid. The most

common subtype is the type 1 composed of one or more large (1–10 cm) cysts.
• On chest radiographs and CT, these lesions most frequently appear as a multicystic mass with variable degree of mass effect on surrounding structures, as seen in Figure 11.12a. Contrast should be administered to assess the blood supply of these lesions and exclude the possibility of a sequestration (discussed in the following).

Congenital lobar emphysema
Congenital lobar emphysema (CLE) exists on the spectrum of bronchial atresia and is thought to be due to an abnormally formed bronchus preventing normal egress of air from the affected segment of the lung. Most frequently, these are found in the upper lungs, left more frequently than right:
• As with CPAM, immediately after birth, these may appear as a solid mass due to the presence of retained fluid. As the fluid clears, the lung will appear hyperlucent with varying degrees of mass effect on the surrounding structures, as seen in Figure 11.12b.
• CT is frequently used to make the definitive diagnosis with the lung appearing hyperlucent (darker) than the normal lung with spreading out and decreased caliber of the feeding vessels; as with the CPAM, IV contrast should be administered to assess for aberrant blood supply.
CLE are frequently resected due to problems with mass effect but, if asymptomatic, may be observed.

Sequestration
Sequestration consists of abnormal lung parenchyma with aberrant connections to the bronchial tree and pulmonary arteries. It is divided into two forms, intralobar and extralobar. Extralobar sequestrations are present since birth, have their own pleural investment and venous drainage, and are frequently associated with other congenital anomalies. The intralobar subtype is postulated to be due to recurrent infections and is frequently found in an older patient population.

Both are most frequently seen in the lung bases and may contain a variable number of cystic and solid components:
• The most helpful feature distinguishing a sequestration from other congenital lung anomalies is the presence of a systemic artery feeding the lesion, thus illustrating the importance of an IV contrast-enhanced CT in the evaluation of congenital lung masses.
Due to the risk of recurrent infection, sequestrations are frequently resected. These lesions (CPAM, CLE, and sequestrations) may exist in complete isolation or occur with one another in which case the lesion is termed a "hybrid" lesion. While imaging findings can suggest the specific diagnosis, frequently, pathology is needed for the final diagnosis.

Congenital diaphragmatic hernia
Congenital diaphragmatic hernia (CDH) is extrusion of abdominal contents into the thoracic cavity, typically through a posterior defect (Bochdalek hernia). This most frequently occurs on the left-hand side with extension of bowel into the left hemithorax; less frequently seen is herniation of liver and other intra-abdominal contents into the right hemithorax. Due to the presence of abdominal contents in the thoracic cavity, the lungs do not form normally. Depending on the gestational age in which the herniation occurred, there is a variable degree of pulmonary hypoplasia present not only

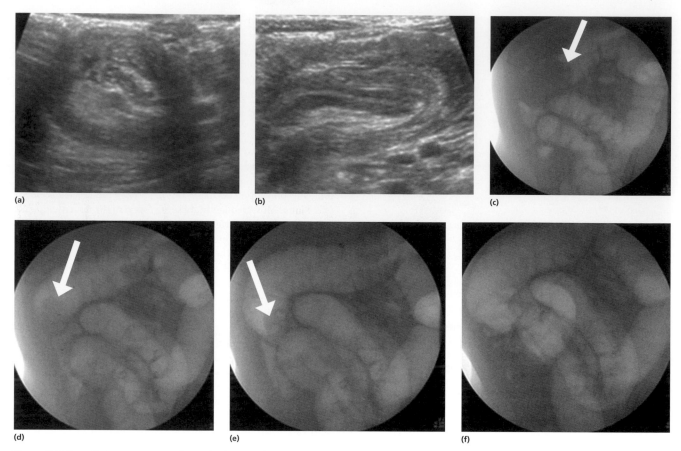

Figure 11.5 Ileocolic intussusception. Grayscale ultrasound images in the axial (a) and sagittal (b) planes in a 2-year-old with intermittent colicky abdominal pain found to have an ileocolic intussusception. The axial image shows the classic targetoid appearance of the bowel telescoped on itself. The sagittal image shows the relative length of the intussuscepted bowel (a–b). Images obtained during fluoroscopic-guided air-reduction enema of the intussusception. On (c), the intussuscepted bowl is seen as a soft tissue mass filling the right colon. The progression of images shows reduction of the bowel with the final image (f) demonstrating resolution of the soft tissue mass with an increase in the amount of small bowel gas. Both of these findings are typically seen after a successful reduction (c–f).

due to mass effect from the abdominal contents on the affected side but also the contralateral lung due to shift of the mediastinal contents. The degree of pulmonary hypoplasia is the primary determinant of patient outcome:

- The diagnosis is frequently made in utero with either US or MRI. A chest radiograph performed early in the neonatal course will show abdominal contents (most frequently gas-filled bowel) in the thorax with shift of the mediastinum. The abdomen is typically scaphoid or flat with a paucity of intra-abdominal bowel gas.
- Cross-sectional imaging, most frequently with CT, may be used to assess the size of the diaphragmatic defect and help with surgical planning.

RDS/surfactant deficiency

A near ubiquitous diagnosis in the premature patient (<36 weeks) population, the imaging findings of RDS, and its complications are important for pediatricians and radiologists alike to recognize. RDS occurs due to a lack of surfactant in the immature lung. Clinically, this manifests as poorly compliant lungs, which may be difficult to ventilate:

- Radiographically, there are low lung volumes (in the absence of positive pressure ventilation) with diffuse opacities that can range from fine and granular to diffuse whiteout of the lungs. These opacities improve when exogenous surfactant is administered. Due to the poorly compliant lungs, these patients are at risk for various air leaks, including pneumothorax, pneumomediastinum, and pulmonary interstitial emphysema (PIE), in which air dissects through the bronchial tree creating branching lucencies in the opacified lung.
- After 4 weeks of age, patients in this group are deemed to have chronic lung disease. This entity is thought to be due to the prolonged need for positive pressure ventilation and supplemental oxygen and manifests radiographically as coarse interstitial opacities with varying degrees of cystic change and regions of atelectasis and hyperinflation.

Transient tachypnea of the newborn

In a term infant, a frequent cause of respiratory distress is transient tachypnea of the newborn (TTN), thought to be due to retained fetal fluid. TTN occurs more frequently in infants born via c-section:

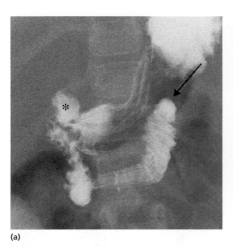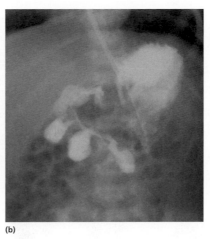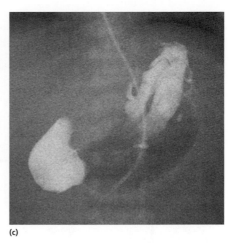

(a)   (b)   (c)

Figure 11.6 Midgut volvulus. Upper GI from a normal child showing an appropriately positioned DJJ indicated by the arrow. Note that it is to the left of the spine and at the same level as the duodenal bulb that is indicated by the asterisk. Both of these findings are necessary to ensure that the patient is properly rotated; additionally, a lateral view is needed to show that the duodenum extends retroperitoneally (a). Upper GI in a patient with malrotation with volvulus indicated by the classic "corkscrew" or "apple peel" (arrow) appearance to the duodenum (b). Upper GI in a different patient with malrotation. The contrast bolus stops abruptly near the second portion of the duodenum and during the course of the exam was not seen to proceed further. This finding can be seen in a variety of causes of duodenal obstruction but in this case was secondary to midgut volvulus (c).

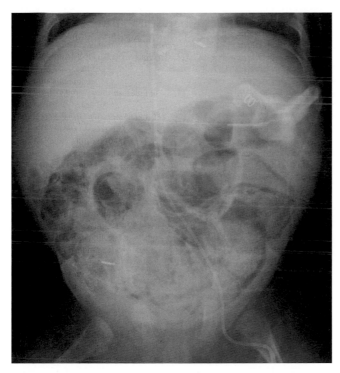

Figure 11.7 Necrotizing enterocolitis. Single frontal radiograph of the abdomen in an infant with massive pneumatosis in the setting of necrotizing enterocolitis. The lucent rings outlining the bowel contents represent pneumatosis or gas within the bowel wall. No free air or portal venous gas is identified.

- Chest radiographs obtained soon after birth are frequently normal but may show mild hyperinflation. A small amount of pleural fluid may be present, as well as hazy or interstitial opacities due to the fetal fluid.

The diagnosis is primarily a clinical one, with resolution of the respiratory distress 24–48 h after birth.

Meconium aspiration

Meconium aspiration most frequently occurs in the term or post-term infants. The diagnosis is suspected when meconium is present in the amniotic fluid coupled with severe respiratory distress in the neonate:

- On radiographs, the classic findings are coarse, ropelike opacities radiating out from the hila, frequently in the presence of hyperinflation. However, the radiographic appearance may overlap with infection, edema, or even RDS, and therefore clinical correlation with the birth history is key to correctly diagnosing this entity.

Positive pressure ventilation is frequently needed, and due to poor compliance of the underlying parenchyma, air leak phenomena similar to those in the RDS-affected lung are frequent complications.

Congenital heart disease

The wide array of congenital heart diseases is beyond the scope of this chapter. Chest radiographs are very nonspecific aside from several "classic" findings that are not frequently manifest. Therefore, echocardiography remains the mainstay in the diagnosis of the various forms of congenital heart disease. Nevertheless, chest radiographs can be complementary to echocardiography particularly in determining the pulmonary vascularity and edema:

- Based on the radiographic appearance, congenital heart disease can be divided into those with decreased, normal, or increased pulmonary vascularity. Vascularity is determined by the number and size of the vessels present.
- With diminished vascularity, the lungs appear darker with fewer apparent vessels radiating from the hila. The converse is true with increased vascularity—the lungs appear whiter with more vessels apparent. Decreased vascularity occurs in those conditions in which the blood is unable to leave the right side of the heart to enter the lungs. These may include tetralogy of Fallot, as well as pulmonary and tricuspid atresia. Increased vascularity occurs when there is too much blood in the lungs most frequently due to the presence of a shunt, such as an atrial

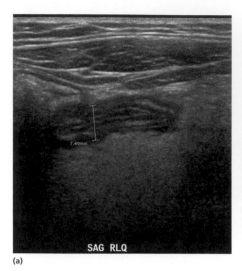
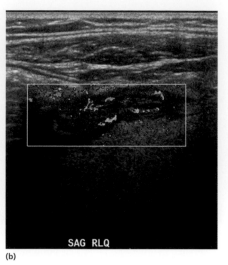

(a)   (b)

Figure 11.8 Acute appendicitis. Grayscale and color ultrasound images of the appendix. Note that the calipers measure this blind-ending tubular structure as greater than 6 mm. Additionally, the mucosa of the appendix is hyperemic. Both of these findings are concerning for acute appendicitis (a and b).

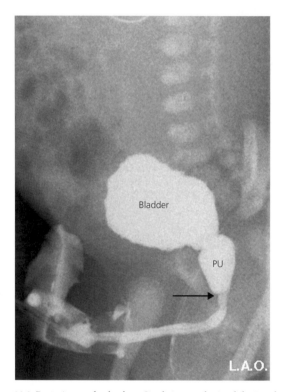

Figure 11.9 Posterior urethral valves. Single image obtained during the voiding portion of a voiding cystourethrogram in a male with posterior urethral valves. PU indicates the dilated posterior urethra and an arrow indicates the level of the valves where there is an abrupt change in the caliber with a faint linear filling defect, likely representing the valves.

septal defect (ASD), ventricular septal defect (VSD), or patent ductus arteriosus (PDA).

Pulmonary edema may occur from a wide variety of causes, and the presence or worsening of edema may dictate a change in the management of the patient:

- Early indicators of pulmonary edema include peribronchial cuffing (in which the on-end bronchiole resembles a donut) and indistinctness of the vasculature. This may proceed to

interlobular septal thickening, best seen as Kerley B lines along the lung periphery. The most pronounced edema may be seen as alveolar edema manifesting as fluffy opacities that typically begin in the perihilar region and proceed to the periphery.

Thymus

While not a form of pathology, the appearance of the thymus on radiography can be a source of confusion to radiologists and clinicians alike:

- The thymus in a neonate is its largest size relative to the body and on chest radiographs may mimic a mediastinal mass. It can have a variety of configurations as seen in Figure 11.13a–f.
- Ultrasonography using a high-frequency linear transducer can be a good problem-solving tool when there is a particularly atypical radiographic appearance. The echotexture of the thymus is predominantly hypoechoic when compared to the liver and spleen with punctate and linear echogenic foci representing fatty tissue interspersed among the thymic tissue.

GI

Neonatal bowel obstruction is a frequently encountered problem in pediatric radiology. Bowel obstruction can be divided into two broad categories of upper and lower obstruction. Differentiating between dilated small bowel and colon is not possible in an infant, so the level of obstruction is determined primarily on the number of dilated bowel loops present on radiographs as seen in Figure 11.14a–c. Depending on the level of obstruction, bowel obstruction may present clinically with feeding intolerance, bilious emesis, failure to pass meconium, and abdominal distension. The differential diagnosis for both upper and lower bowel obstructions is broad, and only the most frequently encountered entities will be discussed in the following.

Esophageal atresia

Esophageal atresia with or without a tracheoesophageal fistula is the most proximal of the bowel obstructions and has a number of different forms, based on the configuration of the esophagus with variable fistulous connections to the trachea. The most common

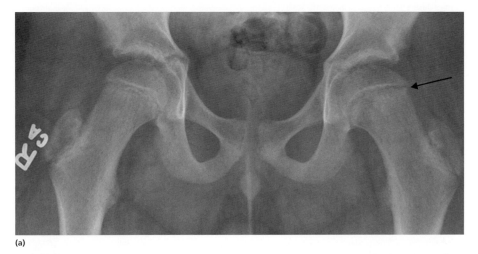

(a)

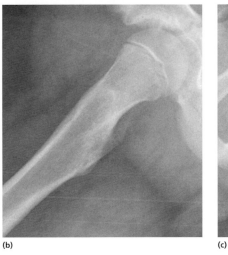

(b)

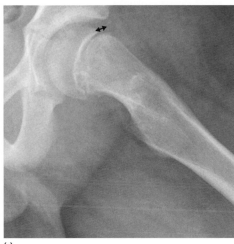

(c)

Figure 11.10 Slipped capital femoral epiphysis. Frontal radiograph of the pelvis in a male with an early slipped capital femoral epiphysis who presented with left-sided hip pain. The arrow indicates subtle widening of the physis when compared to the right side (a). Frog leg lateral view of the normal right hip shows appropriate alignment of the femoral head and neck (b). Frog leg lateral view of the affected left hip shows the offset capital femoral epiphysis. The findings are much more apparent on this view reinforcing the fact that two views are needed to make this diagnosis (c).

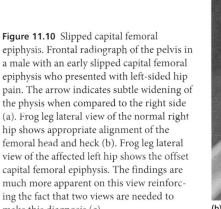

(a)

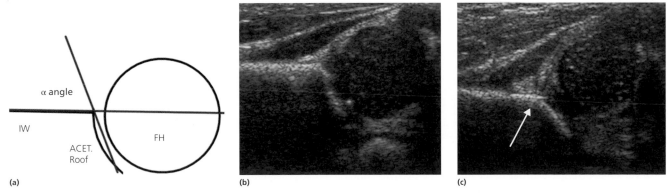

(b)

(c)

Figure 11.11 Normal and dysplastic hip. Illustration indicating the structures obtained during a coronal view of the hip in an infant. The black horizontal line labeled IW indicates the iliac wing that is contiguous with the sloping acetabular roof labeled Acet roof. The angle between these two structures should be 60° or greater. Additionally, the horizontal line extending from the iliac wing should bisect the femoral head labeled FH, and the femoral head should be greater than 50% covered (a). Grayscale ultrasound image of a normal neonatal hip in the coronal plane (b). Grayscale ultrasound image of a dysplastic hip in a neonate. While not measured on this figure, the alpha angle would measure less than 60°, and the femoral head coverage is approximately 25%. Additionally, the arrow indicates blunting or rounding ilium/acetabular roof angle (c).

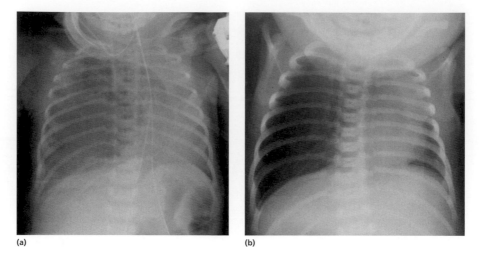

(a) (b)

Figure 11.12 Congenital Pulmonary Airway Malformation (CPAM) and congenital lobar emphysema (CLE). Frontal radiograph of a neonate with a large multicystic mass filling the right hemithorax and displacing the mediastinum to the left with compression of the left lung. This mass has a complex internal architecture and is most compatible with a type 1 congenital pulmonary airway malformation (CPAM) (a). Frontal radiograph of a neonate with hyperinflation of the right hemithorax resulting in displacement of the mediastinum to the left with compression of the left lung. In contrast to (a), the hyperinflated lung looks homogeneously dark. This appearance is typical for CLE (b).

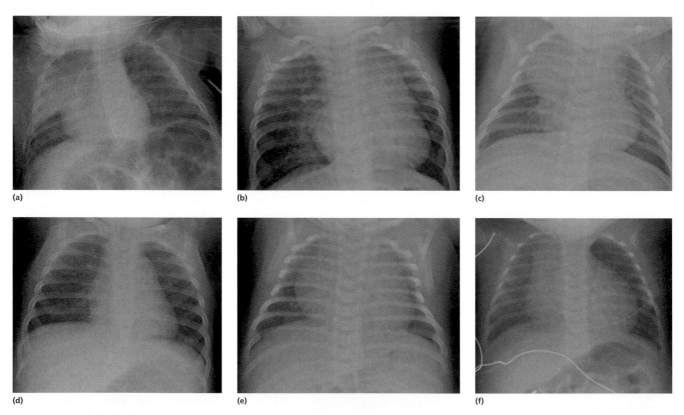

(a) (b) (c)

(d) (e) (f)

Figure 11.13 Normal appearance of the thymus in six neonates. (a–f) Note that the thymus can vary widely in appearance and resemble a mass. If there is question of a mass versus normal thymus, ultrasound should be the first-line imaging modality used.

form consists of complete atresia of the proximal esophagus with a fistula between the trachea/carina and distal esophagus; this fistula accounts for the presence of distal bowel gas in this patient population:
- The diagnosis of complete esophageal atresia may be first suggested with the inability to pass a feeding tube and subsequent radiograph demonstrating the tube coiling in the proximal esophageal pouch.

- Cross-sectional imaging plays little role in the workup of esophageal atresia.
- Tracheoesophageal fistulas with a patent esophagus may present later in life due to recurrent episodes of aspiration. These may be identified on a UGI, either via visualization of the direct fistulous connection or indirectly with contrast noted in the tracheobronchial tree.

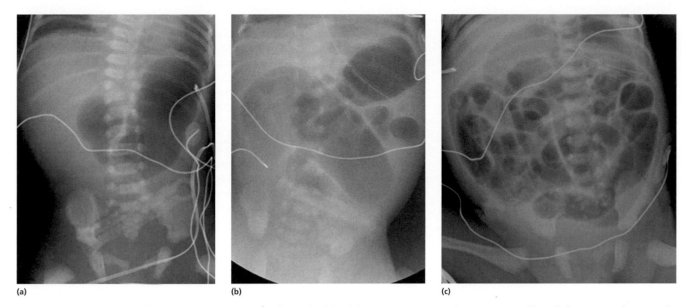

(a)   (b)   (c)

Figure 11.14 Varying levels of bowel obstruction. Frontal radiograph of the abdomen in a neonate with a very proximal bowel obstruction. The stomach and proximal duodenum are dilated creating a "double-bubble" appearance. This sign classically refers to duodenal atresia but can be seen in other forms of duodenal obstruction (a). Frontal radiograph of the abdomen in a neonate with a proximal bowel obstruction. Only a few dilated loops of bowel are identified. This neonate was found to have jejunal atresia at surgery (b). Frontal radiograph of the abdomen in a neonate with a distal bowel obstruction. Numerous dilated loops of bowel are identified with a relative paucity of bowel gas overlying the rectum in a patient with Hirschsprung's disease. Note that one cannot differentiate small bowel and colon in neonates based on the appearance of the gas-filled loops, as the small bowel lacks its normal folds and the colon lacks the distinctive haustra (c).

Duodenal atresia

Duodenal atresia is one of the more frequently encountered causes of UGI obstruction in neonates. The etiology of this condition is unknown but is frequently seen in conjunction with other anomalies; up to one third of patients with duodenal atresia have trisomy 21. The classic imaging finding is a "double bubble" resulting from dilatation of the stomach and duodenal bulb, although this sign is nonspecific and can be seen in other causes of duodenal obstruction such as annular pancreas or duodenal web:

- The double bubble can be seen on fetal imaging (both US and MRI) as well as on postnatal radiographs. In the setting of complete atresia, no bowel gas will be seen distally. Although a UGI can confirm the suspected diagnosis, frequently, no further imaging beyond a radiograph is required to make the diagnosis prior to surgical intervention.
- As with esophageal atresia, cross-sectional imaging has little role in the setting of duodenal atresia but may be used to evaluate the possibility of other congenital anomalies.

Jejunal, ileal, and colonic atresias

Atretic segments in the more distal small bowel as well as the colon are most frequently due to a vascular accident in utero. The appearance of these atresias varies, depending on the level of obstruction, with the more distal obstructions resulting in more dilated loops of bowel:

- A proximal jejunal atresia may present with a "triple-bubble" sign in which the stomach, duodenum, and proximal jejunum are all dilated. Contrast enemas may be performed prior to surgical intervention to assess for the presence of multiple atresias.

- Depending on how distal the atresia is, microcolon may be present. Microcolon develops when there is nonuse of the colon in antenatal life, that is, when no succus is able to make its way into the colon, it will remain small. Thus, the more distal the obstruction, the greater the chances are for microcolon.

Hirschsprung's disease

Hirschsprung's disease is a developmental anomaly due to a lack of ganglion cells in the colonic wall. As a result, the affected segment of bowel remains in a fixed, narrow configuration causing varying degrees of bowel obstruction. In the neonatal period, most patients present with the inability to pass meconium within the first 24 h after birth. A variable length of bowel may be affected but most frequently is limited to the rectum and distal sigmoid colon; rarely, the entire colon may be affected:

- Radiographs typically show multiple loops of dilated bowel with a lack of rectal gas. The study of choice to assess the presence of Hirschsprung's is a contrast enema. The enema will show persistent area of narrowing involving the affected segment. If the aganglionic segment is limited to the rectum and distal sigmoid, there will be a rectosigmoid ratio of less than one due to the relatively small caliber of the rectum when compared to the normal-caliber colon (in normal children, the rectum is of larger caliber than the colon).
- There may also be a sawtooth/serrated appearance to the bowel wall of the affected segment. A normal enema does not exclude the diagnosis of Hirschsprung's disease, and a suction rectal biopsy is needed for definitive diagnosis.

Meconium plug/functional immaturity of the colon/small left colon

These entities exist on a spectrum and all relate to immaturity of the colon resulting in delayed passage of meconium. Factors predisposing to this condition are gestational diabetes and magnesium administration during labor:

- Radiographs will show multiple dilated loops of bowel. Contrast enemas can be both diagnostic and therapeutic. The hallmark findings are a small-caliber left colon with a change in caliber near the splenic flexure with multiple filling defects due to the presence of meconium.

  This is a benign, self-limited entity in the vast majority of cases.

Meconium ileus

Although the names are similar, meconium plug and meconium ileus are distinct entities with vastly different clinical implications. Meconium ileus primarily affects the distal ileum with secondary effects seen in the colon. Meconium ileus is seen almost exclusively in patients with cystic fibrosis. Due to the tenacious meconium seen in this patient population, the ileum becomes obstructed resulting in underuse of the colon in antenatal life with subsequent microcolon. Older patients can experience a similar form of bowel obstruction known as meconium equivalent syndrome or distal intestinal obstruction syndrome (DIOS):

- Postnatally, dilated loops of small bowel are seen on abdominal radiographs. A "mass" representing the inspissated meconium may be seen in the right lower quadrant.
- A contrast enema is the primary test used to make the diagnosis. The enema will show a diffusely small-caliber colon or "microcolon." Variably, contrast may reflux into the ileum outlining the meconium pellets.

Biliary atresia

Biliary atresia is a rare congenital anomaly consisting of a severe deficiency or absence of extrahepatic biliary tree manifesting clinically as neonatal jaundice. US is frequently used as a screening test to exclude other possibilities of neonatal jaundice. However, it is very insensitive in the evaluation of biliary atresia. Even the presence of a gallbladder does not exclude the diagnosis of biliary atresia. CT and MRI have little role in this diagnosis:

- The appropriate imaging modality is hepatobiliary imaging in the nuclear medicine department. Using a radionuclide such as mebrofenin that is excreted by the biliary system, the patency of the extrahepatic biliary system can be ascertained. To increase the sensitivity of this test, phenobarbital is administered for 5 days prior to the examination. The imaging will demonstrate normal uptake of the radiotracer in the hepatic parenchyma with no excretion into the small bowel. Prompt diagnosis is important as the Kasai procedure or hepatoportojejunostomy is the palliative procedure used to drain the bile and is more efficacious the earlier in life it is performed.
- The role of MRI with a hepatobiliary agent, Eovist, has not yet been established, but should be promising.

GU
PUV

PUV is a developmental anomaly, seen only in males, consisting of a membrane of tissue that causes varying degrees of obstruction of the urethra. This flap of tissue arises near the base of the verumontanum, a raised area in the posterior aspect of the urethra, through which the seminal vesicles empty. With the improvements in prenatal imaging, this diagnosis can be suggested in utero. Relevant imaging findings seen on prenatal imaging are a distended urinary bladder and posterior urethra creating a "keyhole" appearance. This may coexist with unilateral or bilateral hydronephrosis. Depending on the severity of the valves, there may be oligohydramnios and pulmonary hypoplasia:

- Postnatally, a VCUG is the test of choice to make the diagnosis. The patient is positioned such that the penis can be imaged obliquely while he is voiding. The presence of the valves, demonstrated as a linear filling defect at the base of the verumontanum, may be difficult to visualize.
- The primary imaging finding is the marked dilatation of the posterior urethra with abrupt narrowing as seen in Figure 11.9. A trabeculated bladder is seen manifested by an irregular bladder contour.
- Vesicoureteral reflux (VUR) is a frequent coexisting diagnosis and is discussed in the subsequent section. On US and during the VCUG, a thickened trabeculated bladder may be seen due to the hypertrophied detrusor muscle contracting against the obstruction. As in utero, hydronephrosis may be present on US but is not required to make the diagnosis.

  If this diagnosis is missed, renal failure may develop due to long-standing obstructive uropathy.

VUR

VUR is a common diagnosis in the pediatric population. It may occur in conjunction with other anomalies such as PUV and duplicated kidneys but most frequently occurs in isolation. The etiology of this condition is unknown but is thought to be due to an abnormally short course of the ureter through the bladder wall resulting in an incompetent insertion.

Reflux of urine up the ureter and into the kidney is thought to predispose affected individuals to pyelonephritis with subsequent renal scarring and renal insufficiency. The diagnosis may be suspected antenatally by visualizing intermittent dilatation of the renal pelvis. Postnatally, the diagnosis is considered clinically in the setting of febrile UTIs. When to pursue imaging studies in the setting of febrile UTIs is a subject of considerable debate:

- When imaging is pursued, most frequently, a renal US and VCUG are performed concurrently. The US can look for evidence of renal scarring, hydronephrosis, or other renal anomalies.
- The VCUG is performed by instilling contrast into the bladder. The bladder is then filled to capacity to look for the presence of reflux up the ureters. On VCUGs, VUR is graded from 1 to 5 with the higher the number, the more severe the reflux.
- Radionuclide cystography may also be performed with installation of radiotracer through the bladder. This may be a more sensitive exam for the presence of VUR as the patient can be imaged for a longer period of time, although anatomic detail is lacking specifically of the urethra. Thus, its use is limited in making the initial diagnosis of VUR, especially in males due to the concern of PUV; however, it can be used for follow-up imaging to assess whether the reflux has resolved.

MSK
DDH

One of the more frequently encountered developmental anomalies in the neonatal population is DDH. Factors predisposing to this condition include female gender, breech presentation, and firstborn. Infants are screened clinically with the Ortolani and Barlow maneuvers performed at birth and during follow-up well-child exams. If these tests are positive, that is, a click or clunk is felt or if there are enough risk factors, a hip US may be performed starting at approximately 6 weeks of age:

- The hips are imaged in a coronal and transverse plane at rest and with stress maneuvers. The percentage of coverage of the femoral head is determined as well as the alpha angle, a measurement of how shallow the acetabulum is. Less than 50% femoral coverage or an alpha angle of less than 60° is considered abnormal. A rounded appearance of the acetabulum is also a subjective indicator of DDH; these findings are demonstrated in Figure 11.11.
- After approximately 5 months of age, the US becomes more difficult due to the femoral head becoming ossified, at which point in time radiographs can be used to determine the relationship between the femoral head and acetabulum.

This is an important diagnosis to make as the long-term consequences, if left untreated, may be severe, including avascular necrosis and early-onset osteoarthrosis.

Osteogenesis imperfecta

There are a variety of forms of osteogenesis imperfecta (OI) that range drastically in severity. The most severe form is type II, which is fatal in utero or soon after birth. The most common mild form is type 1:

- Radiographs are the primary imaging modality used in suggesting this diagnosis. There is diffuse demineralization of the bones, giving the bones a darker than normal appearance on radiograph.
- Multiple fractures in various stages of healing may be present. The ribs may have a crinkled appearance due to innumerable fractures. The extent and variations of OI are beyond the scope of this chapter. However, it is an important entity to consider when evaluating a child with multiple fractures.

Fibromatosis colli

The most frequent cause of torticollis in the neonatal period is fibromatosis colli due to hypertrophy/spasm of one of the sternocleidomastoid muscles (SCM). This results in a palpable mass in the neck as well as turning of the head toward the side of the spasming muscle. Symptoms typically present by 2 months of age and resolve by 6 months of age:

- While the diagnosis can be made via physical examination, US can be used to confirm the diagnosis. US demonstrates a mass-like appearance to the SCM. While the mass can vary in echotexture, it follows the expected course of the SCM and respects the fascial planes.
- Care on the use of MR for further imaging studies, as this lesion may be edematous and show enhancement, which if interpreted by less experienced radiologists may suggest a more aggressive disease process. Invasion of the fascial planes, lymphadenopathy, or a delayed age at initial presentation should prompt consideration of other diagnoses, such as rhabdomyosarcoma.

Miscellaneous
Umbilical catheters: UAC or UVC

The appropriate position of umbilical catheters is important for both the clinician and the radiologist to recognize. Radiographs limited to the chest, while helpful in determining the location of the tip of the catheter, may make it difficult to differentiate between a UAC and UVC, especially if there is any rotation of the patient on the film.

The course of the UAC follows that of the umbilical artery as it enters the umbilicus and courses to either common iliac artery and then into the aorta. The preferred location for the tip is the "high position" extending from T6 to T10, but the low position from L3 to L5 is also acceptable. Positioning the tip between T10 and L2 should be avoided due to the risk of a clot at the tip of the catheter extending into the celiac, SMA, or renal arteries.

The UVC takes a more circuitous route as it extends through the umbilicus into the left portal vein, through the ductus venosus into a hepatic vein and into the IVC. The tip should be located near the inferior cavoatrial junction. Not infrequently, the tips of these catheters are malpositioned, most frequently located in one of the portal veins. Due to the risk of thrombosis as well as installation of drugs and TPN into the liver, these catheters must be promptly repositioned. These catheters can also be too long, extending through the right atrium into the SVC and up the jugular vein, through the patent foramen ovale, into the left atrium and into the pulmonary vein, or through the tricuspid valve, out the right ventricular outflow tract and into the pulmonary artery.

Emergencies and trauma in the pediatric setting

Airway
Aspirated or ingested foreign body

Aspiration or ingestion of foreign bodies is a not infrequent diagnosis made in the pediatric population. While classically occurring in the toddler age group, this can also be seen in younger children, most frequently courtesy of older siblings. Older children and even teenagers are not immune to this affliction. Chest radiographs can be used to differentiate whether the foreign body is in the trachea or proximal esophagus; the trachea is more anteriorly located on lateral radiographs and is easily visible as a vertically oriented air column.

Aspirated foreign bodies frequently present with respiratory distress in the acute setting but may also present with recurrent infections due to airway obstruction. The radiographic signs can be subtle when radiolucent foreign bodies are aspirated (e.g., a peanut, one of the most frequently aspirated objects). The most common finding is hyperinflation of the affected lung due to ball-valve phenomenon. This can be further assessed by obtaining bilateral decubitus views (views with the patient on his or her side). In a normal patient, the dependent lung should be smaller than the top lung due to gravity as seen in Figure 11.2. In a patient with an aspirated foreign body in a bronchus, the downward side will not normally collapse due to the pressure of the hyperinflated lung. A similar concept can be employed using chest fluoroscopy, in which there is less movement of diaphragm on the affected side:

- While less immediately life-threatening, foreign objects in the GI tract can be a cause of significant morbidity. The most worrisome ingested objects are batteries, due to the risk of corrosion (which can occur within hours of ingestion), and multiple magnets, due to the risk of perforation should they be on opposite sides of the bowel wall.

- If the object that was ingested is unknown, initial radiographs can be carefully scrutinized to determine what the object was; differentiating between disc batteries/magnets and coins is the most frequent distinction needing to be made.
- Initial radiographs are obtained to see where the object is and whether it is accessible via endoscopy. Follow-up radiographs can be obtained on a case-by-case basis to follow the object through the alimentary tract.
- CT and UGIs can be used to assess potential complications, namely, perforation and possible abscess formation, either in the mediastinum or the peritoneum.

Asthma/reactive airway disease

Asthma and reactive airway disease (RAD) are clinical diagnoses. Imaging studies, however, can be useful in excluding other causes of respiratory distress as well as showing potential complications. On chest radiographs, hyperinflation is seen with varying degrees of bronchial cuffing due to inflammation of the airways. Pneumomediastinum is not infrequently seen in acute asthma exacerbations, thought to be due to alveolar rupture, with resultant air tracking centrally along the bronchovascular sheath:

- This is a benign, self-limited entity and no intervention or follow-up radiographs are required. Roving atelectasis, seen as migrating opacities, is also frequently seen due to mucus plugging the inflamed airways.

GI

Intussusception

Intussusception is the most common cause of intestinal obstruction between the ages of 3 months and 5 years. This occurs when a segment of bowel telescopes into another. In adults, this occurs most frequently secondary to a lead point such as a neoplasm, Meckel's diverticulum, or duplication cyst. In young children, the etiology is unknown but may be due to enlarged lymphoid tissue in the setting of recent illness.

These patients classically present with lethargy, intermittent abdominal pain, and currant jelly stools. An abdominal radiograph can suggest the diagnosis by demonstrating a soft tissue mass in the right abdomen with dilatation of multiple loops of small bowel. An US is the most frequently used test to confirm the diagnosis. On transverse views, the intussuscepted bowel will have a targetoid appearance due to the bowel enveloped on itself. The length of the intussuscepted bowel can be assessed on sagittal views as seen in Figure 11.5a and b:

- After consultation with a pediatric surgeon, the pediatric radiologist can proceed with reduction of the intussusception. In current practice, an air enema is the most frequently employed means of reduction. With this technique, after radiographs are obtained to confirm the lack of free air, the patient is placed in a prone position and a rectal catheter is placed. With the buttocks pressed firmly together to prevent the egress of air, air is slowly pumped into the rectum. Using fluoroscopy, the air is traced through the colon to the level of the obstruction as seen in Figure 11.5c–f, and the intussusception is reduced in real time.

As intussusceptions frequently recur several times within a week after initial presentation, air-reduction enemas may be required multiple times in the same patient.

Appendicitis

As in adults, appendicitis is a frequent cause of abdominal pain. In children, appendicitis and resulting complications are also included in the differential diagnosis of small bowel obstruction. While CT tends to be the mainstay in diagnosis in adults, US is a frequently used modality in the pediatric population:

- The findings with US are similar to those seen on CT including an noncompressible enlarged appendix (>6 mm) with surrounding free fluid, inflammation, and enlarged lymph nodes, as seen in Figure 11.8. When present, an appendicolith can be seen as an echogenic or bright focus that demonstrates posterior acoustic shadowing. Periappendiceal abscesses can also be visualized with US. While free air can be visualized with US, CT is much more sensitive for this diagnosis.
- In situations in which the appendix is unable to be visualized and there is high clinical suspicion for appendicitis, a CT can be pursued. Recent research has made strides in using MRI for the diagnosis of acute appendicitis. The findings are similar as for CT; however, more dramatic evidence of inflammatory enhancement is appreciated on MR images.

Meckel's diverticulum

Included in the differential for lower GI bleeding in children is a Meckel's diverticulum, an omphalomesenteric duct remnant seen in approximately 2% of people. The cause of the bleeding in this entity is the presence of ectopic gastric mucosa found in approximately half of all Meckel's diverticula:

- The most sensitive and specific imaging modality is a pertechnetate nuclear medicine scan. It is important to realize that this scan does not identify the diverticulum itself but localizes to the ectopic gastric mucosa.
- Thus, there may be a Meckel's present, but it would be unlikely to be the source of GI bleeding. CT and MRI can be used to diagnose complications of Meckel's diverticula including intussusception or perforation.

NEC

NEC, while a pediatric emergency, is infrequently encountered in the outpatient setting. This entity most commonly occurs in preterm infants while residing in the NICU. The etiology of this condition is unknown, and a number of factors have been suggested, including infection, ischemia, and early enteral feeding. Clinically, these neonates present with abdominal distention and increasing residuals (the milk or formula left in the stomach after a feeding):

- The earliest signs on radiographs are bowel distension with lack of movement or "fixed" bowel on sequential radiographs. A very specific indicator of NEC is pneumatosis, or gas in the bowel walls, demonstrated in Figure 11.7. Seen with the bowel wall on edge, these appear as tiny bubbles stacked on another. En face, these are harder to delineate from stool as it may appear as bubbly lucencies. The presence of portal venous gas, gas within the portal vein appearing as branching lucencies over the liver, should also be closely monitored. These infants must undergo close radiographic follow-up looking for free air, which upgrades medical NEC to surgical NEC.
- US is an increasingly used modality demonstrating the hypoperistaltic bowel and the echogenic foci in the bowel wall, representing the pneumatosis.

Malrotation with and without volvulus

Malrotation is an anomaly of midgut fixation. In the normal fetus, there is physiologic bowel herniation that occurs at 6 weeks of gestation with subsequent 270° counterclockwise rotation of bowel. The bowel returns to the peritoneal cavity by approximately 10 weeks of gestation. This results in the DJJ in the upper left hand of the abdomen and the ileocecal valve in the lower right of the abdomen with a long mesenteric base bridging the two. In contradistinction, malrotated bowel has a narrow mesenteric attachment due to failure of the bowel to rotate properly. This narrow attachment predisposes the midgut to rotate and undergo volvulus around this short pedicle.

Malrotation can be an incidental finding, seen in children and even adults who present with chronic abdominal pain, presumably from intermittent duodenal obstruction. The emergency occurs when the malrotated bowel twists on its short pedicle, thus compromising blood flow in the SMV and/or SMA, with subsequent bowel ischemia and possible necrosis:

- The diagnosis is often made with a barium UGI study. The contrast bolus is followed through the stomach into the proximal duodenum. Both frontal and lateral views are needed to rule out malrotation. On the lateral view, the contrast is followed into the duodenum. The second, third, and fourth portions of the duodenum are retroperitoneal so the contrast should extend posteriorly and approach the anterior margin of the spine. On the frontal view, the duodenum must cross the midline to at least the left pedicle and continue superiorly to the level of the duodenal bulb seen in Figure 11.6a. If these imaging criteria are not met, then intestinal malrotation cannot be excluded.
- Malrotation with volvulus is a pediatric surgical emergency due to the risk of necrosis of the small bowel. The classic sign seen in malrotation with volvulus is the "corkscrew" or "apple peel" sign in which contrast fills the proximal portion of the twisted bowel demonstrated in Figure 11.6b. However, it may also present as a complete duodenal obstruction as seen in Figure 11.6c. Not infrequently, there may be dilatation of the more proximal duodenum due to obstruction as well as thickening of the bowel wall folds due to ischemia.
- While US is not currently used as a primary means of diagnosing midgut volvulus, it can be suggested based on the relationship of the SMA and SMV. Normally, the SMV is to the right of the SMA. As the mesentery twists, however, the normal SMA/SMV relationship is inverted with the SMV now to the left of the SMV. On both CT and MRI, there may be a whorling of the mesentery surrounding the SMA.

HPS

HPS develops within the first months after birth. The etiology of this condition is unknown, but it is frequently seen in firstborn males with a family history of HPS. The clinical presentation is an infant with progressive projectile emesis (nonbilious, as the obstruction is preduodenal). As the name would suggest, HPS consists of a hypertrophied pylorus resulting in gastric outlet obstruction. The accepted treatment consists of a longitudinal incision of this muscle known as a pyloromyotomy:

- The diagnosis most frequently is made with US. The hypertrophied pylorus is easily identified in the upper abdomen, and the thickness and length of the pylorus are measured. While standards vary, typically, a thickness of one wall of the pylorus greater than 3 mm and a channel length greater than 1.6 cm are consistent with the diagnosis of HPS, demonstrated in Figure 11.4. The pylorus should be visualized with the stomach full to see if any gastric contents pass through the pylorus and to differentiate from temporary pylorospasm. If the duodenal bulb is distended with fluid, this effectively excludes the diagnosis of HPS.

- A UGI can also be used to make the diagnosis, although this technique is less favored due to the associated radiation. There will be a "shoulder" or "nipple" sign as the contrast bolus impresses upon the hypertrophied muscle. The "string sign" may be seen as a wisp of barium courses through the hypertrophied channel.

MSK

There are several fundamental differences between pediatric and adult bones. Skeletal maturity is defined by when the growth plates or "physes" of bones close. Before this point, the pediatric skeleton is composed of multiple ossification centers that become less cartilaginous and more ossified as an individual ages. These ossification centers develop at relatively predictable times during skeletal growth, and this growth pattern is helpful in determining normal from abnormal.

Pediatric bones are more flexible than adult bones; as such, they break differently than adults. Frequently, the fractures manifest as a buckling of the cortex with no discrete fracture line seen. Additionally, these young bones can bend or bow without breaking. They can even break along a single cortex resulting in a "greenstick fracture." Another fundamental difference between pediatric and adult MSK traumas is that frequently the degree of trauma is underestimated by radiographs because injury to the cartilage is unable to be assessed with radiographs. If one were to need to define the extent of cartilaginous injury, an MRI would be required.

Finally, pediatric bone heals much more quickly than adult bone. Signs of healing, such as periosteal reaction and callus formation, are typically seen within 1 week, unlike adult patients where signs of healing may take up to 2 weeks to develop. This fact is important in determining when to obtain follow-up radiographs in the setting of suspected fracture; pediatric radiologists typically recommend follow-up radiographs in 7–10 days.

Salter–Harris fractures

The Salter–Harris system is a special classification based on the relationship of the fracture to the physis or growth plate. Bones are divided by their relationship with the physis. The shaft or central portion of the bone is referred to as the diaphysis. The metaphysis is the flared portion of bone that separates the diaphysis from the physis. The epiphysis is the portion of bone on the other side of the physis, typically along the joint surface:

- A mnemonic to help remember the various types of Salter–Harris fractures is illustrated in Figure 11.15. Salter–Harris II fractures account for the vast majority of physeal fractures, greater than 70%.

Pediatric elbow

Particular attention will be paid to the pediatric elbow as it is a frequent source of confusion due to the number of ossification centers present. The mnemonic CRITOE is used as a reminder as to the order in which the ossification centers appear: *c*apitellum, *r*adial head, *i*nternal/medial epicondyle, *t*rochlea, *o*lecranon, and *e*xternal/lateral epicondyle; these are illustrated in Figure 11.16a. These appear, respectively, at approximately 2, 4, 6, 8, 10, and 12 years of age. It is important to remember, however, that the exact age of appearance is less important than the order in which the ossification centers appear (i.e., the lateral epicondyle should not be present before the trochlea):

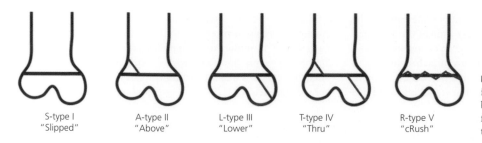

| S-type I | A-type II | L-type III | T-type IV | R-type V |
| "Slipped" | "Above" | "Lower" | "Thru" | "cRush" |

Figure 11.15 Salter–Harris fracture. An illustrated mnemonic helpful in remembering the various forms of Salter–Harris fracture. Note that this figure is drawn with the distal femur in mind.

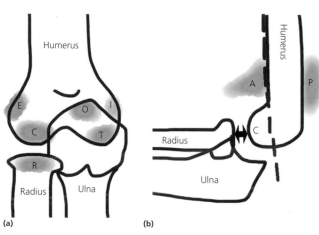

Figure 11.16 Ossification centers. An illustration of an anterior view of an elbow with the red regions indicating the ossification centers. In order of appearance, there are the capitellum (C), radial head (R), internal/medial epicondyle (I), trochlea (T), olecranon (O), and external/lateral epicondyle (E) (a). An illustration of a lateral view of the elbow. The dotted line indicates the anterior humeral line that should intersect with the middle third of the capitellum (C). The black double-headed arrow indicates the appropriate alignment of the radius and capitellum; on all views of the elbow, this relationship should be maintained. The red region labeled A indicates the anterior fat pad sign with a sail or triangular configuration. The red region labeled P indicates the posterior fat pad sign (b).

- The most frequent fracture of the pediatric elbow is the supracondylar fracture. The fracture line may be extremely subtle, especially in the acute setting. Thus, secondary signs are frequently used to suggest the presence of a fracture, such as the presence of an effusion and the alignment of the elbow.
- The presence of an effusion can be ascertained by looking for the anterior and posterior fat pad signs. In a noninjured elbow, the anterior fat pad is frequently seen, but the fat pad should be flush against the distal humerus not uplifted by the effusion, forming a triangle configuration known as the "sail sign."
- The posterior fat pad should never be seen in a normal elbow. The anterior humeral line is drawn vertically along the anterior margin of the humerus and should always intersect with the middle third of the capitellum. If this line intersects the anterior third, this indicates a dorsally angulated fracture. These findings are seen in Figure 11.16b.

SCFE

SCFE is a diagnosis unique to the immature skeleton. It occurs when the femoral head slips posteromedially off of the metaphysis due to a Salter–Harris I-type injury. This occurs most frequently in overweight, adolescent males. This condition presents clinically with hip pain and decreased range of motion:

- Initial radiographs may demonstrate extremely subtle abnormalities, with faint asymmetric widening of the physis, and therefore two views (most frequently frontal and frog leg views) are needed to increase sensitivity of detection as seen in Figure 11.10. With more advanced cases, the slippage is obvious, resulting in the classic description of the "ice cream following off the cone."
- Close inspection of the contralateral hip is needed as SCFE occurs bilaterally in up to 20% of cases. The patients are at high risk for the development of avascular necrosis and early degenerative changes.

Legg–Calve–Perthes disease

Legg–Calve–Perthes (LCP) is a diagnosis unique to the pediatric population consisting of spontaneous avascular necrosis of the capital femoral epiphysis. These most commonly present as a patient with persistent pain and limp. The peak age of incidence is 5–6 years old, and unlike their adult counterpart, many of them will resolve with conservative measures:

- Radiographic findings are those seen with other forms of avascular necrosis. Initially, the radiographs may be subtle, with a smaller femoral epiphysis on the affected side.
- As the condition progresses, there may be widening of the joint space with subchondral fracture resulting in the crescent sign. There may also be areas of increased sclerosis.
- In later stages, there will be broadening, flattening, and irregularity of the femoral head. Ultimately, secondary degenerative changes may occur.

Osteochondritis dissecans/osteochondral defect

Osteochondral defects can affect a number of bones throughout the skeleton, most commonly the knee. The capitellum of the elbow and talar dome of the ankle are also frequent sites for this condition. Despite the varying locations, the underlying pathology of these entities is thought to be the same, although the etiology is not well understood. Various etiologies have been proposed including repetitive microtrauma, vascular insult, or hormonal factors:

- Radiographs are the screening test of choice. In early cases, they may be normal, but as the disease progresses, the subchondral bone becomes more irregular and lucent with regions of sclerosis and may eventually become fragmented with loose bodies in the joint.
- CT can be used for the evaluation of loose bodies, but the most sensitive examination is MRI, which depicts the focal area of edema as increased T2 signal with a defect in the overlying

cartilage. If T2 signal completely surrounds a fragment of bone, this lesion is considered unstable and surgery is indicated. Otherwise, these lesions tend to be treated conservatively.

Cervical spine trauma

Due to the inherent differences in the size of the head relatively to the neck as well as ligamentous laxity and weakness of the neck musculature, injuries to the cervical spine manifest differently in children than adults. The most frequently injured level in infants and children is the upper cervical spine (C1–C4), whereas lower cervical spine injuries occur more frequently in adults:

- Additionally, ligamentous injury in the absence of osseous injuries is frequently seen resulting in a unique entity of spinal cord injury without radiographic abnormality (SCIWORA), meaning that no signs of injury are visible on radiographs or CT.
- Thus, it is of the utmost importance that clinicians pursue an MRI study, even if their index of suspicion is relatively low (especially if this is influenced by relatively unremarkable plain films), especially in the setting of neurological abnormality.

A false-positive that can be a source of confusion in radiographs of the cervical spine in young children is "pseudosubluxation." This is most frequently seen at the C2–C3 level. With pseudosubluxation, the anterior and posterior spinal lines may have up to 3 mm of offset. However, even with this degree of offset, the spinolaminar line remains continuous, as seen in Figure 11.17.

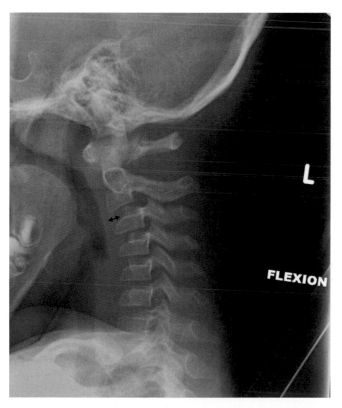

Figure 11.17 Pseudosubluxation. Lateral view of the normal cervical spine in a young child with a history of trauma but a negative neuro exam. The black double-headed area indicates approximately 3 mm of offset along the anterior vertebral body line. The dotted line follows the smooth, intact spinolaminar line. This is an appearance typical for pseudosubluxation.

Miscellaneous
Nonaccidental trauma

Nonaccidental trauma (NAT) is an entity ever present in the mind of a pediatric radiologist. There are a number of injuries that suggest the diagnosis of NAT affecting a variety of organ systems.

In the brain, hemorrhage is the primary finding. Subarachnoid hemorrhage can be seen in greater than 50% of victims. The presence of subdural hematomas of varying ages has been suggested as an indicator of child abuse, but caution should be exercised when trying to ascertain the age of a hematoma. Retinal hemorrhages and sheer injuries at the gray/white matter interface and at the margins of the corpus callosum can be detected with MRI, particularly susceptibility-weighted imaging (SWI):

- A variety of fractures can suggest the possibility of child abuse. To that end, a skeletal survey, consisting of radiographs of every bone in the body, is obtained during the workup of child abuse. Posterior rib fractures, thought to occur during squeezing of the thorax, are highly suggestive of inflicted trauma.
- Metaphyseal corner fractures in which a triangular or bucket handle-shaped (depending on the obliquity of the film) fragment of bone is noted adjacent to the metaphysis are also suggestive of abuse. These are most frequently seen in children less than 1 year of age and are commonly located in the distal femur and tibia but can be seen in the upper extremities as well. The mechanism of injury is thought to be due to shaking with the end of the bone sheared off.
- Other fractures that are considered highly suggestive of abuse are sternal, spinous process, and scapula fractures. In addition to skeletal surveys, bone scans can be considered to assess the possibility of multiple fractures.

Within the abdomen, solid organ injury involving the liver, pancreas, and spleen can occur as with any trauma. The classic abdominal injuries associated with child abuse are pancreatitis and duodenal hematomas:

- When child abuse is suspected, it is incumbent upon radiologists and clinicians to promptly relay their suspicion to the provider caring for the patient so that an appropriate workup can be pursued. This is considered both an ethical and medicolegal mandate.

Vascular or ischemic diagnoses in the pediatric population

Testicular torsion/torsion of the appendix testis

As in adults, testicular torsion is a urologic emergency, and the quicker the diagnosis is made, the more likely the testis is able to be salvaged:

- US with Doppler is the most sensitive tool to make the diagnosis. Findings include an enlarged testicle with a heterogeneous echotexture and asymmetric blood flow of the affected testicle. It is important to realize that the presence of blood flow using Doppler does not exclude the diagnosis of testicular torsion, particularly intermittent torsion.

A testis may infarct in utero, resulting in a firm scrotal mass on physical exam in the newborn, with no blood flow seen with US. When the infarcted testis cannot be salvaged, urgent orchiopexy of the contralateral testis is typically performed.

Another cause of testicular pain that US can be helpful in diagnosing is torsion of the appendix testis. The appendix testis is a small tongue of tissue that extends from the superior surface of the testicle, which can twist and undergo torsion, thereby cutting off its vascular supply. On physical exam, one may see a small blue dot on the skin representing the torsed, necrotic appendix:

- On US, there is heterogeneous, hypovascular mass noted adjacent to a normal-appearing testicle. Over time, this may calcify and become a scrotal pearl.

Ovarian torsion

In the pediatric population, ovarian torsion represents a rare but important cause of abdominal pain. As in adults, US is the imaging modality of choice. The most sensitive finding is an enlarged ovary. Frequently, there will be peripheral displacement of the follicles, and the ovary will be located more medially in the pelvis. Free fluid is a frequent coexisting finding. As in testicular torsion, the presence of blood flow using Doppler does not exclude the diagnosis of ovarian torsion. The diagnosis should be made promptly to increase the odds of discovering a viable ovary at the time of surgery.

Inflammatory or infectious diagnoses in the pediatric population

Airway
Croup

Croup or laryngotracheobronchitis, classically caused by the parainfluenza virus, is a frequently encountered illness in the pediatric population and is the most common cause of upper airway obstruction in children between 6 months and 3 years of age. Clinically, it presents with a barking cough, stridor, and respiratory distress. When the patient presents in a typical fashion, no imaging is required to make the diagnosis. If imaging is pursued, both neck and chest radiographs can be suggestive of this diagnosis:

- On frontal radiographs of both the neck and chest, croup can be seen as a thickening subglottic trachea resulting in the steeple sign with loss of the normal shoulders of the subglottic trachea, as seen in Figure 11.1d and e. Lateral radiographs will demonstrate ballooning of the hypopharynx, a nonspecific sign seen in the setting of a variety of causes of upper airway obstruction.

Epiglottitis

In recent years, the incidence of epiglottitis has dramatically decreased due to the introduction of the H. influenza vaccine. However, due to the life-threatening nature of this condition, it is an important entity to recognize both clinically and radiographically. Clinically, the patient will be in respiratory distress and may be drooling:

- The primary imaging finding is thickening of the epiglottis resulting in the "thumbprint sign" seen on a lateral radiograph of the neck (Figure 11.1g). Thickening of the aryepiglottic folds is frequently present as well as ballooning of the hypopharynx. The edematous epiglottis serves as a potential airway obstruction so it is of the utmost importance not to lay the patient in a supine position (e.g., for a CT examination) prior to intubation for protection of the airway.

Retropharyngeal abscess

Another infectious cause of airway obstruction in the pediatric population is a retropharyngeal abscess. These infections are thought to represent a complication of a primary infection elsewhere in the head and neck (e.g., otitis media with ensuing suppuration of retropharyngeal nodes). Patients present with fever, neck swelling, frequent lack of appetite, and stridor:

- Lateral radiographs of the neck are frequently the initial imaging study ordered. Radiographs will show thickening of the prevertebral soft tissues (the soft tissue immediately anterior to the spine), as demonstrated in Figure 11.1h. At the level of C2, greater than 7 mm is considered thickened, and at the level of C5, greater than 14 mm is considered thickened. An internal standard that can be used is that the thickness should not be greater than the vertebral body.
- Due to the redundant soft tissue in the necks of small children, particularly prominent with the neck flexed, it is important that the X-ray technologist appropriately position the patient so that the redundant soft tissue does not cause a false-positive appearance.
- CT of the neck with contrast is typically the next imaging study performed to assess the size and extension of the retropharyngeal abscess as well as help guide the surgical approach.

Chest
Round pneumonia

An entity unique to the pediatric patient population is round pneumonia. Due to the immature lung, that is, underdeveloped pores of Kohn and channels of Lambert, the infection cannot disperse as easily through these airflow collaterals. The infection is thus confined and assumes a rounded configuration:

- On chest radiographs, it will present as a well-defined, rounded, parenchymal opacity, frequently with air bronchograms as seen in Figure 11.3. The appearance may be alarming due its mass-like appearance. However, in the appropriate clinical context such as the presence of a fever and cough, the radiologist and clinician alike can be reassured about the benign, infectious etiology of this appearance. If there is any doubt as to the nature of this "mass," follow-up radiographs can be obtained 4–6 weeks after the conclusion of the illness.

Bronchiolitis

Viral bronchiolitis is a frequent cause of respiratory distress in infants and young children due to inflammation of the respiratory tract with resultant airway obstruction. Premature infants are particularly susceptible to infection by respiratory syncytial virus (RSV):

- The diagnosis is based primarily on clinical criteria, but chest radiographs play an important role in excluding other causes of respiratory distress. The most sensitive imaging finding for bronchiolitis is hyperinflation of the lungs. Streaky perihilar opacities are also frequently present. Due to the obstruction of airways, regions of platelike or lobar atelectasis may also be seen.

GI
Inflammatory bowel disease

Both ulcerative colitis and inflammatory bowel disease (IBD) frequently present in adolescence. Frequently, the clinical manifestations are nonspecific and may include abdominal pain, weight loss, and diarrhea. A variety of imaging modalities can be used to diagnose IBD as well as assess complications of IBD:

- Radiographs are relatively insensitive in the diagnosis of IBD and are not a mainstay in the evaluation in patients suspected of having this diagnosis, although occasionally they may reveal obstruction or segmental bowel wall thickening. SBFTs are frequently used, particularly in conjunction with spot radiographs of the terminal ileum.
- Historically, CT enterography has been used to assess the presence and extent of bowel wall inflammation including potential response to therapy.

- MRI is playing an increasing role, however, with specific MR enterography protocols developed to specifically address this clinical question. Findings seen on CT and MRI include bowel wall thickening, inflammatory stranding of the mesentery, fibro-fatty proliferation, the presence of strictures with or without obstruction, and fistulae.

Hemolytic uremic syndrome

Rarely after an infection, most frequently with the Shiga toxin-producing strain of *E. coli*, hemolytic uremic syndrome (HUS) may develop. This toxin causes a microangiopathy in the kidney, thus producing varying degrees of renal failure.

The patients typically present with classic colitis symptoms including fever, abdominal pain, and diarrhea. Imaging studies will demonstrate the typical findings of colitis including thumbprinting of the colonic wall due to the edematous haustra, thickening of the wall, and stranding in the adjacent fat due to the presence of inflammation. While these symptoms are resolving, a patient with HUS will develop oliguria or anuria and subsequent rise in creatinine:

- US of the kidneys is the mainstay in evaluation showing increased echogenicity (brightness) of the renal cortex. Doppler imaging will show loss or even reversal of diastolic flow to the kidney.
- Of note, iodinated and gadolinium-based contrast agents should be avoided in these patients. These patients are typically managed conservatively, but some may progress to needing dialysis.

GU

Pyelonephritis

As in adults, pyelonephritis is a clinical and laboratory diagnosis including the presence of fever, flank pain, and a positive urinalysis. Imaging can be used to assess the complications of pyelonephritis, namely, a renal/perirenal abscess:

- When found as an incidental finding during the workup of abdominal pain, on US, the kidney may be enlarged and demonstrate a region of diminished blood flow on Doppler imaging. There will be loss of the normal corticomedullary differentiation in the affected portion of the kidney.
- On contrast-enhanced CT, the kidney may again be enlarged with stranding of the adjacent fat. A "striated nephrogram" may be present in which there is inhomogeneous contrast enhancement of the renal cortex resulting in a vaguely striated appearance; this is nonspecific and can be seen in the setting of urinary obstruction or renal vein thrombosis. Focal involvement of the renal parenchyma can have a mass-like appearance and should be differentiated from a neoplastic process.
- MRI will demonstrate an enlarged kidney that may demonstrate regions of increased T2 signal due to the presence of edema. Enhancement related to inflammation and infection is more dramatic on MR than CT images.

Epididymitis/orchitis

Epididymitis and orchitis are a common cause of testicular pain in the pediatric patient population. It can be infectious (viral or bacterial) or sterile (due to reflux of urine during voiding). The most concerning differential possibility is testicular torsion, and therefore, the diagnosis is most frequently made with US:

- Sonographic findings include a hyperemic and swollen epididymis with varying involvement of the testis. A reactive hydrocele is frequently seen, as is thickening of the scrotal wall.

MSK

Osteomyelitis

While osteomyelitis seen in adults is frequently seen in the setting of trauma or diabetes, acute osteomyelitis in infants and young children is predominantly not related to trauma. Osteomyelitis is most frequently caused by hematogenous spread of bacteria. In infants, due to the presence of vessels crossing the physis, the infection can involve both the metaphysis and epiphysis; however, these vessels involute early in childhood, and until the physis fuses late in adolescence, infection is typically limited to the metaphysis:

- Radiographs obtained early in the course of the disease may be normal. The earliest evidence on radiographs may be soft tissue swelling and subtle lucency involving the metaphysis. If osteomyelitis is suspected clinically with negative radiographs, further imaging should be pursued.
- MRI is currently the test of choice and will show edema of the involved bone (diminished T1 signal intensity and increased T2 signal intensity) with patchy enhancement. Regions of nonenhancement are concerning for areas of necrosis, which is an indication for surgical debridement. Subperiosteal abscesses may also form and require open drainage.
- Radionuclide bone scans, particularly a three-phase bone scan, can be obtained to evaluate for the presence of osteomyelitis, but this exam provides limited information regarding the need for possible surgical intervention, namely, the presence of necrotic bone or periosteal abscesses.

Inadequately treated acute osteomyelitis may evolve into subacute or chronic osteomyelitis. Subacute osteomyelitis classically manifests on radiographs as a Brodie's abscess seen as a lucent lesion with sclerotic margins:

- For chronic osteomyelitis, the bone may become progressively more sclerotic. A sequestrum (a necrotic piece of bone) may be present within an involucrum serving as a nidus of infection. A cloaca may also be present in which the infection extends through the cortex.

Septic arthritis

Septic arthritis constitutes a pediatric emergency due to the rapid destruction of the joint in the presence of pus; the orthopedic adage "never let the sun set on an infected joint" remains true. These patients present with fever, elevated inflammatory markers, and pain of the affected joint:

- Radiographs are relatively insensitive to the diagnosis but may demonstrate the presence of an effusion. US is much more sensitive in the evaluation of joint fluid, and in the same setting, US-guided aspiration can be performed to assess for the presence of septic arthritis.
- Rarely, an aspiration cannot be performed or is inadequate, in which case an MRI may be a valuable adjunct to the workup. MRI findings will show increased fluid in the joint with edema surrounding the joint space (increased signal on T2 and STIR sequences) and associated enhancement of the synovium on postcontrast images. Lymph nodes in the surrounding soft tissue may be enlarged.

Toxic synovitis

A frequent cause of hip pain in children less than 10 years of age is toxic or transient synovitis and is classically seen after a viral infection:

- Radiographs are frequently normal although there may be widening of the joint space secondary to an effusion. Sonography of the hip may also reveal a hip effusion.

Distinguishing between septic arthritis and toxic synovitis is based primarily on clinical and laboratory data as no features on imaging studies are capable of differentiating these two entities. Despite the name, these patients are rarely toxic, presenting with low-grade fever and minimal elevation of inflammatory markers.

Neoplastic diagnoses in the pediatric population

Wilms' tumor

Wilms' tumor (WT) is the most common primary renal tumor in the pediatric population and the sixth most common tumor of childhood. WTs are most frequently seen in children between 1 and 5 years of age. They are frequently found incidentally by the parent due to the presence of a large mass or abdominal swelling. A number of syndromes predispose children to the development of WT such as Beckwith–Wiedemann and Wilms' tumor, aniridia, genitourinary malformation, and mental retardation (WAGR). This tumor most frequently occurs sporadically.

Included in the differential diagnosis of solid pediatric renal masses are congenital mesoblastic nephroma, malignant rhabdoid tumor, and clear cell sarcoma of the kidney. Unfortunately, at the time of presentation, these masses may be so large as to make it difficult to delineate their organ of origin. The other childhood tumor that it must be distinguished from is neuroblastoma (NB):

- Radiographs may be normal or may demonstrate a nonspecific soft tissue mass displacing normal abdominal contents.
- US may frequently be the initial imaging test to evaluate the etiology of the abdominal mass. On US, WT will appear as a heterogeneous abdominal mass with internal vascularity; grayscale and color Doppler interrogation of the renal vein and IVC may be helpful in determining the presence of vascular invasion.
- Cross-sectional imaging with either CT or MRI is useful in delineating which organs are involved and in helping stage the disease. When determining the organ of origin, it is useful to look for a "claw sign" in which the normal contour of the organ is disrupted and the organ appears to cup or grip the tumor.

- In the case of WT, a renal claw sign is frequently present. This mass tends to be heterogeneous but does not frequently calcify. It has a propensity to invade or displace the vasculature and most frequently metastasizes to the lung and liver. Many of these findings are illustrated in Figure 11.18a. Close inspection of the contralateral kidney is important as the presence of bilateral renal disease greatly impacts treatment.

NB

NB is the most common extracranial solid tumor in children. The affected age group is slightly younger than that seen in WT with a peak age of incidence of 2 years. As with WT, patients most commonly present with a palpable abdominal mass, but the symptoms at the time of presentation can vary greatly, ranging from Horner's syndrome due to a neck mass to opsomyoclonus secondary to paraneoplastic syndrome. NB may arise anywhere along the sympathetic chain but most frequently arises from the adrenal glands:

- As with WT, radiographs are insensitive to the diagnosis of NB, although the presence of calcifications in an area of suspected soft tissue mass is suggestive.
- US can demonstrate a heterogeneous, frequently partially calcified suprarenal mass.
- Cross-sectional imaging is used to aid in staging. As opposed to WT, these tumors frequently calcify (up to 90%) and tend to encase vessels as opposed to invading them, as seen in Figure 11.18b.
- Metaiodobenzylguanidine (MIBG) is a radiotracer taken up by the majority of NB tumors, and MIBG scintigraphy is routinely performed to assess the presence of osseous metastases and soft tissue disease that may be occult on CT or MR.

Hepatoblastoma

Hepatoblastoma is the most common malignant hepatic tumor in young children, with most cases presenting before 4 years of age. These tumors are more frequently seen in extremely premature and low-birth-weight infants. Patients typically present with a painless abdominal mass with an elevated alpha-fetoprotein noted on lab values. Included in the differential for a hepatic mass in a child are

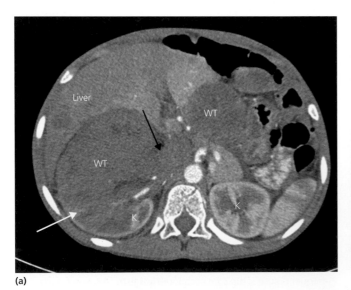

(a)

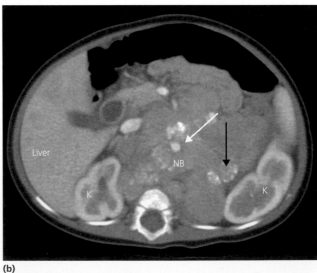

(b)

Figure 11.18 Wilms' tumor (WT). Axial contrast-enhanced CT in a young child with WT. The white arrow indicates the "claw sign" of the residual renal parenchyma (K) partially encasing the tumor. The black arrow indicates invasion of the renal vein, a finding typical for WT (a). Neuroblastoma (NB). Axial contrast-enhanced CT in a young child with NB. The black arrow indicates a region of calcification. The white arrow indicates the contrast-filled aorta that is encased by the tumor. Both of these features are frequently seen with NB. Note also that both kidneys (K) have a normal appearance (b).

mesenchymal hamartoma, a benign predominantly cystic lesion found in children less than 2 years of age, and hepatocellular carcinoma, typically seen in older children with an underlying disorder such as biliary atresia or hemochromatosis:

- As with the other abdominal tumors, radiographs play little role in the workup of hepatoblastoma. US will frequently be used as the initial imaging modality to assess the origin of a palpable abdominal mass.
- With US, the mass will be predominantly hypoechoic relative to the surrounding liver, but due to the presence of internal hemorrhage, calcifications may be shown as regions of increased echogenicity. With Doppler, the mass is typically hypervascular.
- CT performed with contrast will demonstrate a predominantly hypodense, heterogeneous mass that demonstrates heterogeneous enhancement but with less enhancement than the adjacent liver.
- MRI will show a mass centered in the liver that is predominantly T1 hypointense and T2 hyperintense with variable and heterogeneous enhancement. As with CT, the mass tends to enhance less than the adjacent liver. Staging is performed using the PRETEXT system and depends on which liver segments are free of tumor.

GU rhabdomyosarcoma

In the pediatric population, rhabdomyosarcomas may arise anywhere along the GU tract, from the vagina to the bladder and to the prostate, and are thought to arise from primitive muscle cells. Most cases are seen in children between 2 and 6 years of age. The differential for a pelvic mass in a child includes a sacrococcygeal teratoma, a germ cell tumor arising from the coccyx, and ovarian tumors in girls. Patients may present with a painless abdominal mass but not infrequently may present with bladder outlet obstruction secondary to mass effect. These masses tend to be heterogeneous, containing both cystic and solid components.

A classic form of rhabdomyosarcoma is sarcoma botryoides in which the tumor consists of multiple cysts, resembling a bunch of grapes. This form may arise from the bladder wall as well as the vaginal wall in which case it may prolapse through the introitus, becoming evident on physical exam:

- Ultrasonography can be used as the initial imaging modality. The appearance can vary considerably depending on the tumor composition. They are typically large at the time of presentation and heterogeneous if solid, with multiple septations if predominantly cystic.
- These tumors can be seen initially during fluoroscopy studies, most commonly for the workup of urinary obstruction. It will present as a filling defect in the bladder and can be confused for a ureterocele or polyp.
- CT will show a heterogeneous mass with enhancing portions that appears locally aggressive. MRI will show similar findings with moderately high signal intensity on T2-weighted images and heterogeneous enhancement noted on the postcontrast scans.

Lymphoma/leukemia

Lymphoma and leukemia are two of the three most common malignancies in children. The most common form of leukemia in children is acute lymphoblastic leukemia (ALL). Imaging plays little role in the workup of leukemia. However, the initial diagnosis can be suggested on the basis of imaging findings. These can be seen as leukemic lines consisting of radiolucent (dark) horizontal lines through the metaphyses of long bones. These tend to be multifocal involving the large joints; they are thought to not represent involvement by leukemia but are a manifestation of systemic illness. Leukemia can also manifest as focal areas of bone destructive resulting in a permeative-appearing bone lesion most frequently in the metaphysis; as opposed to the leukemic lines, these lesions do represent an actual focus of disease.

Lymphoma can be divided into Hodgkin lymphoma and non-Hodgkin lymphoma (NHL); NHL can be subdivided into numerous subtypes including but not limited to diffuse large B-cell lymphoma (DLBCL) and Burkitt's lymphoma (BL):

- Depending on the various subtype, the imaging appearance of these entities can vary widely. While nodal disease is a frequent manifestation, the solid organs that tend to be involved include the liver, spleen, and kidneys.
- Some disease appearances suggest one diagnosis over another. For instance, Hodgkin lymphoma frequently manifests as a lobulated, homogeneous mediastinal mass, while BL typically presents as a rapidly growing abdominal mass.

MSK

Osteosarcoma

Osteosarcomas are the most common primary bone tumors in children and are found predominantly in the metaphyses of long bones. Children usually present with persistent pain. Radiographs are typically used in the initial evaluation. While multiple subtypes of osteosarcomas exist, conventional osteosarcomas, composing approximately 80% of all osteosarcomas, will be the focus of this description:

- Osteosarcomas are osteoid- or bone-forming tumors. Due to the presence of this osteoid matrix, these lesions will have a sclerotic or cloud-like, fluffy appearance. The edges of the mass will have a wide zone of transition, defined as the segment of bone that extends between completely normal bone and definitely abnormal bone. In contrast, in a benign lesion such as a bone cyst, the zone of transition will be very short (1–2 mm), but in more aggressive lesions, the zone of transition will be much longer.
- Additionally, there will be aggressive periosteal reaction, classically described as a sunburst appearance. A concomitant soft tissue mass containing osteoid matrix is present in the majority of cases.
- MRI of the entirety of the affected bone is performed for staging purposes and operative planning. On MRI, the lesion will be T1 hypointense and T2 hyperintense. The areas of osteoid matrix/calcification will appear as diminished signal on all sequences. There will be heterogeneous enhancement on the postgadolinium images. The entirety of the bone is imaged to assess for skip lesions that are not apparent on radiographs.
- Included in the staging of osteosarcomas is a bone scan to look for the presence of distant osseous metastases. A chest CT without contrast is also performed to look for lung metastases, the most frequent extraosseous site of disease spread. These nodules frequently contain punctate calcifications and can be a cause of pneumothorax.

Ewing's tumors

Ewing's tumors fall in the category of primitive neuroectodermal tumor (PNET) and are the second most common primary bone tumor of children. As opposed to osteosarcomas, Ewing's are more frequently found in the diaphysis of long bones with a predilection for the flat bones, particularly of the pelvis.

Rarely, extraskeletal origin of Ewing's sarcomas may be seen:

- These tumors manifest on radiographs as a poorly defined, lytic lesion with a wide zone of transition. A soft tissue mass is frequently present but may be more difficult to appreciate on radiographs than osteosarcomas due to the lack of a radiodense matrix. These tumors also possess an aggressive periosteal reaction, classically described as a lamellated "onion skin" appearance creating a Codman triangle.
- The MR appearance of Ewing's sarcoma is difficult to differentiate from osteosarcoma and infection. It will be hypointense on T1-weighted images and hyperintense on T2-weighted images with variable extent of enhancement depending on the degree of necrosis.

Osteoid osteoma

Osteoid osteoma is a benign bone lesion. This often becomes manifest as persistent pain that is worse at night and that is relieved by NSAIDs. In reality, most pain is relieved by NSAIDs and can be worse at night so these signs may not be very helpful in differentiating this from other causes of MSK pain:

- A variety of imaging modalities can be used when the diagnosis of osteoid osteoma is suspected. Most frequently, radiographs are the initial imaging test and will show a region of thickening of the cortex and smooth periosteal reaction, classically with a central lucent nidus. CT will show similar findings but the nidus may be more apparent.
- An MRI performed in isolation of a radiograph can present a confusing picture as there may be profound edema (increased signal on T2-weighted images), which can obscure the nidus; this reinforces the concept that radiographs should be the initial test of choice when MSK pathology is suspected.
- Bone scan will show a focal area of uptake, which is nonspecific and can be seen in the setting of infection, trauma, or tumor. Treatment has classically been with surgical resection.

More recently, radiofrequency ablation under CT guidance has essentially replaced surgery as the standard of care.

Langerhans cell histiocytosis

Langerhans cell histiocytosis (LCH) is due to monoclonal proliferation of Langerhans cells. There are a variety of eponymous classifications for this heterogeneous disease entity that are a frequent source of confusion. A more straightforward method of classification of LCH is based on how extensive the disease is: a single lesion (referred to as an eosinophilic granuloma when involving the bone), multiple sites within a single organ, or multiple sites within multiple organs:

- The primary manifestations recognized on imaging studies involve the lung and bone, and while the diagnosis may be suspected by its appearance on imaging studies, a histologic specimen is required to establish the diagnosis. In the lung, LCH may present as pulmonary nodules that eventually undergo cavitation and with progressive interstitial thickening and scarring. In the bone, LCH can be included in the diagnosis of virtually any lytic lesion.
- Classic imaging signs attributed to LCH include vertebra plana (flattening of a vertebral body), typically in the thoracic spine, and a lytic lesion in the skull with beveled edges (the inner table is involved to a greater extent than the outer table creating the appearance of a bevel).
- Skeletal surveys in which radiographs are taken of every bone are useful in determining the extent of disease; alternatively, bone scintigraphy may be used.

Suggested reading

Blickman, J.G., Parker, B.R. & Barnes, P.D. (2009) *Pediatric Radiology: The Requisites.* Mosby/Elsevier, Philadelphia, PA.

Brant, W.E. & Helms, C.A. (2012) *Fundamentals of Diagnostic Radiology.* Wolters Kluwer/Lippincott Williams & Wilkins, Philadelphia, PA.

Coley, B.D. & Caffey, J. (2013) *Caffey's Pediatric Diagnostic Imaging.* Saunders, Philadelphia, PA.

Donnelly, L.F. (2009) *Pediatric Imaging: The Fundamentals.* Saunders/Elsevier, Philadelphia, PA.

Donnelly, L.F. (2012) *Diagnostic Imaging.* Amirsys, Inc, Salt Lake City, Utah.

Keats, T.E. & Anderson, M.W. (2013) *Atlas of Normal Roentgen Variants that may Simulate Disease.* Elsevier/Saunders, Philadelphia, PA.

Link, H.E. & Gooding, C.A. (2010) *Essentials of Pediatric Radiology: A Multimodality Approach.* Cambridge University Press, Cambridge, New York.

Siegel, M.J. (2011) *Pediatric Sonography.* Wolters Kluwer/Lippincott Williams & Wilkins, Philadelphia, PA.

CHAPTER 12

Interventional Radiology

Ari J. Isaacson, Sarah Thomas, J.T. Cardella, and Lauren M.B. Burke
University of North Carolina, Chapel Hill, USA

Introduction

Interventional radiology (IR) differs from other radiology subspecialties in that imaging is primarily used to guide minimally invasive procedures. In this chapter, we will focus on describing the spectrum of procedures that comprise IR.

IR is traditionally employed as a consultation service to perform procedures at the requests of other physicians; however, currently, the practice of IR is progressively becoming more of an independent hospital service, admitting patients and providing their care throughout their stay. In addition to performing procedures, interventional radiologists also see patients in clinic to discuss possible treatment options and to provide follow-up care postprocedurally.

The conventional training pathway for IR includes an internship of any type, 4 years of diagnostic radiology residency, and 1 year of IR fellowship. In the next few years, the training pathway will be transitioning to a surgical internship and 5 years of IR residency. The residency years will incorporate diagnostic radiology, critical care, and IR procedural rotations. This will allow for future interventionalists to have more clinical experience during their training while still gaining proficiency in image interpretation and performance of procedures. Both of these training pipelines lead to diagnostic radiology and IR dual certification.

Types of imaging

Fluoroscopy: The advantage that fluoroscopy provides is that many images can be obtained in rapid sequence without exposing the patient to high radiation doses. This allows for real-time imaging guidance with X-ray-like "video." To augment the information that fluoroscopy provides, high-density contrast can be used to highlight structures of interest. For example, imaging of the vasculature obtained after the injection of iodinated contrast material is called *angiography*. In addition, contrast material can be injected into the biliary system, gastrointestinal (GI) tract, and urinary tract when performing fluoroscopic procedures. One more common technology used in conjunction with fluoroscopy is *digital subtraction angiography (DSA)*. This process subtracts all dense structures such as bones that are present at the initiation of imaging, allowing vessels that subsequently become opacified after contrast injection to be clearly viewed without obstruction from overlying structures.

Ultrasound (US) creates images by transmitting and receiving sound waves that are modified in characteristic patterns by the tissues they encounter. The result is grayscale images that can be utilized in real time to provide procedural guidance without exposing the patient to radiation. Additionally, when evaluating blood vessels, the Doppler phenomenon can be used to either create waveforms that represent the velocity of blood flow or color images that denote the direction in which the blood is flowing. Other advantages of US include the portability of the units themselves allowing for easier bedside procedures as well as the lower cost of the devices in comparison to other imaging modalities. Disadvantages included the inability to see deeper structures consistently, interference caused by bowel gas and bone on the US waves, and limited differentiation of certain types of tissues.

In addition to conventional US, *intravascular ultrasound (IVUS)* has become a powerful tool utilized by some interventional radiologists. In this method, a US transducer is mounted onto a catheter and generates intraluminal images. It allows for more accurate measurement of vessel diameter than fluoroscopy. This is very helpful when determining appropriate stent size before deployment or evaluating the stent "fit" after deployment. Importantly, it also provides information that would otherwise be obtained with fluoroscopy, but without the radiation exposure. This can be particularly helpful in pregnant women and in children. The downside of IVUS is that the transducer catheters are not reusable and are costly.

Computed tomography (CT) provides outstanding overall display of anatomy and is used for a variety of purposes in IR. It is important however, to be cognizant of radiation exposure to the patient. CT images can be obtained in rapid sequence to provide real-time guidance for more difficult procedures. This is termed *CT fluoroscopy*. However, this results in even higher exposure to the patient, as well as the interventional radiologist, if not properly shielded.

Critical Observations in Radiology for Medical Students, First Edition. Katherine R. Birchard, Kiran Reddy Busireddy, and Richard C. Semelka.
© 2015 John Wiley & Sons, Ltd. Published 2015 by John Wiley & Sons, Ltd.
Companion website: www.wiley.com/go/birchard

Other modalities such as magnetic resonance imaging (MRI) and positron emission tomography (PET) are starting to be used to guide procedures in which other modalities are inadequate for visualization. However, fluoroscopy, US, and CT provide useful imaging for the vast majority of IR procedures.

IR tools

Catheters are small-caliber tubes that come in many sizes and can be used for multiple purposes throughout IR. The types that are used in blood vessels have varying shapes at the tips, allowing them to be navigated through tortuous vasculature (Figure 12.1). Once in place, they allow for the injection of contrast or can serve as a conduit for delivering embolic material to a desired location. Angioplasty balloons and stents are also mounted on the end of catheters. Central venous catheters (CVCs) are placed to allow for the delivery of medication and for easy collection of blood. Nonvascular catheters can be used for drainage, whether placed in an abscess, the biliary system, the kidneys, or the bladder. Gastric catheters are used to deliver nutritional formulas.

Sheaths are stiffer tubes that catheters are inserted through (Figure 12.2). Sheaths placed at vascular access sites, such as the common femoral artery, eliminate the trauma associated with repetitive insertion and removal of catheters directly into blood vessels. Sheaths also stabilize access into vessels that are difficult to catheterize because of the vessel shape and stiffness.

Guidewires are very narrow wires made of radiopaque materials that act as "rails" for catheters (Figure 12.3). Once a guidewire has been placed in a desired location under fluoroscopic guidance, catheters can be placed over the wire and easily guided to the target without the challenge of renavigating from the skin entry site. Guidewires vary in size, stiffness, and slipperiness for use both in vascular and nonvascular structures.

Balloons are used to dilate narrowed areas within blood vessels as well as other nonvascular structures. They are mounted on catheters and are compressed to allow delivery through narrow passages. Once in place, they are inflated with dilute contrast material so that they can be visualized with fluoroscopy and inflated to the extent of the desired level of lumen expansion. Following the procedure, they are then deflated to near their starting size in order to be removed. They are made in various sizes and from materials of various strengths to accommodate different inflation pressures. When balloons are used in vessels to dilate narrowed segments, it is called *angioplasty*.

Stents are mounted on catheters and then deployed to maintain dilatation of a narrowed structure. They can be used both in the vasculature and in other structures such as the common bile duct (CBD) or GI tract. They range in complexity from bare metal framework to metal struts with a variety of outer coverings, depending on their intended use. Stents are packaged in their collapsed

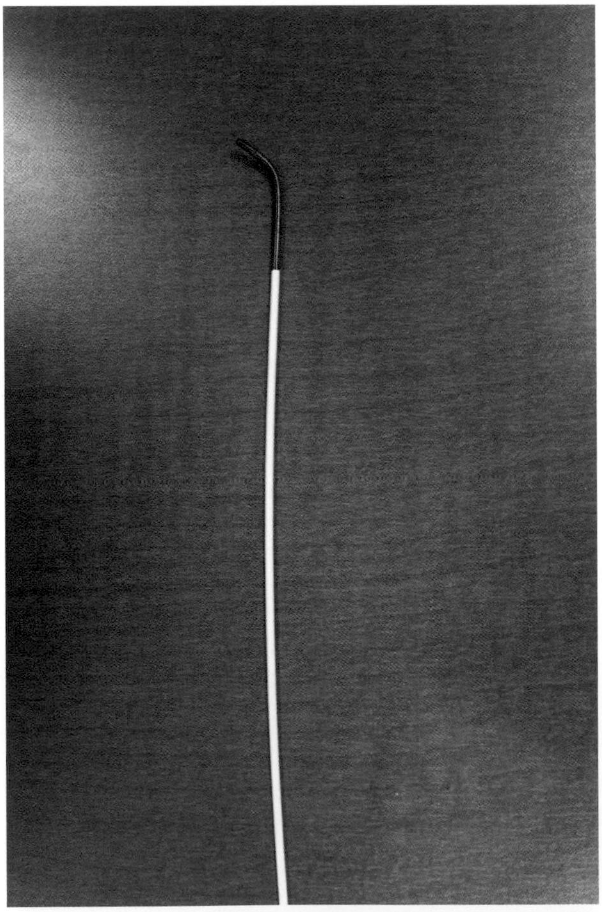

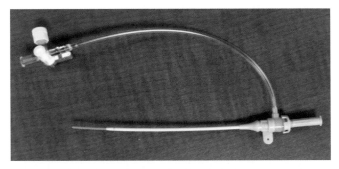

Figure 12.2 Sheath—vascular entry sheath with diaphragm, preventing backflow of blood during catheter exchange.

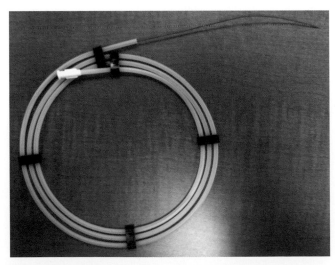

Figure 12.3 Guidewire—commonly used guidewire with floppy tip to prevent trauma to blood vessels during insertion.

Figure 12.1 Intravascular catheter—commonly used intravascular catheter with angled tip allowing for a guidewire to be manipulated through tortuous vessels.

configuration in order to be easily delivered to the target location. However, once the stent is maneuvered into the desired position, it is "deployed" into its expanded configuration. Some stents self-expand after the removal of an overlying sheath. Other stents come mounted on a balloon catheter and require inflation of the balloon for expansion of the stent.

Embolic materials are used within blood vessels to either temporarily or permanently stop the flow of blood within them. Depending on the size of the agent, embolization occurs more proximally within the arteries and large arterioles or more distally at the small arteriole level. Delivery to the target location occurs through catheters under fluoroscopic guidance. Selection of the appropriate embolic material is based on the condition that is being treated.

Anesthesia is provided for most IR procedures in the form of moderate sedation that includes short-acting intravenous (IV) anxiolytic and analgesic medications. Additionally, local anesthesia is given in the form of a lidocaine injection. Radiology nurses, under the supervision of the IR physician, administer IV medications and monitor the patients throughout the procedure. Occasionally, general anesthesia is required, most commonly for pediatric patients.

Procedures

Venous interventions

CVCs are positioned with the catheter tip in the superior vena cava (SVC) or right atrium to allow for the delivery of medications and the aspiration of blood without damaging the peripheral veins. There are four main types of CVCs including nontunneled catheters, tunneled catheters, peripherally inserted central catheters (PICCs), and implanted ports.

Nontunneled catheters traverse the skin and immediately enter a large vein. These are temporary vascular access devices designed to be used only while a patient remains in the hospital. Examples of these include "triple lumen catheters" and temporary dialysis and apheresis catheters.

Tunneled catheters traverse the skin and then travel through a 5–7 cm subcutaneous tunnel before entering a large vein. The tunnel makes the catheter less likely to accidentally be withdrawn and also acts as a barrier between skin bacteria and the accessed vein. Therefore, tunneled central catheters are designed for long-term use both during hospital stay and after discharge. Examples of these catheters include permanent dialysis and apheresis catheters, Hickman catheters, and Broviac catheters (Figure 12.4a).

PICCs are placed into a smaller vein, most commonly in the upper arm. They traverse the skin and immediately enter a superficial vein. Although the access is peripheral, the tip of the catheter is still placed centrally. These catheters have the advantage of a lower risk of bleeding during placement and a lower risk of associated cellulitis compared to tunneled catheters. They can be used for weeks to months for multiple purposes.

Implanted ports are ideal devices for patients requiring long-term repetitive venous access and are most commonly placed in patients needing chemotherapy. The port itself is a small cylindrical or triangular device that is placed in the subcutaneous tissue and serves as the vascular access site. It is accessed through a specialized diaphragm that can accommodate repetitive needlesticks without becoming damaged (Figure 12.4b).

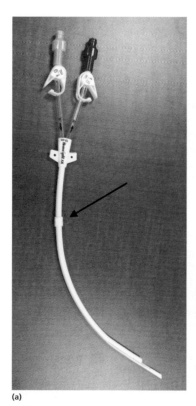

(a)

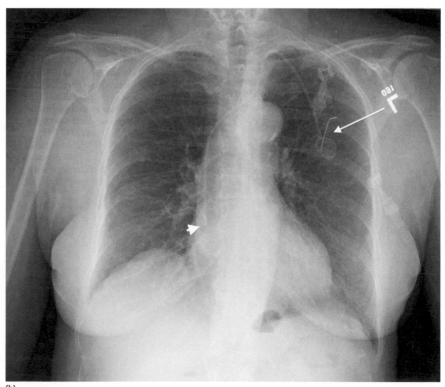

(b)

Figure 12.4 Central venous catheters—tunneled dialysis catheter with retention cuff (arrow) that incorporates into the subcutaneous tissue preventing accidental withdrawal (a).Chest X-ray demonstrating a left-sided implanted chest port with access needle in place (arrow). The tip of the catheter is located at the cavoatrial junction (arrowhead) (b).

Insertion involves surgically creating a subcutaneous pocket, most often in the upper chest. The port is placed in the pocket and then attached to a catheter that courses through a subcutaneous tunnel before entering the accessed vein. Once the port pocket incision has healed, implanted ports provide several advantages over other vascular access devices. Since there is no catheter protruding from the skin, patients do not have any limitations on their physical activities. Additionally, because the skin barrier overlying the port remains intact, the risk of infection is low. Ports can be used for years without malfunctioning if maintained properly. When they are no longer needed, they can be removed during a short procedure performed with only local anesthesia.

Placement of all of the CVCs described in the section "Central Venous Catheters (CVCs)" begins with the insertion of a needle into the target vein under US guidance. A guidewire is then inserted and advanced into the right atrium or inferior vena cava (IVC) under fluoroscopic guidance. If a tunneled catheter is being placed, a very small skin incision is made, and the catheter is then passed through the subcutaneous tissue toward the venotomy site. If a port is being placed, the port pocket is created, and then the catheter is advanced through the subcutaneous tissue toward the venotomy site. The final step involves advancing the catheter into the vein, either directly or through a peel-away sheath. Many catheters have to be cut to the appropriate length, and therefore, fluoroscopically measuring the correct intravascular length is necessary before catheter insertion.

Venous thrombolysis/thrombectomy is performed in IR for the treatment of *deep venous thrombosis (DVT)*. Emerging research has suggested that the treatment of DVT with anticoagulation alone often results in the development of *postthrombotic syndrome* involving chronic pain and swelling of the involved limb. To prevent this, more aggressive treatment has been suggested to eliminate the clot before these long-term symptoms develop. The most common method is called *catheter-directed thrombolysis*:

- This procedure involves placing a specially designed catheter with numerous holes in its distal segment into the vein containing the thrombus. A thrombolytic agent such as tissue plasminogen activator is then slowly infused via this catheter over multiple hours. The patient is then reevaluated with angiography to determine whether the clot has cleared or additional infusion time is necessary.

    Mechanical thrombectomy can also be performed with a variety of devices that physically disrupt the clot and evacuate it through a catheter.

When the right common iliac artery compresses the left common iliac vein resulting in thrombosis, it is called *May–Thurner syndrome*. This condition is treated with thrombolysis followed by stenting of the left common iliac vein (Figure 12.5).

IVC filters are placed fluoroscopically to prevent lower extremity or pelvic vein clots from migrating to the lungs and resulting in potentially fatal *pulmonary embolism (PE)*. The majority of the time, anticoagulation alone is sufficient to prevent PE. However, IVC filters may be indicated in the following settings in some patients:

1 Who have a contraindication to anticoagulation such as concurrent hemorrhage or recent major surgery
2 Have had a recent stroke
3 Who have developed worsening DVT or PE despite anticoagulation
   ◦ To place an IVC filter, either the internal jugular vein or common femoral vein is accessed. A catheter containing the collapsed filter is then advanced into the IVC and positioned

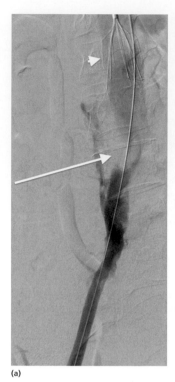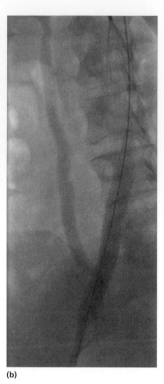

(a) (b)

Figure 12.5 Venous thrombolysis—DSA image demonstrating an area of nonopacification in the left common iliac vein resulting from compression by the overlying right common iliac artery (arrow) in a patient with May–Thurner syndrome. IVC filter (arrowhead) is also present (a). Fluoroscopic image after stenting of the left common iliac vein (b).

just below the most inferior renal vein using fluoroscopic guidance. The filter is then unsheathed, allowing it to expand and become lodged in the IVC. It will then trap all large blood clots that are migrating superiorly toward the pulmonary arteries. Placing the filter below the renal veins is important to avoid causing thrombus formation in the renal veins, which can lead to renal failure (Figure 12.6).

Because of potential complications associated with IVC filters including extracaval migration, fracture, and IVC thrombosis, it is recommended that they be removed as soon as the patient can be anticoagulated or is no longer at risk of DVT/PE.

Over recent years, removable IVC filters are routinely employed for this reason:

- Retrieval is performed by first gaining access to the internal jugular vein. A catheter is positioned just superior to the filter using fluoroscopic guidance. A snare that has a small retractable loop is advanced through the outer catheter and used to "lasso" the hook at the top of the filter. Once snared, the outer sheath is advanced over the filter, causing it to collapse back to its narrow width, similar to before it was deployed. The filter contained within this outer sheath is then removed from the patient.

SVC angioplasty/stenting can be performed in the setting of *SVC syndrome*. SVC syndrome is the result of SVC narrowing and manifests as neck and upper extremity swelling. The narrowing can be caused by a long-term indwelling catheter, previous radiation therapy, or compression from adjacent tumor.

- If initial balloon angioplasty does not result in resolution of the stenosis, a stent can be placed to reduce symptoms (Figure 12.7).

Venous sampling can be performed to localize hormone-producing tumors. The procedure is most commonly performed on patients who have hypertension as a result of elevated serum aldosterone. Blood work and diagnostic imaging alone cannot always identify the site of a hormone-producing adrenal tumor.

Since confirmation of the side of the involved adrenal gland is critical prior to surgery, this procedure plays an important preoperative role:

- Catheters are used to collect blood samples from both adrenal veins and the IVC. The aldosterone concentration of the samples is then analyzed in the laboratory providing confirmation of the side of the adrenal adenoma. This procedure can also be used to locate pancreatic endocrine tumors as well as parathyroid adenomas prior to resection.

Arterial interventions

Peripheral artery angioplasty/stenting is a treatment option for *peripheral arterial disease (PAD)*. PAD is characterized by narrowing of pelvic and lower extremity arteries, resulting in gluteal and lower extremity pain after walking. More severe disease can threaten limbs, occasionally requiring amputation. Treatment of PAD by endovascular methods is currently performed by interventional radiologists and, depending on the center, may also be provided by vascular surgeons and cardiologists:

- Pelvic and lower extremity angiography is performed to evaluate the number and length of the narrowed arterial segments. Severe disease is more effectively treated with surgically placed bypass grafts, while less severe disease can be treated with angioplasty and stenting under fluoroscopic guidance (Figure 12.8).
- Endovascular aortic repair (EVAR) is performed to treat aortic aneurysms and dissections:
- Covered stents are placed within the diseased portion of the aorta to recreate a normal lumen. To deliver stents large enough to fit the aorta, a surgical cut down is necessary for arterial access. Because of the surgical aspect of this procedure, these treatments are performed by an IR in conjunction with a surgeon, or solely by a surgeon. Fluoroscopy is used to guide stent placement.

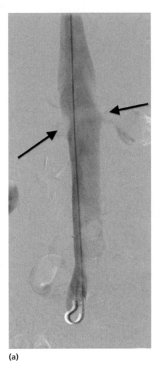 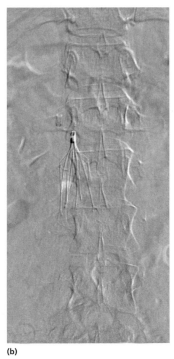

(a)   (b)

Figure 12.6 Inferior vena cava (IVC) filters—IVC venogram demonstrating the level of the renal veins as evidence by mixing artifact of nonopacified blood (arrows) (a). DSA image after IVC filter placement below the renal veins (b).

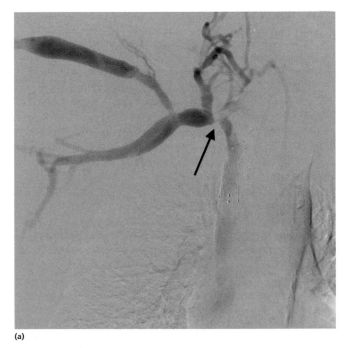 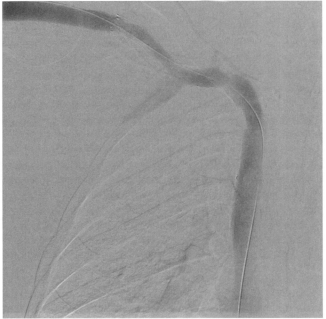

(a)   (b)

Figure 12.7 Superior vena cava (SVC) stenting—DSA image of a patient who had multiple stents placed for SVC syndrome. There is residual stenosis at the edge of a stent in the right subclavian vein (arrow) (a). Improved appearance with less opacification of collateral veins after placement of an additional stent across the stenosis (b).

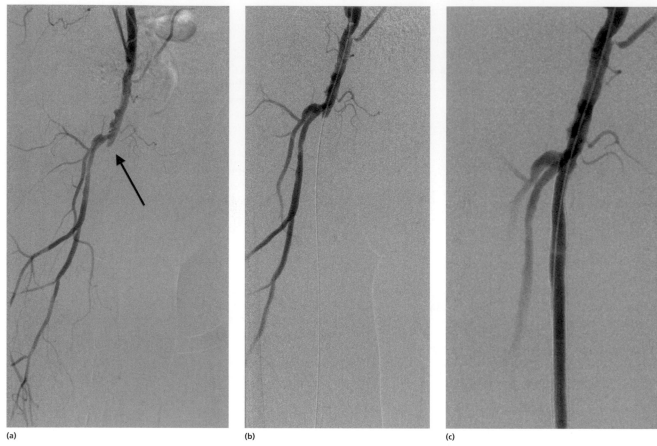

(a)   (b)   (c)

Figure 12.8 Peripheral artery stenting—DSA image of occluded right superficial femoral artery (arrow) due to atherosclerotic disease in a patient with claudication (a). Same vessel now with traversal of the occlusion with a guidewire (b). Same vessel that is now patent after stenting (c).

Occasionally, after placement of an aortic stent, blood is still able to flow into the aneurysm sac, causing it to expand. This puts the patient at risk of aneurysm rupture despite the presence of a stent:

- This undesirable flow of blood into the aneurysm sac is called an *endoleak* and can be treated in IR guided by multiple imaging modalities including fluoroscopy, CT, and occasionally US. Embolization of vessels feeding the aneurysm sac or embolization of the sac itself is performed to eliminate the risk of rupture.

Posttraumatic arterial embolization is a common procedure that interventional radiologists are called upon to perform urgently. Patients appropriate for IR treatment must be hemodynamically stable; otherwise, they should undergo immediate surgery. Stable patients with recognized ongoing hemorrhage, based on imaging findings of either *contrast extravasation* or *pseudoaneurysm,* may undergo this minimally invasive treatment avoiding the morbidity associated with surgery. The most common sites of posttraumatic bleeds occur in the pelvis, spleen, and liver:

- Embolization is performed by first placing a catheter into the common femoral artery. Then, using a guidewire, the catheter is directed to the site of hemorrhage. Often, a microcatheter is utilized to navigate through smaller vasculature.

Once angiography has confirmed that the catheter is located at the bleeding site, an embolic agent is injected to reduce flow through the bleeding vessel. In the posttraumatic setting, a liquid mixture of gelatin foam and contrast is the most commonly used embolic agent. It is temporary, undergoing reabsorption after approximately 2–4 weeks, once the bleeding vessel has healed.

Pulmonary intervention

Pulmonary angiography/thrombolysis for PE is a procedure provided by IR. Although most PEs can be effectively treated with long-term anticoagulation, there are clinical scenarios that require immediate intervention. Hemodynamically unstable patients or patients demonstrating evidence of right heart strain should be treated with thrombolysis or thrombectomy:

- Thrombolysis in this setting is similar to the description in the DVT section in that an infusion catheter is placed into the pulmonary artery(ies), coursing through the blood clot. A thrombolytic agent is then slowly infused with the goal of dissolving the thrombus. Alternatively, a widemouthed catheter can be placed within the clot, and it can be physically removed by applying suction to the catheter.

Pulmonary arteriovenous malformation (AVM) embolization is most commonly performed for patients with hereditary hemorrhagic telangiectasia, a condition that affects small blood vessels throughout the body. An AVM is an abnormal tangle of vessels that is fed by one or more arteries, immediately draining through a vein, bypassing the capillary bed (Figure 12.9). There are multiple reasons for treating pulmonary AVMs. Once they reach a certain size, the risk of bleeding increases. Also, patients may report fatigue because of low systemic oxygen tension secondary to blood bypassing the lungs. Finally, brain abscesses can form when blood-borne bacteria bypass the normal filtration provided by the lungs and travel to the brain:

- Embolization of a pulmonary AVM is performed by advancing a catheter through the right heart into the pulmonary artery. Angiographic

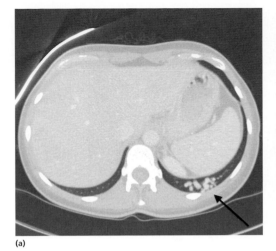
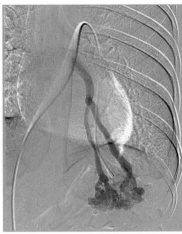

Figure 12.9 Pulmonary arteriovenous malformation (AVM)—axial noncontrast CT image demonstrating a tangle of vessels at the left lung base (arrow) typical of a pulmonary AVM (a). AP DSA image demonstrating the venous drainage of the same pulmonary AVM (b).

(a)

(b)

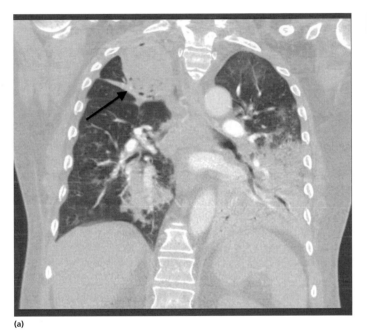
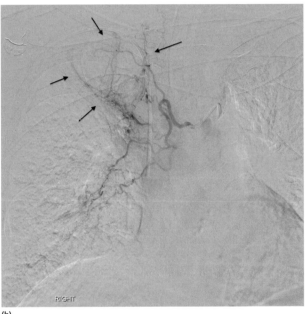

(a)

(b)

Figure 12.10 Bronchial artery embolization—coronal chest CT showing a right apical fungus-filled cavity (arrow) that was causing hemoptysis in this patient (a). DSA image with a catheter in the right bronchial artery that arises from the thoracic aorta. Branches are seen supplying the right apical mycetoma (arrows). Embolization was performed after microcatheter insertion (b).

images are then obtained to identify the feeding pulmonary artery branch. The catheter is then placed into this branch, and embolic agents such as coils are deployed to block the feeding artery.

Bronchial artery embolization can be performed to treat *hemoptysis* secondary to various chronic lung conditions (Figure 12.10). Bronchial artery embolization is indicated if hemoptysis results in a large amount of blood loss or if it becomes a lasting problem over the course of several days:

- This is performed by gaining common femoral artery access and guiding a catheter to the bronchial arteries that arise from the descending thoracic aorta. A microcatheter is then advanced into the bronchial artery, and embolic particles are injected until there is no further blood flow in the vessel from which bleeding has been fluoroscopically identified. Particles are mixed with contrast, and injection is observed under fluoroscopy to ensure that there is no backflow of these particles to nontargeted vessels.

Biliary intervention

Percutaneous transhepatic biliary drain (PTBD) placement creates drainage of an obstructed biliary system or in other settings diverts bile from a transected CBD:

- This procedure is performed using US or fluoroscopy to guide a small-caliber needle percutaneously through the liver into an intrahepatic biliary duct. Once the needle is in place, a guidewire is inserted and the intrahepatic tract is dilated. A catheter is then advanced over the wire in the biliary system.

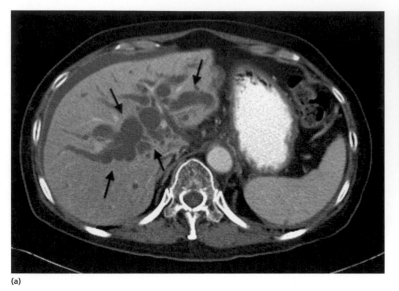
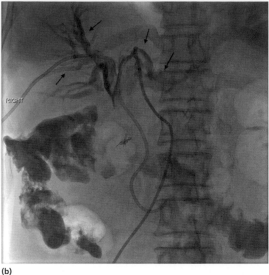

(a) (b)

Figure 12.11 Percutaneous transhepatic biliary drain (PTBD)—axial contrast-enhanced CT image demonstrating intrahepatic biliary ductal dilatation (arrows) secondary to a pancreatic tumor that is not seen on this image (a). Fluoroscopic spot image after placement of a right external biliary drain and a left internal/external biliary drain. The dilated intrahepatic biliary ducts can still be seen (arrows) (b).

An internal/external drain is designed to be advanced through the CBD into the duodenum. It has holes at its tip as well as more proximally, allowing bile to drain from the intrahepatic ducts into the small bowel, traversing a CBD obstruction or injury. An external drain does not traverse the CBD, but remains in the intrahepatic biliary system and drains bile from the liver to a bag outside the patient's body.

During this procedure, contrast is injected into the biliary system allowing for a fluoroscopic cholangiogram to be obtained. This image provides diagnostic information about the location and severity of the obstruction as well as about any abnormalities involving the remainder of the biliary tree (Figure 12.11).

CBD stent placement can be performed in the setting of cancer in which the tumor narrows the CBD and impedes biliary drainage into the bowel. Covered stents are used to delay the invasion and subsequent narrowing of the stent by the tumor.

Because the stent cannot be reopened after obstruction by an invading tumor, CBD stents are only placed palliatively for patients with poor prognoses.

Cholecystostomy drain insertion is a treatment alternative for patients with cholecystitis who are unable to undergo surgery due to comorbidities:

- This is performed by percutaneously placing a needle through the liver and into the gallbladder under US guidance. A guidewire is then advanced through the needle and coiled in the gallbladder. The needle is removed over the wire, and a drain is placed into the gallbladder.

  Verification of appropriate placement can be performed under fluoroscopy with a small-volume contrast injection. The drain is then attached to an external bag, allowing the gallbladder to remain decompressed until the patient is a candidate for definitive surgery or the inflammation has subsided.

Portal venous hypertension interventions

Transjugular intrahepatic portosystemic shunt (TIPS) is a procedure performed in patients experiencing symptomatic sequelae of portal venous hypertension, such as bleeding esophageal varices that cannot

be treated with endoscopy or ascites or pleural effusion that does not respond to diuretics. The purpose of the procedure is to decrease the pressure differential between the portal vein and the hepatic veins. This is achieved by creating a false passage through the liver tissue, connecting one of the portal veins with one of the hepatic veins:

- Initial access is obtained through the internal jugular vein, and a catheter is passed through the right atrium into the IVC under fluoroscopic guidance. The catheter is then directed into a hepatic vein, most commonly the right hepatic vein.

  A guidewire is inserted and the catheter is exchanged for a long needle that can be advanced over the wire. The wire is then removed and this needle is used to puncture from the hepatic vein through the liver parenchyma into a portal vein, most commonly the right portal vein. Once the needle is through, the wire is reinserted and coiled in the main portal vein.

  A covered stent is then advanced over the wire and deployed in the newly created passage connecting the portal vein and hepatic vein. Final angiography is then performed, demonstrating blood flowing easily from the portal vein, through the TIPS stent and into the right atrium (Figure 12.12). Patients are subsequently followed with US examinations to monitor for TIPS stent narrowing.

Balloon occlusion retrograde transvenous obliteration (BORTO) of varices is a treatment option for patients with bleeding gastric varices (as opposed to esophageal varices as discussed earlier). Chronic portal hypertension results in physiologic vascular changes as the body attempts to compensate. One commonly seen change is the formation of a gastrorenal shunt in which blood from enlarged gastric veins, which normally would flow into the portal venous system, finds a path of less resistance into the left adrenal vein. The blood then flows to the left renal vein and then to the IVC and returns to the heart. The presence of a gastrorenal shunt makes a BORTO procedure feasible:

- The procedure is performed by gaining access to the common femoral vein and guiding a catheter through the IVC into the left renal vein under fluoroscopic guidance. A balloon occlusion catheter is then advanced into the left adrenal vein that is dilated because it is shunting high-volume blood flow from the varices to the systemic circulation.

The balloon is then inflated, occluding the left adrenal vein, and a sclerosing agent is injected through the catheter into the gastric varices. It is then allowed to dwell for several hours, irritating the walls of the varices, resulting in thrombosis.

GI interventions

Gastrostomy tubes (G-tubes) allow for the administration of nutritional formulas directly into the stomach for patients who cannot take food by mouth. They also can be put to suction for gastric decompression:

- The night before G-tube placement, barium is given to the patient either by mouth or through a nasogastric tube. A radiograph of the abdomen is obtained the following morning to determine if the barium has opacified the transverse colon. Visualization of the transverse colon is important during fluoroscopic gastric

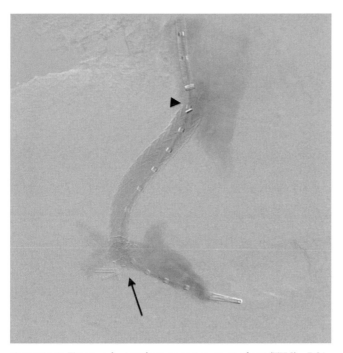

Figure 12.12 Transjugular intrahepatic portosystemic shunt (TIPS)—DSA image of a TIPS stent coursing from the right portal vein (arrow) to the IVC (arrowhead) via the right hepatic vein.

puncture to ensure that the colon is not inadvertently injured. A nasogastric tube is required to be in place, prior to the procedure.

An initial US examination of the abdomen is performed to identify and mark the liver margins. This is to prevent inadvertent passage of the access needle through the nonradiopaque liver. The stomach is then inflated with air through the nasogastric tube to make it easier to puncture.

A needle is advanced into the stomach under fluoroscopy, and its position is verified by aspirating air as well as injecting a small amount of contrast that outlines the gastric rugae. A gastropexy tack is then deployed that pulls the anterior stomach wall up to the anterior abdominal wall.

This is repeated so that two tacks are placed several centimeters apart. Between the two tacks, a third needle puncture is made into the stomach. A wire is then passed through the needle and coiled in the stomach. The needle is exchanged for a peel-away sheath, and the gastrostomy tube is advanced through the sheath into the stomach. The sheath is removed, and a retention balloon on the tube is inflated with dilute contrast. The tube is withdrawn until the balloon is snugly positioned against the anterior stomach wall.

An outer disc is then cinched down on the skin, preventing movement of the tube as well as the passage of gastric fluid out to the skin. A final contrast injection through the tube under fluoroscopy verifies proper placement (Figure 12.13).

Gastrojejunostomy tubes (G-J tubes) are indicated for patients who have difficulty with being fed into their stomachs. These include patients with delayed gastric emptying and gastroesophageal reflux:

- The initial steps for placing a G-J tube are identical to the placement of a G-tube. However, the additional step of using an angled catheter to pass a wire into the small bowel is required to place a G-J tube.

Arterial embolization for GI bleed is often performed to avoid surgical treatment:

- The location of the hemorrhage within the bowel should be identified on imaging prior to attempting embolization. Once the affected segment of bowel is identified, the appropriate mesenteric artery is catheterized.

  Angiography is performed to confirm the bleeding site, and then an embolic agent is used to block blood flow to that segment of bowel.

Although this description makes bowel ischemia seem likely, it is a rare occurrence due to the rich network of collateral vessels supplying the intestines (Figure 12.14).

Figure 12.13 Gastrostomy tubes (G-tubes)—a G-tube on the back table with retention balloon inflated (arrow) (a). Abdominal radiograph demonstrating a G-tube within an air-filled stomach. The retention balloon (arrow) is opacified with dilute contrast, and the gastropexy tacks (arrowheads) are also seen (b).

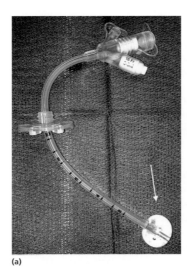

(a)

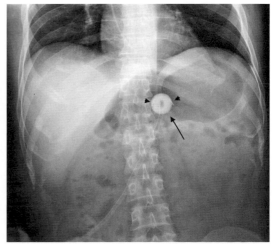

(b)

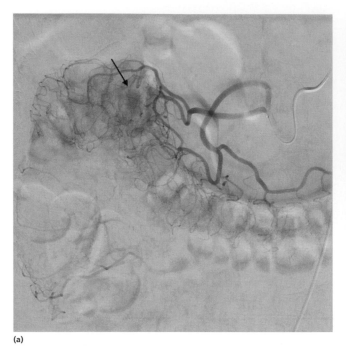
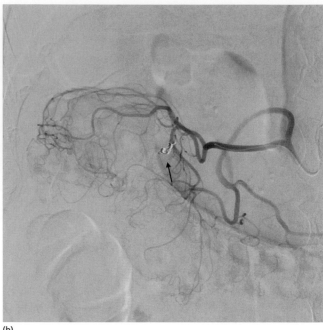

(a)   (b)

Figure 12.14 Arterial embolization for GI bleed—DSA image of contrast extravasation (arrow) in the proximal transverse colon demonstrating the site of bleeding in this patient with diverticulosis (a). Postembolization DSA image with coils present (arrow) and no residual contrast extravasation (b).

Renal/urinary interventions

Nephrostomy tubes are catheters that are placed through the skin into the renal pelvis to allow for drainage of obstructed kidneys, to divert urine away from an injured lower urinary tract to promote healing, or to provide access for further treatment of renal stones:

• Patients are initially given antibiotics to protect against bacteria that might be introduced into the blood from the urine during the procedure. The patient is positioned prone and US is used to identify the kidney with a dilated collecting system.

   If there is no hydronephrosis, fluoroscopy can be used to identify the kidney either by targeting a radiopaque stone or by administering IV contrast and waiting until it opacifies the renal collecting system.

   Once the kidney is identified on imaging, a long thin needle is inserted through the skin into a renal calyx. Because of the embryological development of the renal vasculature, a posterolateral approach allows for the lowest risk of bleeding as the needle and subsequent tube traverse the renal parenchyma. Also, entry through the lower pole is preferred because of the risk of penetrating the pleura and causing a pneumothorax with an upper pole approach.

   Once the needle is positioned in the collecting system, a wire is advanced under fluoroscopy into the renal pelvis or ureter. The needle is then removed, the tract is dilated, and the nephrostomy tube is advanced over the wire. Contrast can then be injected, creating a fluoroscopic image called a *nephrostogram*.

   This is useful in demonstrating the degree of renal collecting system dilatation; identifying filling defects such as thrombus, tumor, or radiolucent stones; and evaluating for obstruction within the ureter (Figure 12.15).

   Ureteral stents or "JJ" stents can be placed in an antegrade fashion through percutaneous access into the renal collecting system. The stents are actually catheters that have holes proximally and distally providing a conduit for urine to drain from the renal pelvis to the bladder. This is useful when there is intrinsic narrowing or external compression of the ureters limiting passage of urine:

• Procedurally, placement of ureteral stents is similar to nephrostomy tubes, and often, nephrostomy tubes are placed in conjunction with ureteral stents.

   Once access into the collecting system is obtained with US or fluoroscopic guidance, a stiff guidewire is advanced into the bladder.

   The appropriate length ureteral stent is then advanced over the wire until the distal end is located in the bladder and the proximal end is in the renal pelvis.

Suprapubic catheters are better solutions than long-term Foley catheters due to lower risk of infection and injury to the urethra:

• They are placed by first distending the bladder with saline through a Foley catheter. Under US guidance, a needle is then advanced through the skin into the bladder.

   A wire is then inserted through the needle and coiled in the bladder under fluoroscopy. The tract is dilated and the catheter is then inserted over the wire. The final step is to inject contrast to ensure proper placement.

Pelvic interventions

Uterine fibroid embolization (UFE) has proven to be an attractive alternative to surgery for the purpose of relieving symptoms associated with fibroids. The procedure is only indicated when the fibroids are hypervascular, and therefore, a preprocedural MRI is necessary:

• The procedure is performed by gaining access into the common femoral artery and guiding a catheter into the internal iliac artery from which the uterine artery arises.

   A microcatheter is then advanced into the uterine artery beyond branches that could supply the cervix, and particles are injected until there is sluggish blood flow. Embolization is then performed in the contralateral uterine artery as well.

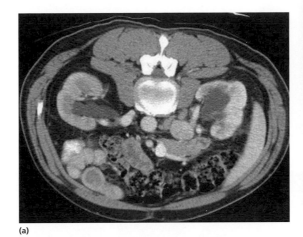

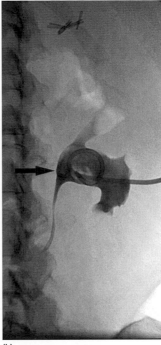

(a)

(b)

Figure 12.15 Nephrostomy tubes—axial contrast-enhanced CT image showing bilateral dilatation of the renal collecting systems (a). Fluoroscopic image demonstrating a nephrostomy tube with pigtail (arrow) in the renal pelvis (b).

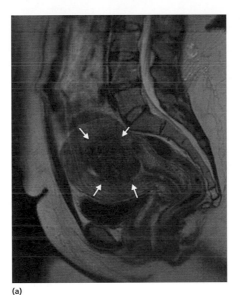

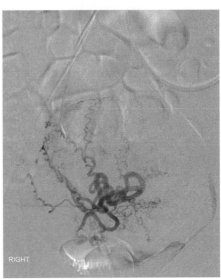

(a)

(b)

Figure 12.16 Uterine fibroid embolization (UFE)—sagittal T2-weighted MR image of the pelvis demonstrating large submucosal uterine fibroids (arrows) (a). DSA image of a catheter in the right uterine artery with numerous abnormal corkscrew vessels typically seen with fibroids. These arteries were embolized with tiny particles causing shrinkage of the fibroids over time (b).

Patients are admitted to the hospital overnight in order to be treated for symptoms of *postembolization syndrome* that include pain, fever, and nausea. Relief from symptoms associated with the fibroids does not occur immediately, but rather full therapeutic benefit is usually seen after several months (Figure 12.16).

Gonadal vein embolization is performed to treat women suffering from *pelvic congestion syndrome*, characterized by chronic dull pelvic or lower back pain that can be exacerbated by standing or menstruation. The pain is a result of engorged pelvic veins that do not drain normally due to valvular dysfunction:

- Treatment involves catheterization of the ovarian veins that arise from the IVC on the right and the renal vein on the left. Coils and sclerosant are then placed in these veins to cause thrombosis, alleviating the symptoms of pelvic congestion syndrome.

A similar procedure is performed in men for the treatment of varicocele, a condition of engorged scrotal veins that can cause pain and/or infertility. Both of these procedures can be treated without overnight hospital stay.

Musculoskeletal interventions

Vertebral augmentation is divided into *vertebroplasty* and *kyphoplasty*:

- Both procedures involve injection of specialized cement into a fractured vertebral body for stabilization and reduction of pain. The difference is that in kyphoplasty, a balloon is inflated during cement injection in order to gain vertebral body height.

Both procedures are performed by using fluoroscopy to guide cannulae through the skin and vertebral pedicles into the vertebral body.

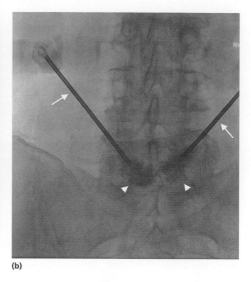

(a)

(b)

Figure 12.17 Vertebral augmentation— sagittal T1-weighted MR image demonstrating multiple vertebral compression fractures (arrows) (a). Fluoroscopic image of cannulae (arrows) coursing through the pedicles into the vertebral body during vertebroplasty. Cement (arrowheads) has been injected resulting in immediate pain relief from fixation of a compression fracture (b).

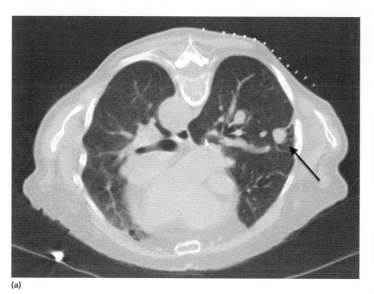

(a)

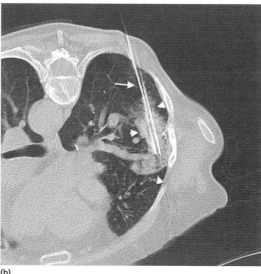

(b)

Figure 12.18 Percutaneous thermal ablation—axial CT image demonstrating a metastatic nodule in the lower lobe of the right lung (arrow) (a). Intraprocedural CT with ablation probes (arrow) placed in the lesion. Inflammation can be seen in the surrounding lung (arrowheads) (b).

Injection of cement is then performed under fluoroscopy to ensure that it does not extrude from the vertebra affecting adjacent structures. This is performed as a same-day procedure and often results in immediate pain relief (Figure 12.17).

Osteoid osteoma ablation can be performed to alleviate the characteristic nighttime pain associated with this benign bone tumor that occurs in young people:

- The procedure is performed by placing an ablation probe through the skin, into the bone lesion under CT guidance. The probe is then used to heat the lesion for several minutes.

 The probe is then removed with minimal bleeding and the puncture site is dressed.

 Once the pain from the procedure subsides, usually within 1 week, the majority of patients no longer have pain from the lesion.

Interventional oncology

Percutaneous thermal ablation is an effective treatment for eliminating smaller tumors, most commonly in the liver, lungs, and kidneys:

- Both radiofrequency and microwave generators can be used to heat probes that are placed within target tumors under CT or US guidance.

 Ablation can also be performed using freezing agents that tend to be less painful but are associated with higher bleeding risks. These procedures can be performed without overnight hospital stay and without general anesthesia (Figure 12.18).

Transarterial chemoembolization (TACE) is a procedure to treat tumors in the liver (Figure 12.19):

- Following arterial access via the common femoral artery, a catheter is directed superiorly through the abdominal aorta into the celiac artery. A microcatheter is then inserted through the initial catheter and guided into the hepatic artery branches that are supplying the tumor(s).

 The initial description of this procedure involved injecting liquid chemotherapy mixed with contrast agent followed by particles to block the blood supply and trap the chemotherapy agent in the small blood vessels supplying the tumor.

 More recently, the technique has evolved to use tiny embolic beads soaked in the chemotherapeutic agent and mixed with contrast agent.

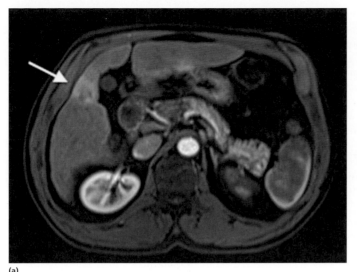

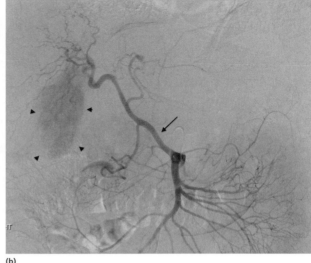

(a)   (b)

Figure 12.19 Transarterial chemoembolization (TACE)—axial T1-weighted postcontrast MR image in arterial phase demonstrating an area of early enhancement in the liver (arrow) compatible with hepatocellular carcinoma (a). DSA image of the same patient demonstrating a replaced common hepatic artery (arrow) arising from the superior mesenteric artery and an area of early tumor blush (arrowheads) corresponding to the MRI findings (b).

The effect of this treatment is to decrease the size of tumors, extending patient life. It does not eliminate the tumor completely, except in uncommon circumstances of multiple small hypervascular tumors. Patients are often admitted overnight after this procedure to treat symptoms of postembolization syndrome.

Transarterial radioembolization (TARE) is similar to TACE, but instead of chemotherapy-soaked beads, beads impregnated with the radioactive isotope yttrium-90 are injected. There is risk during any embolization procedure that the embolic agent may travel to an unwanted location instead of the target, resulting in "nontarget" ischemia. When radioactive beads are being used, there is additional risk of radiation injury with nontarget embolization:

- In order to minimize this risk, a pretreatment angiogram is performed to evaluate for arterial flow from the hepatic vessels to nontarget organs such as the lungs, stomach, and bowel.

  If a branch of the hepatic artery is seen coursing to the stomach or bowel, it should be embolized with coils prior to treatment to prevent possible radiation injury during treatment. Similar to TACE, TARE results in decreasing the size of tumors in the liver and extending patient life.

Portal vein embolization is performed when a patient is to undergo a partial liver resection to remove tumor, and the future liver remnant will be too small to provide compensatory hepatic function:

- In this circumstance, the portal vein branch feeding the hepatic lobe to be resected is embolized, most often using coils and particles. This redirects all of the portal blood flow to the future liver remnant, causing it to hypertrophy significantly over the course of several months.

Fiducial placement is performed prior to patients undergoing external beam radiation to treat tumors:

- Under CT or US guidance, a needle is used to deploy small radiopaque markers in a triangle around the lesion to be targeted. Once in place, the radiation oncologists use the fiducials for treatment planning.

Abscess treatment

Image-guided abscess drainage is a very common procedure, performed most often in postsurgical patients. Fluid collections can be treated with drainage throughout the body, but this treatment is most frequently performed in the abdomen and pelvis:

- Either CT or US is used to guide placement of a needle through the skin into the collection, with aspiration of fluid confirming appropriate placement.

  A guidewire is then passed through the needle and coiled in the collection. The tract is dilated and a drain is then placed over the wire into the abscess. The drain is usually attached to a suction bulb.

  Follow-up *sinograms* are performed at 1–2-week intervals after drain placement. This involves injecting a small amount of contrast agent through the drain and obtaining fluoroscopic images to determine if the abscess has resolved and the drain can be removed. Occasionally, a drain has to be exchanged because it is clogged or has to be manipulated into an undrained component of the initial collection.

Other interventions

Image-guided biopsy is performed on a routine basis to identify the nature of unknown lesions and to characterize the type of disease affecting failing organs, such as the liver or kidney:

- The procedures are either performed with US or CT guidance. Most commonly, a coaxial approach is used in which an outer needle is positioned at the margin of the tissue to be sampled. A thinner needle is then inserted through the outer needle and used to obtain the biopsy.

  Both fine needle aspirations and core samples can be obtained in this manner. The advantage of a coaxial technique is that multiple samples can be obtained without needing to reposition the needle each time. This is especially important when sampling tissue that is difficult to access.

Image-guided thoracentesis/paracentesis is performed in IR when these procedures cannot be performed blindly:

- US is the modality of choice for imaging guidance. A needle with an outer cannula is inserted into the peritoneal or pleural space, and the outer cannula is then advanced off of the needle. This technique reduces the chance of inadvertently puncturing underlying organs. The outer cannula is attached to suction, and the volume of remaining fluid can be monitored periodically with US.

Following thoracentesis, the needle is removed and an occlusive dressing is placed, taking care not to allow air to leak into the puncture site. A follow-up chest X-ray is obtained to evaluate for pneumothorax.

Tunneled pleural/peritoneal catheters are placed when patients have recurrent pleural effusion or ascites, most commonly from malignancy:

- The catheters allow the patients to evacuate the fluid at home as needed without having to come into the hospital to undergo the procedure.

   The tunneled catheters have cuffs that adhere to the subcutaneous tissue preventing inadvertent dislodgment and also protecting against the spread of skin bacteria into the pleura or peritoneum. Placement is very similar to tunneled CVCs.

Dialysis access intervention is vital to ensure that patients with end-stage renal disease maintain their dialysis schedule. Internal accesses, including surgically created arteriovenous fistulae (AVFs) and arteriovenous grafts (AVGs), often become narrowed, and the flow of blood across them is slowed:

- In these situations, angiography is performed to identify the location of the narrowing, and angioplasty is subsequently performed. If angioplasty is ineffective, stents can be placed.

   Occasionally, the blood flow through AVFs and AVGs becomes so stagnant that they clot off altogether. In these situations, thrombolysis is performed followed by angioplasty to restore flow.

   These procedures are performed using fluoroscopy for guidance. Occasionally, US guidance is necessary to access an AVF or AVG that is not easily palpable.

Thoracic duct embolization can be performed to treat postsurgical leakage of lymphatic fluid into the pleural space:

- To identify a target, imaging is performed by injecting a contrast agent into the lymphatic system, either in the web spaces of the toes or into the inguinal lymph nodes visible on US.

   After some hours, the contrast is transported superiorly within the lymphatic ducts and potentially opacifies the thoracic duct. It then can be targeted using fluoroscopy.

   A long, narrow needle is passed through the superior abdomen until the tip is seen to puncture it. Coils can then be deployed preventing further accumulation of lymphatic fluid in the pleural space.

Celiac block is performed in the setting of chronic pain, often from mesenteric malignancy, commonly pancreatic cancer:

- Under CT guidance, two long, narrow needles are positioned on either side of the celiac artery. Contrast is injected to ensure proper positioning.

   A long-acting analgesic and steroid is then injected to ameliorate pain caused by irritation of the neural plexus that overlies the celiac artery. Additionally, alcohol can be injected to destroy these nerves resulting in more permanent pain relief.

Noninvasive vascular imaging

The preceding section on IR refers to techniques that are generally termed "minimally invasive," as they involve the use of various forms of sharps and catheters to enter the patient's body and, in the case of vasculature, the vessels themselves. In this section, we will describe methods of visualizing the vasculature that do not involve direct cannulation of vessels. Some techniques involve the IV administration of contrast agents, whereas others rely on the physical differences of moving blood to generate images. We will be describing techniques based on CT, MRI, and US that have allowed for noninvasive imaging of the vasculature.

Normal anatomy

Systemic blood flow is achieved via arteries and veins. Arteries take blood away from the heart and have thick, muscular walls. Blood flow within end organs is via capillaries; capillaries have a large surface area and have thin, permeable walls to exchange nutrients and waste products with the tissues. After blood has passed through the capillary bed, it reaches the veins. Veins carry blood back to the heart and have thinner walls with less smooth muscle than arteries. They also have valves to prevent backflow of blood, as the pressure is not as high as in arteries to sustain forward flow.

Arteries and veins both have three layers in their walls. The innermost layer is called the intima, and it is in this layer that calcium deposits in atherosclerotic disease. The middle layer is called the media, and this contains smooth muscle and elastic tissue that give vessels the ability to change size in response to various stimuli. The outermost layer is called the adventitia and is the strongest layer, made of tough connective tissue.

Imaging modalities

US can be a useful way to evaluate blood vessels, without the risk of radiation exposure. Vessels that are best seen by US are close to the surface of the body, as sound waves do not penetrate well through air or through a large amount of soft tissue. In addition to grayscale ultrasound imaging, color Doppler flow (wherein flow is colorized based on the direction of flow) and spectral Doppler flow (a graphic tracing of the velocity of blood flow over time) are useful to evaluate vascular flow. Veins and arteries can be distinguished from one another in several ways on US: first, direction of flow is helpful—if flow is away from the heart, the imaged vessel is likely an artery, and vice versa. Veins have thinner walls and valves, and they flatten with compression. Arteries have thicker walls, and the pressure in their lumen is high enough that they will not flatten with compression. Finally, a spectral Doppler tracing in a normal artery shows a sharp increase in velocity in systole, followed by a rapid deceleration as systole ends; in contradistinction, a vein shows a gentle rise and fall in velocity.

Common applications of vascular US include evaluation for DVT in the extremities and evaluation for carotid artery atherosclerotic disease. In thin patients, US can be used as a screening tool for abdominal aortic aneurysm (AAA), but full evaluation of AAA requires computed tomography angiography (CTA) or magnetic resonance angiography (MRA).

CTA has become a workhorse in evaluating vascular anatomy (Figure 12.20). CTA requires a large-bore (at least 20 gauge) IV in a medium- to large-sized vein—usually within a few centimeters of the antecubital fossa—and rapid injection of iodinated contrast (approximately 4–5 ml/s). Once the contrast bolus is in the veins, accurate timing is needed to make sure the contrast is within the vessel of interest. With different timing, different vessels can be highlighted; for instance, an early timing will highlight the pulmonary arteries, which allows radiologists to evaluate for pulmonary arterial embolus. Slightly later, timing with the contrast bolus in the aorta allows evaluation for aortic trauma, dissection, or aneurysm. Even later timing allows evaluation of the veins, for deep venous thrombus in the pelvis or abdomen, where it is difficult for US to penetrate.

MRA is increasing in its use because of the lack of ionizing radiation and slightly greater flexibility in administration of IV contrast (Figure 12.21). Gadolinium-based contrast agents can be used safely down to a glomerular filtration rate (GFR) of 30 ml/min. This is because gadolinium-based contrast agents, unlike iodinated contrast, are not directly nephrotoxic in the doses in clinical use.

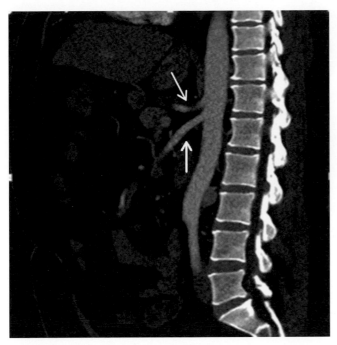

Figure 12.20 Normal CTA—*sagittal* reformatted image from a normal CTA of the abdomen and pelvis demonstrating the celiac axis (superior arrow) and superior mesenteric artery (inferior arrow) arising from the aorta.

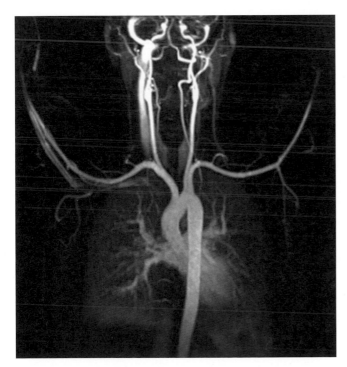

Figure 12.21 Normal MRA—coronal MRA of the chest with normal anatomy. This image can be reconstructed into axial, coronal, and sagittal slices to better view suspected abnormalities.

The main risk of gadolinium is nephrogenic systemic fibrosis (NSF), which only occurs in patients with severe renal disease (GFR < 30 ml/min). NSF is a lethal scleroderma-like reaction to gadolinium deposition in the soft tissues. However, MRA provides the advantage of still being able to view the vasculature with certain

noncontrasted data acquisitions (termed sequences). Therefore, noncontrasted MRA can still be performed for this population, but the images are typically inferior to contrasted MRA. Common applications of MRA include vascular imaging in children, patients with mild-to-moderate renal insufficiency, and neurologic vascular imaging (covered in another chapter).

Congenital anomalies

There are many congenital variants of vascular anatomy, some of which can cause pathology. The focus of this section will be narrowed to congenital anomalies of the aortic arch. However, there are congenital variants of many different systemic and pulmonary arteries and veins.

Aberrant subclavian artery

Embryologically, there are many aortic arches that fuse during development into two main left and right arches, with the right and left carotid and subclavian arteries arising from their respective arch. In normal development, the distal connection between the right common carotid artery and the descending aorta regresses, leaving the right common carotid artery to arise from a common trunk with the right subclavian artery, known as the innominate or brachiocephalic artery.

If a different connecting artery regresses or if there is no regression, then several different arch anomalies can occur. For instance, if the connection between the right subclavian and carotid arteries regresses, the right subclavian artery will have an anomalous origin from the descending aorta, which is known as an aberrant right subclavian artery (Figure 12.22). It will take a posterior course through the mediastinum and can make an impression on the esophagus. In some cases, this can cause dysphagia, also known as "dysphagia lusoria."

Trauma/emergency

There are many emergency conditions that involve the vessels, including PE, traumatic aortic injury, aortic dissection, aneurysms, and pseudoaneurysms. PE, dissection and traumatic aortic injury are covered in the chest chapter, so this section will concentrate on aneurysms and pseudoaneurysms.

Aneurysms

A true aneurysm is defined as a dilatation of the lumen of a vessel, greater than 1.5 times its normal diameter, with all three layers of the vessel wall (intima, media, and adventitia) intact. A false aneurysm, or pseudoaneurysm, is dilatation of the vessel lumen when fewer than three of those layers are intact. In many cases, the only layer keeping the pressurized blood within the lumen is a thin layer of adventitia, and thus, a pseudoaneurysm can be thought of as a contained perforation or transection of a vessel.

One of the most common places for true aneurysms to develop is the abdominal aorta. AAAs often coexist with diffuse atherosclerotic disease and may be related to inflammation in atherosclerosis that weakens the aortic wall. The abdominal aorta is considered aneurysmal at 3 cm and at a high enough risk of rupture to require treatment at 5 cm. Rupture of an AAA can be rapidly fatal, so prompt diagnosis and treatment is crucial:
- Imaging findings of AAA rupture include hematoma in the retroperitoneum or active extravasation of contrast from the aorta (Figure 12.23).

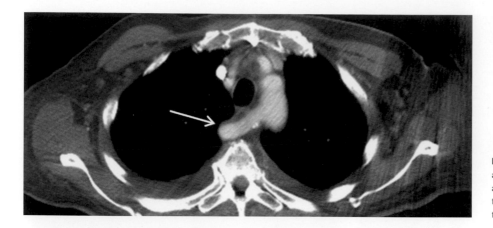

Figure 12.22 Aberrant right subclavian artery—note the aberrant right subclavian artery (arrow) arising from the distal transverse aorta and traveling posterior to the esophagus.

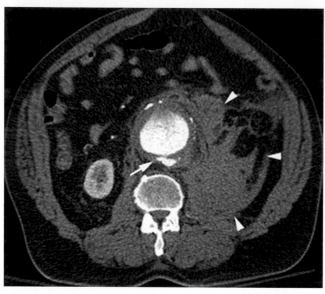

Figure 12.23 AAA rupture—note the retroperitoneal hemorrhage (arrowheads) and active extravasation of IV contrast from the posterior aorta (arrow).

Findings on CT that are worrisome for impending rupture include rapid enlargement, hematoma within the wall of the aneurysm, focal interruption of an otherwise continuous ring of calcium in the intima, and draping of the aorta over the adjacent psoas muscle.

There are several other types of true aneurysms in addition to those associated with atherosclerosis. Vasculitis, or inflammation of blood vessels, can cause narrowing and/or dilatation of a vessel's lumen; vasculitis is characterized by multiple areas of abnormality within a single vessel or several similar-sized vessels. Infected blood vessels can also become dilated, leading to mycotic aneurysms:

- Imaging features of a mycotic aneurysm include rapid growth, eccentric location, and perivascular fat stranding.

Pseudoaneurysms

Pseudoaneurysms, or false aneurysms, can be traumatic, iatrogenic, or inflammatory in nature. Traumatic pseudoaneurysms, such as traumatic aortic injury, are covered elsewhere. Iatrogenic pseudoaneurysms often occur after puncture of an artery, which

could be during placement of an arterial line for angiography or cardiac catheterization:

- Common imaging features of pseudoaneurysms include eccentric location, contrast enhancement of the lumen of the pseudoaneurysm, surrounding hemorrhage, and a "yin–yang" sign of flow into and out of the pseudoaneurysm on color Doppler US (Figure 12.24).

DVT

DVT is common in areas of relative venous stasis, especially the lower extremities. The extremity veins' superficial location is conducive to US imaging:

- Common US imaging findings in acute DVT include expansion of the vessel lumen, hypoechoic (dark gray) thrombus centrally within the vessel lumen, and noncompressibility of the vein—remember that normal veins should flatten out with compression (Figure 12.25).

Chronic DVT occurs when there has been occlusive thrombus that has scarred over time and partially recanalized; imaging findings include a small vessel lumen and eccentric or circumferential thrombus in the vessel lumen.

Spectral Doppler tracings can suggest upstream occlusion in the pelvis, even if the lower extremity veins are clear of thrombus. In these cases, CT venography (CTV) or MR venography (MRV) of the pelvis and IVC is the study of choice.

Use of a longer intravascular dwell time contrast agent in MRA, such as MultiHance or ABLAVAR, renders MRV images to have much more intense opacification of venous structures than CTV and hence is generally preferable.

Ischemia

Ischemia is an insufficiency of oxygen and nutrients to tissue due to poor blood flow. Although most ischemia is due to arterial insufficiency, venous blockage can also cause poor blood flow and ischemia as well. This section will focus on arterial ischemia, as it is more common.

Atherosclerosis

The most common reason for arterial insufficiency to an organ is due to arterial narrowing or occlusion from atherosclerosis in small- or medium-sized arteries. The clinical syndrome depends on the ischemic tissue; for ischemia in the lower extremity or pelvic arteries, the clinical manifestation is claudication; for the renal arteries, hypertension; and for the visceral arteries, postprandial abdominal pain and weight loss:

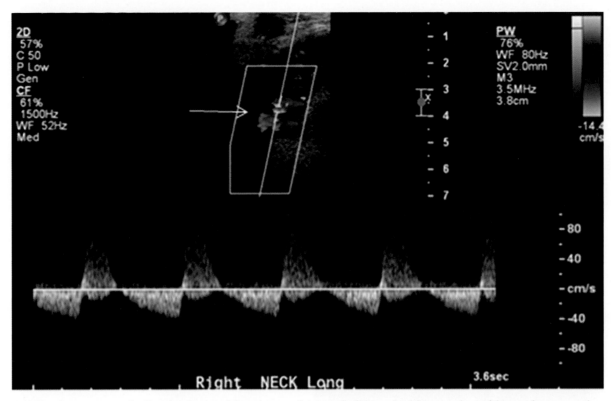

Figure 12.24 Pseudoaneurysm—color Doppler ultrasound demonstrates a "yin-yang" of blue and red flow in and out of the pseudoaneurysm (arrow). The spectral tracing beneath demonstrates flow above and below the baseline that corresponds to the color image.

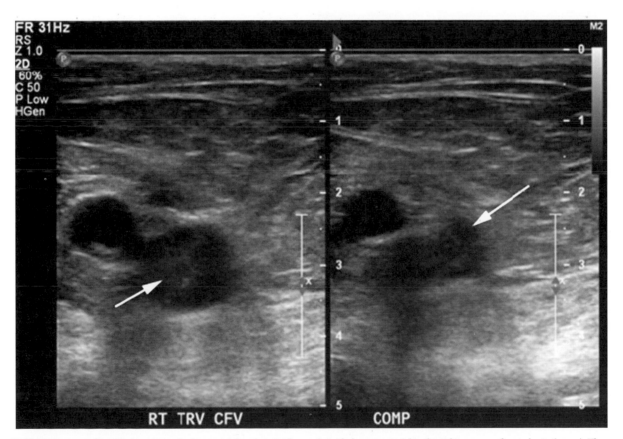

Figure 12.25 Deep venous thrombosis—grayscale ultrasound demonstrates hypoechoic/dark gray material in the right common femoral vein (arrow). The picture on the right, taken while compression was applied, shows that the vein does not efface fully with compression. These findings indicate thrombus in the vein.

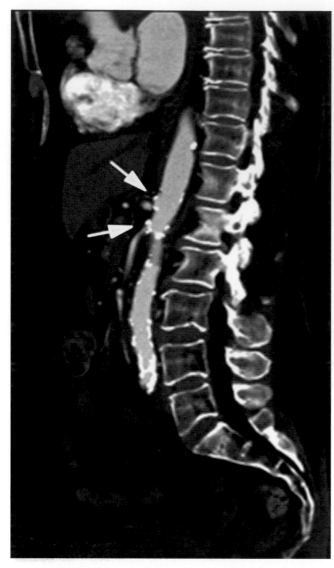

Figure 12.26 Visceral arterial stenosis—notice that the celiac artery (superior arrow) and superior mesenteric artery (inferior arrow) both demonstrate calcified atherosclerotic plaque and luminal narrowing. This can cause symptoms of postprandial abdominal pain, or "abdominal angina."

- Imaging findings of atherosclerosis in the vessels include calcified or noncalcified mural thrombus and narrowing of the vessel lumen (Figure 12.26).

Chronically occluded or narrowed vessels may also show enlarged collateral vessels in the surrounding tissues.

End organs can also possess findings of ischemia, with wedge-shaped areas of nonenhancement in the solid organs like the kidneys and spleen, or wall thickening and stranding of the bowel.

Embolism

Another common reason for ischemia is acute blockage of blood flow due to embolism of thrombus from elsewhere. Common sources for embolus include the heart and aorta; a right-to-left shunt like a patent foramen ovale may also allow venous thrombus to embolize to the systemic capillary beds. Embolism often lodges at branch points in vessels:

- Imaging findings of embolic disease include central filling defect within the vessel, located at a vascular branch point. Often, there will be a meniscus of contrast that surrounds the filling defect, which protrudes into the vessel lumen.

Suggested reading

Adusumilli, S., et al. The efficacy of selective arterial embolization in the management of colonic bleeding. *Techniques in Coloproctology* (2013): 1–5. (http://www.sciencedirect.com/science/article/pii/S0093775410002332).

Angel, L.F. *et al.* (2011) Systematic review of the use of retrievable inferior vena cava filters. *Journal of Vascular and Interventional Radiology*, **22** (11), 1522–1530.

Boyer, T.D. & Haskal, Z.J. (2010) The role of transjugular intrahepatic portosystemic shunt (TIPS) in the management of portal hypertension: update 2009. *Hepatology*, **51**, 306. doi: 10.1002/hep.23383.

Fraser, J. et al.. Deep venous thrombosis: recent advances and optimal investigation with ultrasound. *Radiology*. 1999;**211**:1, 9–24. http://pubs.rsna.org/doi/full/10.1148/radiology.211.1.r99ap459.

Schwartz, S. et al., CT findings of rupture, impending rupture, and contained rupture of abdominal aortic aneurysms. *American Journal of Roentgenology*. 2007;**188**: W57–W62. http://www.ajronline.org/doi/abs/10.2214/AJR.05.1554.

Sedghi, Y., Collins, T.J. & White, C.J. (2013) Endovascular management of acute limb ischemia. *Vascular Medicine*, **18** (5), 307–313.

Singh, H. & Neutze, J.A. (2012) Percutaneous nephrostomy placement. In: *Radiology Fundamentals*, pp. 273–275. Springer, New York.

Smith, Kevin A., Hyun S. Kim, Interventional radiology and image-guided medicine: interventional oncology, *Seminars in Oncology*, **38**, 1, 2011, 151–162, ISSN 0093-7754, http://dx.doi.org/10.1053/j.seminoncol.2010.11.011.

Walser, E.M. (2012) Venous access ports: indications, implantation technique, follow-up, and complications. *Cardiovascular and Interventional Radiology*, **35** (4), 751–764.

Index

aspirated, 214, 216f, 225–6
  ingestion, 215
Le Fort fractures, 139
fractures, 105. *See also specific fractures*
free air, 73f, 74f
frontal sinuses, 136

gadolinium-based contrast agents
    (GBCAs), 4, 7, 9
gallbladder, 70
gangrenous cholecystitis, 82f
gastric cancer, 94–5
gastric polyp, 72f
gastrointestinal system, 15–17, 68–71
  interventions, 243
  malignancies of, 94–5
  pediatric imaging, 214–17, 220, 226–7, 230–1
gastrojejunostomy tubes, 243
gastrostomy tubes, 243
GBCAs. *See* gadolinium-based contrast agents
GCS. *See* Glasgow Coma Scale
genitourinary system, 17–20, 70–1
  pediatric imaging, 216, 231
Glasgow Coma Scale (GCS), 22
glioma, 108, 113f
  optic nerve, 150f
glomus jugulare tumors, 153
gonadal vein embolization, 245
gout, 191, 192f
gradient coils, 4
granulomas, 46
Graves ophthalmopathy, 148
great cardiac vein, 50
guidewires, 236, 236f

hamartomas, 46
hangman's fracture, 121
HCC. *See* hepatocellular carcinoma
headache
  brain imaging, 115
  imaging role and workup algorithms, 22
head and neck imaging
  anatomic considerations, 136, 137f, 143–5
  anatomic variants, 138f
  critical observations, 138, 145
  degenerative conditions, 139–42
  infectious conditions, 139–42
  inflammatory conditions, 139–42
  neoplasms, 142–3, 148–51
  squamous cell carcinoma, 156–8
  trauma, 20–1, 138–9
helical acquisition mode, 3
hemangioblastomas, 135
hematoma
  epidural, 101, 105
  extramedullary, 124
  hypertensive thalamic, 109f
  intramural, 54
  subdural, 101, 105
  subgaleal, 105
hematuria, 19
hemochromatosis, 62, 77
hemolytic uremic syndrome, 231
hemoptysis, 11
hepatoblastoma, 232–3
hepatocellular carcinoma (HCC), 77, 87–8, 89f
heterotaxy, 79
HIE. *See* hypoxic ischemic encephalopathy
high-intensity focused ultrasound (HIFU), 4
hip pain, 24
Hirschsprung's disease, 223
HIV. *See* human immunodeficiency virus
Hodgkin lymphoma, 233
horseshoe kidney, 77–8

HPS. *See* hypertrophic pyloric stenosis
human immunodeficiency virus (HIV), 129
hydrocephalus, 102
hyperextension injuries, 121
hypertensive thalamic hematoma, 109f
hypertrophic obstructive cardiomyopathy, 61
hypertrophic pyloric stenosis (HPS), 214, 218f, 227
hypopharynx, 155
hypoxic ischemic encephalopathy (HIE), 22

idiopathic interstitial pneumonias (IIPs), 42
idiopathic orbital inflammatory syndrome, 148
idiopathic pulmonary fibrosis (IPF), 42
IIPs. *See* idiopathic interstitial pneumonias
ILD. *See* interstitial lung disease
ileal atresia, 223
infectious conditions
  abdominopelvic imaging, 80–6
  brain imaging, 111
  chest imaging in, 34–40
  head and neck imaging, 139–42
  MSK imaging, 170–2
  orbits, 148
  pediatric imaging, 230–2
  soft tissue, 170–2
  spine imaging, 130
  temporal bone, 153
inferior blowout fracture, 145
inferior vena cava (IVC) filters, 238, 239f
inflammatory conditions
  abdominopelvic imaging, 80–6
  brain imaging, 111–14
  chest imaging in, 34–40
  of female pelvis, 86
  head and neck imaging, 139–42
  inflammatory bowel disease, 230–1
  orbits, 148
  pediatric imaging, 230–2
  polyps, 140–2
  spine imaging, 126–9
  temporal bone, 153
infrahyoid neck, 155–6
inner ear, 151
interatrial septum, 49
interstitial lung disease (ILD), 42
interventional radiology
  abscess treatment, 247
  arterial, 239–40
  biliary, 241–2
  CT in, 235
  DSA, 235
  fluoroscopy, 235
  gastrointestinal, 243
  MSK, 245–6
  oncology, 246–7
  pelvic, 244–5
  portal venous hypertension, 242–3
  procedures, 237–48
  pulmonary, 240–1
  renal, 244
  tools, 236–7
  types of imaging, 235–6
  ultrasound, 235
  venous, 237–9
interventricular septum, 50
intestinal malrotation, 78–9
intra-abdominal infection, 75
intradural-extramedullary tumors, 132–5
intrahepatic cholangiocarcinoma, 90f
intramedullary AVMs, 125
intramedullary tumors, 135
intramural hematoma, 54
intraparenchymal hemorrhage, 105
intravascular ultrasound (IVUS), 235

intravenous urogram (IVU), 17–18
intraventricular hemorrhage (IVH), 105
intussusception, 214, 218f, 226
inverted papilloma, 142–3, 144f
iodine-based contrast agents, 8–9
ionizing radiation modalities, 7
IPF. *See* idiopathic pulmonary fibrosis
ischemic cardiomyopathy, 61
IVC filters. *See* inferior vena cava filters
IVH. *See* intraventricular hemorrhage
IVU. *See* intravenous urogram
IVUS. *See* intravascular ultrasound

jaundice, 17
jejunal atresia, 223
joint-centered disease, 173–4
joint injections, MSK imaging, 197
juvenile nasopharyngeal angiofibroma, 143

kidney neoplasms, 89–92
kidneys, ureters, and bladder (KUB)
  ultrasound, 18
  X-ray, 17
Klatskin tumor, 91
knee pain, 24
KUB. *See* kidneys, ureters, and bladder

LAD artery, 50
Langerhans cell histiocytosis (LCH), 234
large cell carcinoma (LCC), 48
laryngeal squamous cell carcinoma, 157–8, 157f
laryngocele, 159–60
larynx, 155
last image hold (LIH), 2
lateral blowout fracture, 145
LCC. *See* large cell carcinoma
LCH. *See* Langerhans cell histiocytosis
LCP. *See* Legg-Calve-Perthes disease
LCx artery, 50
lead-pipe colon, 85f
left atrium, 49
left lower quadrant (LLQ), 16, 65, 66f
left upper quadrant (LUQ), 65, 66f
left ventricle, 50
Legg-Calve-Perthes (LCP) disease, 228
leukemias, 132
  acute lymphoblastic, 233
  pediatric, 233
ligament, 167f
  MSK imaging, 166–7
ligamentum flavum, 117
LIH. *See* last image hold
LIP. *See* lymphoid interstitial pneumonia
lipohemarthrosis, 174
lipoma, 44
liver, 70
  laceration, 80f
  metastases, 87
  neoplasms, 87–9
LLQ. *See* left lower quadrant
LMCA, 50
low-back pain, 24
lower GI series, 15
lower urinary tract trauma, 19
lung abscess, 39–40, 41f
lung cancer, 29, 46
  imaging role and workup algorithms, 13
  non-small cell, 47
  small cell, 47
LUQ. *See* left upper quadrant
lymphangiomas, 146
lymphoid interstitial pneumonia (LIP), 34f, 42
lymphoma, 75, 93–4, 94f, 132, 148
  pediatric, 233